Pathology
of
Heart Valve Replacement

For my wife, children and parents

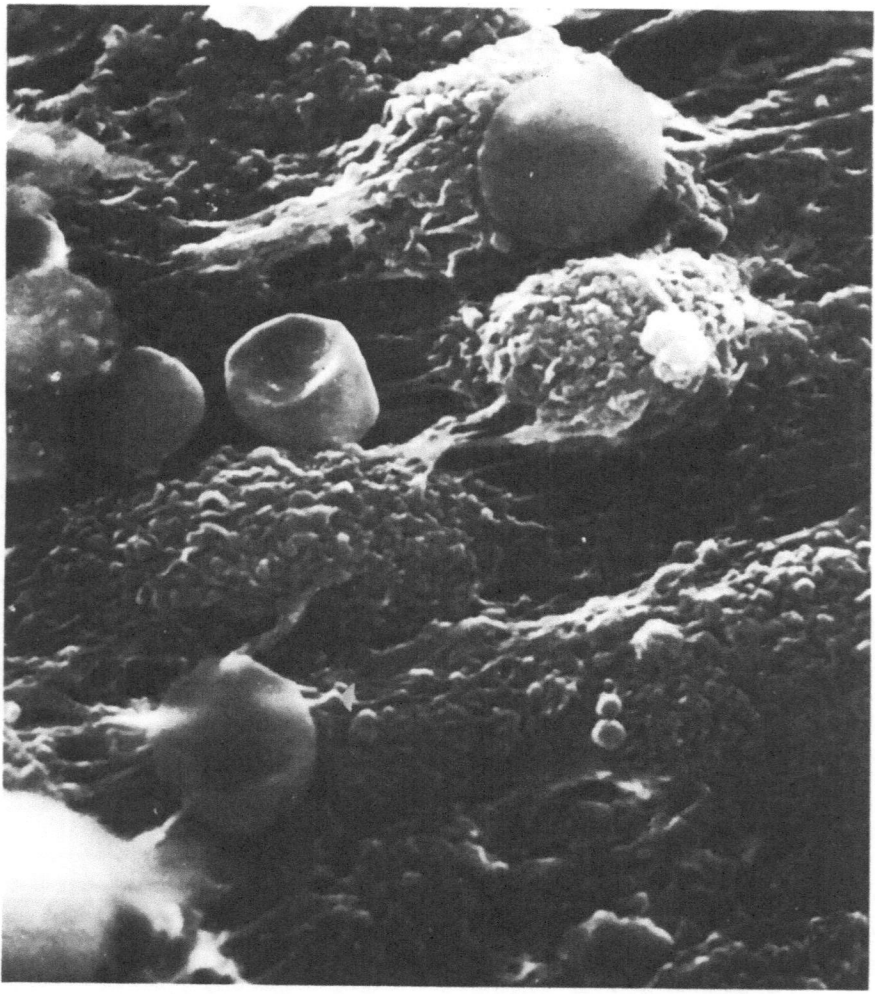

Scanning electron microscopy of a Mitroflow bovine pericardial heart valve, which had been implanted in the mitral position in a baboon for 36 days. Mesothelial covering cells have been lost exposing bare collagen, which is partially covered by histiocytes (cells with ruffled cytoplasmic processes), erythrocytes and scanty fibrin. (Uranyl acetate and lead citrate × 3400)

Pathology of Heart Valve Replacement

Alan G. Rose
MBChB, MD, M.Med (Path), MRCPath, FACC

Senior Specialist, Groote Schuur Hospital, Cape Town, and Associate Professor of Pathology, University of Cape Town Medical School, Cape Town, South Africa

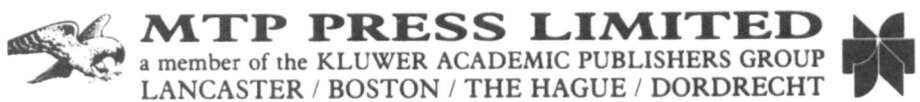

MTP PRESS LIMITED
a member of the KLUWER ACADEMIC PUBLISHERS GROUP
LANCASTER / BOSTON / THE HAGUE / DORDRECHT

Published in the UK and Europe by
MTP Press Limited
Falcon House
Lancaster, England

British Library Cataloguing in Publication Data

Rose, Alan G.
   Pathology of heart valve replacement.
   1. Heart valve prosthesis
   I. Title
   617'.412   RD598
   ISBN-13: 978-94-010-7948-8   e-ISBN-13: 978-94-009-3227-2
   DOI: 10.107/978-94-009-3227-2

Published in the USA by
MTP Press
A division of Kluwer Academic Publishers
101 Philip Drive
Norwell, MA 02061, USA

Typeset by Speedlith Photo Litho Ltd., Thomas Street, Manchester, England.

Contents

COLOUR PLATES

Colour Plates A–M will be found between pages 54 and 55; Colour Plates N–X between pages 118 and 119.

Foreword

Dr Rose honoured me with a request for a Foreword. I am delighted to oblige.

The treatment of valvular heart disease has improved remarkably in the past 40 years. Many factors have contributed; not least being the introduction of artificial heart valves for treatment, more than 25 years ago. Their use has shown that they are good, but not an ideal substitute for native valves.

A galaxy of pathological changes are associated with the insertion and malfunction of artificial heart valves. Each has to be defined, classified and related to clinical procedures or problems with a prosthesis; then a means sought to prevent them. Often, in understanding their cause, investigative procedures have/will improve patient care and broaden knowledge in other spheres.

Dr Rose has been a student of this pathology for many years and has made many contributions. No doubt his interest in the area was whetted by colleagues in Cape Town, leaders in the field of cardiovascular medicine and surgery. This monograph provides a collected review of his experience. In it one finds lessons in geographic pathology, in considering the causes of valvular heart disease in Cape Town and valuable information regarding the identification of artificial heart valves and a means of examining a heart bearing one. Dr Rose's detailed analyses of the causes of death, and of the related pathology in the heart and other organs of patients bearing different types of heart valve prostheses at different locations, are well documented and discussed. The findings are beautifully illustrated.

The monograph will be a valuable addition to the literature. Also, it provides a gauge, not only of Dr Rose's past experience in Cape Town, but one against which future endeavours there and elsewhere may be measured. One would hope that most, if not all of the complications mentioned will disappear and become of historical interest, as indeed some have during the past 25 years. This will happen only if there is an interaction between scientists of many different backgrounds who seek to overcome the problems represented by the complications Dr Rose discusses. I am sure that this will occur.

Malcolm D. Silver, MD, PhD
Professor and Chairman
Department of Pathology, University of Toronto
Chief of Pathology, Toronto General Hospital

Preface

No prosthetic valve as perfect as the normal human heart valve has yet been devised. Replacement valves, although generally helpful in restoring patients to normal life, may also cause significant complications. Many serious problems in this connection remain unsolved: their solution will depend on collaboration between the disciplines of biomedical engineering, material science, biochemistry, pathology and related fields. Whilst abundant information is available regarding the clinical and haemodynamic effects of various valvular prostheses, there is a relative paucity of pathological data on patients with such prostheses. Clear identification of serious complications following heart valve replacement is very important in planning means of lowering the postoperative mortality rate. An autopsy provides substantial evidence as to whether or not a death is valve-related.

Many pathologists are unfamiliar with the various types of prosthetic heart valves that are available. Some are also uncertain as to how to examine either a heart containing a prosthesis, or an explanted valve prosthesis, as well as what complications to look for at autopsy. It is hoped that this book will be of assistance to pathologists, and that it will also interest clinicians caring for patients with prosthetic heart valves.

Acknowledgements

I am grateful to Professor Golda Selzer for initially kindling my interest in cardiac pathology, and to Dr Jesse E. Edwards for providing an inspiring example of excellence in the field of cardiovascular pathology. Professor V. Schrire and Professor W. Beck and staff of the Cardiac Clinic, as well as Professor C. N. Barnard and Professor B. A. Reichart and staff of the Department of Cardiothoracic Surgery, Groote Schuur Hospital, Cape Town, kindly allowed access to the clinical records of their patients with prosthetic heart valves studied in this work. Professor P. J. Commerford and Mrs C. Lawley kindly supplied data regarding the survival and embolism event-free status of all of the Groote Schuur Hospital patients who received valve prostheses between 1962 and 1985. Mr J. R. P. Dale and Mr M. Emms provided electron microscopical technical assistance. Photographic assistance was provided by Ms J. Rose, Ms H. Earp-Jones and Ms C. Bilobrk. Ms M. Stansfield created the uncredited line drawings of mechanical and tissue valves. I am most grateful to the various valve manufacturers, and to several authors and publishers, who have allowed me to use their photographs and diagrams as acknowledged in the text of this work. Grant support from the Chris Barnard Fund and the Medical Research Council of South Africa is also acknowledged. Last, but not least, I am grateful to Dr Peter Clarke and Mr Phil Johnstone of MTP Press Ltd for help and encouragement during the preparation of this book.

1
History of Cardiac Valve Replacement

INTRODUCTION

Whilst general surgery has progressed steadily over a prolonged period, its younger offshoot, cardiac surgery, has made a dramatic breakthrough about once every 5 years[1]. Each advance has become associated with the names of one or two individuals: treatment of constrictive pericarditis (Churchill, 1933), treatment of the patent ductus arteriosus (Gross, 1938), closed mitral repair (Harken, 1948), the pump oxygenator (Gibbon, 1953), valve prostheses (Hufnagel, 1952; Harken and Starr, 1958), reconstruction of the congenitally malformed heart (Kirklin, 1963), cardiac transplantation (Barnard, 1967), and saphenous vein bypass grafting of coronary arteries (Favoloro, 1970). The principal landmarks in the history of surgical replacement of diseased heart valves are reviewed below.

GENERAL HISTORICAL ASPECTS[2-7]

The pathology of mitral stenosis was first described by Raymond Vieussens at Montpelier in 1715 in a textbook entitled *Traite nouveau de la structure et des causes du mouvement naturel du coeur*. In 1882, Block sutured cardiac wounds in experimental animals. However, cardiac surgery had to contend with the dogma of the day. In 1893 Billroth stated that 'Any surgeon who would attempt an operation on the heart should lose the respect of his colleagues.' Paget (1896) wrote that 'the surgery of the heart has probably reached the limits set by nature to all surgery'.

Despite this, in 1896 Rehn repaired a right ventricular stab wound. In 1898 Samways proposed the surgical relief of mitral stenosis. In 1902 Brunton opened stenosed mitral valves in cadavers and operated on the normal mitral valves of dead cats using a transventricular tenotomy knife. In the same year Sauerbruch and Meyer used pressure chambers to overcome the problem of surgically induced pneumothorax. In 1908, in the first recorded operation for acquired mitral valve disease, Cushing and Branch unsuccessfully operated on a dog with mitral stenosis. In 1909 Meltzer and Auer introduced an endotracheal tube for anaesthesia. In 1910 Carrel suggested that fingers may be used to dilate a stenosed mitral valve. In 1913 Doyen attempted the first operation on a human cardiac valve. The patient died early postoperatively and autopsy revealed muscular subpulmonary rather than valvular stenosis.

1

Tuffier performed the first successful operation on a human heart valve in 1914 using a finger to dilate the stenotic aortic valve.

Important advances also occurred in the ancillary services. In 1929 Forssmann[8] performed the first human cardiac catheterization (on his own heart). This new technique was later used by Cournand[9] and Richards[10] to study patients with congestive heart failure. This work gained these three men the 1956 Nobel Prize for Medicine. However, Bleichroeder[11] had performed the same experiment as Forssmann as early as 1912, at a time when radiological assistance was not yet available. Although this work was acknowledged by Forssmann in an addendum to his publication, Bleichroeder's courageous achievement has been largely ignored. In 1933 Charles and Scott[12] purified heparin so that it could be used clinically for anticoagulation, e.g. for extracorporeal circulation. The first blood bank was established by Fantus[13] in the United States of America in 1937.

MITRAL STENOSIS

Closed heart procedures for mitral stenosis

In 1923 Cutler and Levine[14] at the Peter Bent Brigham Hospital, performed the first 'successful' operation for mitral stenosis using instruments inserted through the left ventricular apex. Mitral regurgitation resulted from this procedure. In 1925 Souttar performed the second successful operation for mitral stenosis using a transatrial approach[15]. He was able to detect severe mitral incompetence and dilated the orifice with his index finger, rather than magnifying the incompetence by cutting into the valve. His patient was the first to have a successful result from this operation. During the period 1930–45 cardiac valve surgery made little progress. Thirty years later Beck[16] noted that the cardiovalvulotome, which he had helped to develop, had probably delayed the development of the mitral valvotomy operation by 20 years.

Indirect surgical techniques for mitral stenosis

In 1913 Jeger proposed inserting a valved vein between a pulmonary vein and the left ventricle in order to decompress the left atrium in mitral stenosis. Litwak created such a graft in a dog, but the graft thrombosed. No such attempt was made in humans. In 1913 Schepelmann linked the two atrial appendages of a rabbit with an aortic graft. In 1926 Dmitrieff perforated the atrial septum both via the jugular vein and at thoracotomy. Such a procedure was performed by Harken et al. in 1948[17] and by Bailey[18] in the following year, but later the efficacy of the operation was questioned.

THE MODERN ERA: 1949 ONWARDS

The starting point for modern cardiac surgery occurred in November 1944 when Alfred Blalock successfully operated upon cyanotic congenital heart disease. The current era of valve surgery began in 1949 when Harken[17],

Bailey[18], and Brock[2,19], all working independently, first successfully repaired stenotic mitral valves. Bailey[18] performed a successful mitral commissurotomy using digital palpation to guide the cutting blade. Harken[17] performed a similar operation 6 days after Bailey, using a valvulotome to cut the fused commissures. Only a few months after the successful operations of Bailey and Harken, Brock[19] performed finger fracture of a stenotic mitral valve.

Between 1950 and 1955 several hundred successful mitral commissurotomies were performed worldwide. In 1954, Dubost et al.[20] described a transatrial mechanical dilator for correcting mitral stenosis. By 1962 he had achieved several hundred valvulotomies with only a 2% mortality rate[21]. The early dilator had a maximum spread of only 3.5 cm, which was often too small to fully open both commissures. An ideal spread of 5 cm was provided by the instrument designed by Mr O. S. Tubbs, which became widely used worldwide.

MITRAL INCOMPETENCE

Although many of the experimental studies on the mitral valve involved the production of mitral insufficiency, the concept of surgically relieving incompetence developed slowly[7]. For many years surgeons erroneously believed that mitral incompetence was not a significant lesion. In 1910 Carrel[22] tried to relieve mitral incompetence in dogs by producing a slight stenosis of the upper part of the left ventricle by resecting part of the mural muscle.

CLOSED-HEART PROCEDURES FOR MITRAL REGURGITATION

Autogenous or plastic materials were inserted blindly to support or augment the posterior mitral leaflet, or a circumferential suture was used to narrow the mitral valve ring. Unfortunately, recurrent incompetence often complicated the operation. In 1949 Templeton and Gibbon[23] reported cardiac valve reconstruction using venous and pericardial grafts. Later, others used atrium for 'transventricular tamponage'. In the 'commissurorrhaphy' operation[24] the valve leaflets were sutured together with pericardial strips. During the 1950s various plastic materials were used to augment the posterior mitral leaflet, e.g. methyl methacrylate (Lucite), Plexiglas and polyvinyl formalinized plastic (Ivalon). In 1955 Jordan and Wible[25] sited a nylon leaflet mounted on an Elgiloy spring frame below the mitral valve to prevent mitral regurgitation. Kay and Cross[26] obtained palliative results using a closed-heart version of what later was called posteromedial annuloplasty[2]. All of the closed techniques for the correction of mitral incompetence were unsatisfactory, and no further surgical advances were made until bloodless field mitral valve surgery became possible.

CLOSED-HEART PROCEDURES FOR AORTIC STENOSIS AND REGURGITATION

In 1948 Smithy et al.[27] described a method of performing transaortic and transventricular aortic valvotomy in experimental animals. Shortly thereafter, Bailey et al.[28] reported their results with retrograde aortic valve incision and dilatation. This approach was abandoned due to arterial dissection and the development of aortic incompetence; a transventricular approach yielded better results. Others made unsuccessful attempts to alleviate aortic incompetence by tying a suture around the base of the aorta to narrow the aortic ring. Campbell[29] and Hufnagel[30] independently designed artificial heart valves composed of a mobile, spherical poppet within a Lucite tube using the caged-ball principle devised by Williams[31] in his bottle-stopper patent of 1858. On 11 September 1952 Hufnagel[32] ushered in the era of prosthetic valve surgery by successfully inserting his caged-ball valve into the descending thoracic aorta of a patient with severe aortic incompetence.

The concept of entirely removing the heart from the circulation had been raised in speculative form in 1812. In 1926 two Soviet scientists proved that animals could be kept alive with a heart–lung machine[33]. John Gibbon of Philadelphia started work on such a machine in 1935, but it was not perfected for humans until 1952.

In 1953 Gibbon[34] dramatically achieved the first successful use of total cardiopulmonary bypass for bloodless field intracardiac surgery in humans. This, together with Hufnagel's surgical success with the caged-ball aortic prosthesis[32] set the stage for future surgical attempts to replace diseased heart valves with artificial substitutes. The next decade opened the floodgates of cardiac surgical progress. The provision of a pump to replace cardiac function was relatively simple compared to the problems faced in developing an artificial lung. The artifical lung developed by Gibbon was subsequently incorporated into the Gibbon-Mayo pump. Lillehei and colleagues[35] in Minnesota initially made use of a human donor to supply oxygenated blood in 30 patients with complicated congenital heart lesions and later developed their bubble oxygenator. Melrose[36,37] published details of his heart–lung apparatus. Later, following a fruitful collaboration with Gerbode, his machine gained worldwide acceptance. Modifications and refinements of the heart–lung machine continued to be made during the 1960s and 1970s and the next major step was the development of the membrane oxygenator.

OPEN-HEART VALVE REPAIR PROCEDURES

As a result of the above-mentioned breakthroughs, surgeons were able to try and correct valvular lesions by directing their attention to the abnormal valve itself.

Open-heart surgery for mitral valve disease

Between 1956 and 1968 the heart–lung bypass machine was used for operative correction of congenital heart diseases[2], but later it was also used for acquired valvular disease[38]. Lillehei and the Minnesota group at first performed

4

paediatric intracardiac surgery using another person as an oxygenator (controlled cross-circulation). The De Wall–Lillehei bubble oxygenator, which was introduced later, was simple to use; it was also cheap and disposable, but perfusion rates were slow. The modern membrane oxygenators have faster perfusion rates. The first successful open-heart operation for acquired mitral valve disease was performed on 29 August 1956 at the University of Minnesota by Dr C. W. Lillehei.

Mitral stenosis

Open-heart surgery for mitral stenosis was used to break down fused commissures or to remove calcium from the edges of the valve. Because the site of commissural fusion was often difficult to localize, some surgeons still used a dilator. However, direct vision was of great assistance in surgical correction of areas of subvalvular fusion[7]. In recent years there has been a swing towards doing open mitral valvotomies in all patients with significant mitral stenosis.

Mitral incompetence

Open reconstructive techniques which have been attempted in order to correct mitral incompetence include: (a) repair by direct suture of cuspal tears or perforations; (b) increasing the surface area of the deficient leaflet; (c) repair of ruptured chordae tendineae by immobilizing the flail area, resuturing chordae to the papillary muscle, plicating the ruptured leaflet with posteromedial annuloplasty, or constructing artificial chordae of silk, Dacron or Teflon; (d) narrowing the mitral annulus increases the area of cuspal apposition.

Lillehei et al.[39] were the first to perform mitral annuloplasty under direct vision. Heavy through-and-through silk sutures were placed in the mitral ring at one or both commissures. Annuloplasty procedures helped 50% of patients with moderate or severe isolated mitral regurgitation, especially those with ring dilatation, but it was less successful if the cusps were severely fibrosed or shrunken[2]. Poor results were obtained using artificial chordae prepared from silk, Teflon or Dacron fibre, but McGoon's plication procedure gave better results[40]. Later failures led to technical modifications such as using Ivalon or Teflon to buttress the sutures and prevent them cutting through the tissues. However, the annuloplasty technique that has provided the best long-term results is posteromedial annuloplasty or modifications thereof.

Various annuloplasty rings have been used to narrow the size of the atrioventricular valve annuli. The first of these was the C-shaped *Morse annuloplasty ring*, which was manufactured in 1963 by American Edwards

Laboratories. The *Puig–Massana–Shiley annuloplasty ring* (manufactured by Shiley Incorporated) is presently available in two sizes. Each has an internal purse-string suture, which enables the diameter to be varied. *Carpentier–Edwards mitral and tricuspid prosthetic valve rings* are manufactured by American Edwards Laboratories. The rings consist of a titanium alloy coated with silicone rubber. The surface layer consists of polyester fabric. From 1980 the rings were made in an open form (Figure 1.1).

Replacement of the mitral valve with a prosthesis

Unfortunately the above-described reconstructive techniques were not applicable to most rheumatic patients with calcified, immobile, stenotic and incompetent mitral valves.

Partial replacement of the mitral valve with an immobile prosthesis

This technique was only applicable to patients with mitral incompetence due to a shrunken, immobile posterior leaflet, with a pliable and mobile anterior leaflet. An immobile Ivalon baffle (see Colour Plate F) could be sutured so as to augment a shrunken posterior mitral leaflet[41]. This operation and related variants thereof gave poor late results due to infection, mitral stenosis and emboli. Mitral valve replacement superseded this operation.

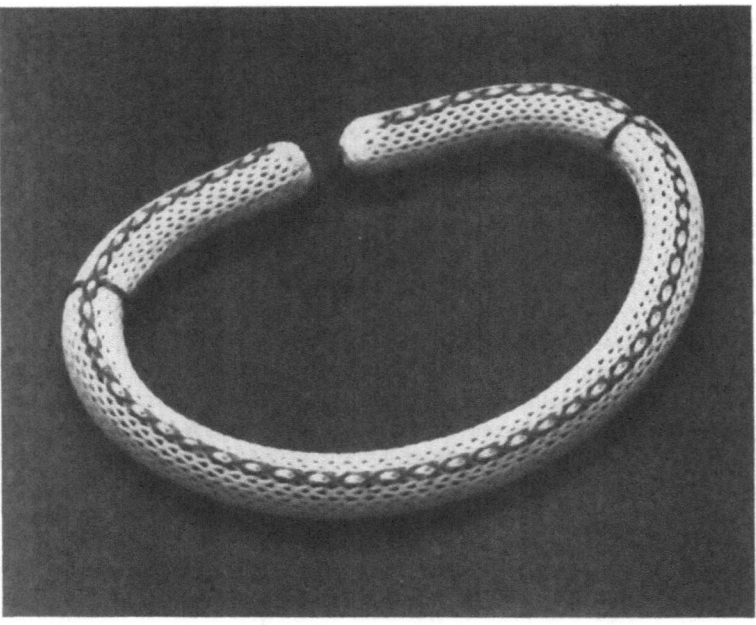

Figure 1.1   Carpentier–Edwards mitral prosthetic valve ring. (Courtesy of American Edwards Laboratories)

Partial replacement of the mitral valve with a mobile prosthesis

Partial replacement of the mitral valve with a mobile prosthesis aimed to avoid the stenosis, which complicated partial replacement of the valve with an immobile prosthesis. Silicone rubber (Silastic) leaflets, Silastic-covered Teflon leaflets with attached chordae tendineae and knitted Teflon leaflets with chordal extensions were unsuccessfully tested in animals and were not used in humans[7]. Instead, knitted Dacron or autologous pericardial leaflets were used to replace the posterior mitral leaflet.

Total replacement of the mitral valve with a prosthesis

Experimental results[42]

Problems with perfusion, operative techniques, poor valve design and inappropriate selection of synthetic materials plagued canine mitral valve replacement experiments[7]. Thromboembolism was a major problem. A variety of *monocuspid flap valves* were evaluated, including some made of stainless steel; a flexible monocusp Mylar valve with multiple hinges, and a Silastic valve. Similarly poor results were obtained with *multicuspid prosthetic mitral valves* made from Silastic, Teflon or polyurethane. In order to try and overcome these poor results, *prostheses with artificial chordae tendineae* were fashioned, which aimed to mimic the normal mitral valve. Such prostheses, made from polyurethane reinforced with Dacron, Dacron mesh infiltrated with fibroblasts[41] or Silastic, also yielded disappointing results.

The first experimentally successful prosthetic *ball valve* had a Lucite ball and a base made of Teflon. Thrombosis and poor mechanical fixation were major problems. Ball valves were also constructed entirely of Lucite, Ivalon or of steel[43]. Starr tried out many materials before selecting a prosthesis having a Silastic ball contained within a Lucite cage.

Clinical results[44–46]

Monocuspid valves: a monocuspid valve made of laminated Mylar covered with knitted Teflon initially gave good results, but late valve dysfunction led to its abandonment.

Multicuspid valves: the Silastic bicuspid valve[46] was the most successful. It had two flexible leaflets made of a silicone-coated Dacron fabric enclosed in a Lexan housing with an antithrombogenic covering layer.

Valves with artificial chordae tendineae: a moulded polyurethane valve with Teflon chordae tendineae yielded poor results[47].

Ball valves: the introduction of the ball-valve prosthesis into clinical surgery by Starr and Edwards[48] was the most notable recent advance in surgery for acquired valvular disease. An early model of the Starr–Edwards prosthesis had a Silastic ball contained within a rigid cage made of Stellite 21 (Vitallium) and attached to a Teflon fabric sewing ring. In recent years a number of modifications were made, mainly to try and obviate cloth wear, but none yielded better results than those obtained with the early design. The latest Starr–Edwards valves use the early design.

OPEN-HEART PROCEDURES FOR AORTIC VALVE DISEASE

In 1956 Murray[49] reported on the use of the homograft aortic valve in the descending thoracic aorta. The incomplete relief obtained by placing the Hufnagel valve in the descending thoracic aorta led cardiac surgeons to operate on the aortic valve itself. In 1958, Lillehei et al.[50] performed one of the first human cardiac valve replacements when they implanted a bicuspid silicone rubber flap valve in the subcoronary position of a 56-year-old woman. The prosthesis functioned satisfactorily for 6 years.

Others treated aortic insufficiency by narrowing the aortic valve ring, e.g. the tricuspid aortic valve was converted into a bicuspid valve by excising or plicating the non-coronary cusp. Attempts were also made to create a flap valve from the aortic wall just above the incompetent aortic valve. Others sutured Ivalon to the free edge of one of the aortic cusps. In 1967 Hurley recommended debridement of calcified material, plus commissurotomy for aortic stenosis. However, restenosis frequently occurred and many valves were too contracted and calcified to obtain significant haemodynamic improvement[2].

Harken, in 1960, was the first to successfully replace a diseased aortic valve with a prosthetic caged-ball valve in the natural position[51]. He reported the survival of two out of seven patients with double-caged-ball valves inserted in the subcoronary position for aortic incompetence. (In September of the same year Starr and Edwards[48] accomplished a similar feat in a patient with mitral valve disease.) Despite the encouraging initial results in dogs, the early caged-ball valves had a high incidence of thromboembolism and they were also noisy. The silicone rubber balls deteriorated and there was a high rate of paravalvular leakage and infection. The design was soon changed.

After the first successful mitral valve replacement with the single-caged Starr–Edwards prosthesis in 1960 this prosthesis soon gained worldwide acceptance. This prosthesis introduced the concept of a sewing ring and foreshadowed the modern era of surgical replacement of diseased heart valves. The overall results were good, and clinicians were able for the first time to compare the natural history of valvular heart disease with the effect of correcting an obstructed or leaking heart valve. Furthermore, a major advance in the understanding of valvular heart disease was achieved now that it was possible to separate valvular dysfunction from myocardial disability[2].

COMMENT

Remarkable progress has been made in cardiac surgery since 1896 when Rehn first sutured the living human heart. Moore[1] points out that, despite these many achievements, the heart remains a most vital organ, acute postoperative disorders are poorly tolerated, and the mortality remains high in several types of cardiac operation. The patient pays a severe price for any technical error, be it valvular insufficiency due to failure of a single suture, hemiparesis due to dislodgement of a smal thrombus, or an arrhythmia from a poorly placed suture in the bundle of His. Cardiac surgery has no place for the careless, hasty or unpractised operator.

REFERENCES

1. Moore, F. D. (1972). In Norman, J. C. (ed.) *Cardiac Surgery*, 2nd edn, pp. xiii-xiv. (New York: Appleton-Century-Crofts)
2. Lefrack, E. A. and Starr, A. (1979). *Cardiac Valve Prostheses*. (New York: Appleton-Century-Crofts)
3. Richardson, R. G. (1969). *The Surgeon's Heart. A History of Cardiac Surgery*. (London: Heinemann)
4. Johnson, S. L. (1970). *The History of Cardiac Surgery 1896–1955*. (Baltimore: Johns Hopkins Press)
5. Zimmerman, L. M. and Veith, I. (1967). *Great Ideas in the History of Surgery*. (New York: Dover Publications)
6. Samways, D. W. (1898). Cardiac peristalsis: its nature and effects. *Lancet*, **1**, 927
7. Ellis, F. H. Jr. (1967). *Surgery for Acquired Mitral Valve Disease*. (London: W. B. Saunders)
8. Forssmann, W. (1929). Die Sondierung des richten Herzens. *Klin. Wochenschr.*, **8**, 2085
9. Cournand, A. and Ranges, H. A. (1941). Catheterization of the right auricle in man. *Proc. Soc. Exp. Biol. Med.*, **46**, 462
10. Richards, D. W., Cournand, A. and Darling, R. C. (1941). Pressure in the right auricle of man, in normal subjects and in patients with congestive heart failure. *Trans. Assoc. Am. Physiol.*, **56**, 218
11. Bleichroeder, F. (1912). Intra arterielle therapie. *Berl. Klin. Wochenschr.*, **49**, 1503D
12. Charles, A. F. and Scott, D. A. (1933). Studies on heparin. I. The preparation of heparin. *J. Biol. Chem.*, **102**, 425
13. Fantus, B. (1937). The therapy of Cook County Hospital : blood preservation. *J. Am. Med. Assoc.*, **109**, 128
14. Cutler, E. C. and Levine, S. A. (1923). Cardiotomy and valvotomy for mitral stenosis: experimental observations and clinical notes concerning an operated case with recovery. *Boston Med. Surg. J.*, **188**, 1023
15. Souttar, H. S. (1925). The surgical treatment of mitral stenosis. *Br. Med. J.*, **2**, 603
16. Beck, C. S. (1940). The technique of opening the stenotic mitral valve. *J. Am. Med. Assoc.*, **156**, 1400
17. Harken, D. E., Ellis, L. B. and Ware, P. F. (1948). The surgical treatment of mitral stenosis. I. Valvuloplasty. *N. Engl. J. Med.*, **239**, 801
18. Bailey, C. P. (1949). The surgical treatment of mitral stenosis (mitral commissurotomy). *Dis Chest*, **15**, 377
19. Baker, C., Brock, R. C. and Campbell, M. (1950). Valvulotomy for mitral stenosis: report of six successful cases. *Br. Med. J.* **1**, 1283
20. Dubost, C., Oteifa, G. and Blondeau, P. (1954). Le problème technique de la commissurotomie mitrale: resultats obtenus par la dilatation instrumentale de la stenose. *Mem. Acad. Chir.*, **80**, 321
21. Dubost, C., Blondeau, P. and Pinwica, A. (1962). Instrumental dilation using the transatrial approach in the treatment of mitral stenosis: a survey of 1,000 cases. *J. Thorac. Cardiovasc. Surg.*, **44**, 392
22. Carrel, A. (1910). On the experimental surgery of the thoracic aorta and the heart. *Ann. Surg.*, **52**, 83
23. Templeton, J. Y. III and Gibbon, J. H. Jr (1949). Experimental reconstruction of cardiac valves by venous and pericardial grafts. *Ann. Surg.*, **129**, 161
24. Bailey, C. P., Bolton, H. E. and Redondo-Ramirez, H. P. (1952). Surgery of the mitral valve. *Surg. Clin. N. Am.*, **32**, 1807
25. Jordan, P. Jr and Wible, J. (1955). Spring valve for mitral insufficiency. *Arch. Surg.*, **71**, 468
26. Kay, E. B. and Cross, F. S. (1955). Surgical treatment of mitral insufficiency. *Surgery*, **37**, 697
27. Smithy, H. G., Pratt-Thomas, H. R. and Deyerle, H. P. (1948). Aortic valvulotomy: experimental methods and early results. *Surg. Gynecol. Obstet.*, **86**, 513.
28. Bailey, C. P., Glover, R. P. and O'Neill, T. J. E. (1950). Experiences with the surgical relief of aortic stenosis. *J. Thorac. Cardiovasc. Surg.*, **20**, 516
29. Campbell, J. M. (1950). An artificial aortic valve. *J. Thorac. Cardiovasc Surg.*, **19**, 312
30. Hufnagel, C. A. (1951). Aortic plastic valvular prosthesis. *Bull. Georgetown Univ. Med. Cent.*, **4**, 128
31. Williams, J. B. (1858). *United States Patent Number 19323*, 9 February

32. Hufnagel, C. A. and Harvey, W. P. (1953). The surgical correction of aortic insufficiency. *Bull Georgetown Univ. Med. Cent.*, **6**, 60
33. McGrew, R. E. (1985). *Encyclopedia of Medical History*, p. 328. (London: Macmillan)
34. Gibbon, J. H. Jr. (1954). Application of mechanical heart and lung apparatus to cardiac surgery. *Minn. Med.*, **37**, 171
35. Lillehei, C. W. (1955). Direct vision intracardiac surgery by means of controlled cross circulation or continuous arterial reservoir perfusion for correction of ventricular septal defects, atrioventricularis communis, isolated infundibular pulmonic stenosis and tetralogy of Fallot, cardiovascular surgery. *Proceedings of the Symposium held at the Henry Ford Hospital, Detroit, Michigan, March 1955*. p. 371. (Philadelphia: W. B. Saunders)
36. Melrose, D. G. (1952). Artificial (extracorporeal) heart–lung apparatus. *Med. Illus.*, **6**, 591
37. Gerbode, F., Osborn, J. J., Melrose, D. G., Perkins, H. A., Norman, A. and Baer, D. M. (1958). Extracorporeal circulation in intracardiac surgery : A comparison between two heart–lung machines. *Lancet*, **2**, 284
38. Nichols, H. T., Blanco, G., Morse, D. P. and Likoff, W. (1962). Open mitral commissurotomy: experience with 200 consecutive cases. *J. Am. Med. Assoc.*, **182**, 268
39. Lillehei, C. W., Gott, V. L. and De Wall, R. A. (1957). Surgical correction of pure mitral insufficiency by annuloplasty under direct vision. *Lancet*, **2**, 446
40. McGoon, D. C. (1960). Repair of mitral insufficiency due to ruptured chordae tendineae. *J. Thorac. Cardiovasc. Surg.*, **39**, 357
41. Barnard, C. N. and Schrire, V. (1968). Ivalon baffle for posterior leaflet replacement in the treatment of mitral insufficiency: a follow-up study. *Surgery*, **63**, 727
42. Merendino, K. A. (1961). *Prosthetic Valves for Cardiac Surgery*, p. 340. (Springfield, Illinois: Charles C. Thomas)
43. Starr, A. (1960). Total mitral valve replacement. Fixation and thrombosis. *Surg. Forum*, **11**, 258
44. Cross, F. S., Gerein, A. N. and Jones, R. D. (1963). Evaluation of two prostheses for total replacement of the mitral valve. *J. Thorac. Cardiovasc. Surg.*, **46**, 719
45. Cruz, A. B., Kaster, R. L., Simmons, R. L., Bruneau, L. and Lillehei, C. W. (1965). A new caged meniscus prosthetic heart valve. *Surgery*, **58**, 995
46. Young, W. P., Gott, V. L. and Rowe, G. G. (1965). Open-heart surgery for mitral valve disease, with special reference to a new prosthetic valve. *J. Thorac. Cardiovasc. Surg.*, **50**, 827
47. Braunwald, N. S., Cooper, T. and Morrow, A. G. (1960). Complete replacement of the mitral valve : Successful clinical application of a flexible polyurethane prosthesis. *J. Thorac. Cardiovasc. Surg.*, **40**, 1
48. Starr, A. and Edwards, M. L. (1961). Mitral replacement: clinical experience with a ball-valve prosthesis. *Ann. Surg.*, **154**, 726
49. Murray, G. (1956). Homologous aortic-valve-segment transplants as surgical treatment for aortic and mitral insufficiency. *Angiology*, **7**, 466
50. Long, D. M. Jr, Sterns, L. P., De Riemer, R. H., Warden, H. E. and Lillehei, C. W. (1960). Subtotal and total replacement of the aortic valve with plastic valve prostheses: experimental investigation and successful clinical application utilizing selective cardiac hypothermia. *Surg. Forum*, **10**, 660
51. Harken, D. E., Soroff, H. S., Taylor, W. J., Lefemine, A. A., Gupta, S. K. and Lunzer, S. (1960). Partial and complete prostheses in aortic insufficiency. *J. Thorac. Cardiovasc. Surg.*, **40**, 744

2
Pathology of Natural Heart Valves and Indications for Heart Valve Replacement

INTRODUCTION

This chapter reviews the diseases leading to heart valve replacement, the clinical indications for valve replacement and the problem of matching prosthesis to patient. Pathological assessment of the aetiology of excised diseased native valves and the incidence of Aschoff bodies in surgically resected atrial appendages are also considered.

PATHOLOGY OF CARDIAC VALVES WARRANTING REPLACEMENT BY VALVE PROSTHESES

This survey of valvular pathology covers 18 132 autopsies performed at the University of Cape Town during the 30-year period 1950–79. The data for acquired valvular disease are consistent with those of a developing country[1] and differ from those in the developed countries of Europe and North America where rheumatic fever is seldom encountered[2–6].

Acquired valvular heart disease

Table 2.1 gives the functional classification of the clinically significant acquired valvular heart diseases encountered in 1225 autopsy patients (6.8% of 18 132 autopsies). Demographic data on these patients have been published elsewhere[7].

In Cape Town the mitral valve (Colour Plates A to C) is the most commonly diseased heart valve (52.1% of acquired valvular diseases), followed by the aortic valve (39.4%), and the tricuspid (8.3%) and pulmonary valves (0.3%). Rheumatic-type valvular disease accounted for 99.8% of the cases of mitral stenosis and 68.9% of patients with mitral incompetence. In the United States, Roberts et al.[6] found at necropsy that aortic stenosis was twice as frequent as mitral stenosis. In Cape Town mitral stenosis is approximately one third more common than aortic stenosis (Table 2.1) and the autopsy incidence of

Table 2.1 Aetiology of acquired valvular heart disease in 1225 necropsy patients

	MS (%)	MI (%)	AS (%)	AI (%)	TVD (%)	PVD (%)
Rheumatic fever	444 (99.8)	133 (69.8)	139 (46.3)	76 (41.8)	8 (79.4)	
Unclassified		3 (1.6)	87 (29)*			
Aortic nodular sclerosis			64 (21.3)			
Infection		34 (17.6)	10 (3.3)	60 (33)	18 (17.7)	2 (66.7)
Syphilis				17 (9.3)		
Medionecrosis				17 (9.3)		
Floppy valve		13 (6.7)**	2 (1.1)	2 (2)		
Restrictive cardiomyopathy		6 (3.1)				
Rupture papillary muscle		3 (1.6)				
Rheumatoid arthritis				3 (1.6)		
Lost commissural support						
(a) Fallot-type ventricular septal defect				2 (1.1)		
(b) Aortic dissection				3 (1.6)		
Whipple's disease	1 (0.2)					
Ankylosing spondylitis				1 (0.6)		
Ehlers–Danlos syndrome				1 (0.6)		
Carcinoid syndrome					1 (1)	1 (33.3)
Systemic lupus erythematosus		1 (0.5)				
Totals	445 (36.3)	193 (15.8)	300 (24.5)	182 (14.9)	102 (8.3)	3 (0.3)

Grand total = 1225 (6.8% of 18 132 autopsies).

*81 of the patients had isolated AS
**One patient had Marfan's syndrome
MS = mitral stenosis, MI = mitral incompetence, AS = aortic stenosis, AI = aortic incompetence, TVD = tricuspid valve disease, PVD = pulmonary valve disease
(Modified from Rose, A. G. (1986). Etiology of acquired valvular heart disease in adults. A survey of 18 132 autopsies and 100 consecutive valve replacement operations. *Arch. Pathol. Lab. Med*, **100**, 385–388. Copyright 1986 by American Medical Association.)

12

mitral stenosis has not diminished over the 30-year period 1950–79[7]. In the United Kingdom and Japan the incidence rate of rheumatic fever is 0.06/1000 inhabitants and in America it is 0.7/1000 persons. A conservative estimate[8] of the incidence of rheumatic fever in South Africa is 7/1000 inhabitants, and in immigrants from India to the Province of Natal it is 11/1000.

Only 46.3% of acquired aortic stenosis (Colour Plates D and E) was due to chronic rheumatic-type deformity. In 81 out of the 87 patients (93%) with unclassified aortic stenosis the aortic valve was the only diseased heart valve. According to Roberts et al.[6] such isolated valvular aortic stenosis is nearly always non-rheumatic in origin and most commonly represents a congenital malformation of this valve[9,10]. Davies[11] states that the predominant cause of isolated aortic valve stenosis is premature calcification of a congenitally bicuspid valve.

Congenital heart disease

The autopsy incidence of congenital heart disease at the University of Cape Town is given in Table 2.2. Diseases not necessarily treated by valve replacement or use of a conduit are included for comparative purposes. Even

Table 2.2   Types of congenital heart disease in 358 autopsy patients comprising 2.0% of 18 132 autopsies encountered over the 30-year period 1950–79

		Totals
Mitral valve		
Stenosis	5 (1.4%)	
Incompetence	4 (1.1%)	29
Atresia	20 (5.6%)	
Aortic valve		
Stenosis	7 (2.0%)	
Atresia	12 (3.4%)	31
Calcified bicuspid	12 (3.4%)	
Incompetence	0	
Tricuspid valve		
Stenosis	10 (2.3%)	
Atresia	12 (3.4%)	30
Straddling	3 (0.8%)	
Ebstein's anomaly	5 (1.4%)	
Incompetence	0	
Pulmonary valve		
Stenosis	24 (6.7%)	
Fallot's tetralogy	82 (22.9%)	146
Atresia	40 (11.2%)	
Common atrioventricular canal	14 (3.9%)	
Subaortic stenosis	9 (2.5%)	
Double-outlet right ventricle	15 (4.2%)	122
Persistent truncus arteriosus	22 (6.2%)	
Complete transposition	62 (17.3%)	
Total	358	

if cases of tetralogy are excluded, congenital pulmonary valve disease was twice as common as other congenital valvular diseases. Congenital mitral incompetence may require mitral valve replacement. Aortic stenosis may be present from birth or it may develop as a result of cuspal calcification in later life, e.g. in a unicommissural aortic valve.

CLINICAL INDICATIONS FOR HEART VALVE REPLACEMENT

Several reports deal with the pathophysiological and clinical aspects of diseases of the natural heart valves[12-15] and others consider the general aspects of heart valve surgery[16,17]. The functional capacity of the heart is assessed by the classification of the New York Heart Asociation (NYHA), which is based on the patient's history of past and present disability[18].

Acquired valvular heart disease

Surgery for acquired valvular disease is palliative only. Working together, the cardiologist and cardiac surgeon must select for operation those patients in whom heart valve replacement (with its attendant operative and long-term risks) offers a better prognosis for health and longevity than continued medical therapy.

Mitral valvular disease

Mitral valvotomy is usually performed on patients with severe mitral stenosis and an aggravation of symptoms, i.e. in class III of cardiac function by the NYHA classification[18] not due to medically remediable causes. Some patients are only referred for surgery once they are totally disabled (class IV). All closed operations are performed with the immediate availability of cardiopulmonary bypass, so that valve replacement may be performed if valvotomy is unsuccessful. If severe cuspal calcification accompanies the stenosis, then mitral valve replacement is usually indicated[19]. Patients with similarly severe disability due to mitral regurgitation may also need valve replacement. Fortunately, patients with both mitral stenosis and mitral insufficiency run protracted courses and the timing of the surgery can be selected deliberately.

Aortic valvular disease

Critical aortic valve stenosis, and mild stenosis associated with severe coronary arterial atherosclerotic narrowing, may give identical symptoms. The first requires aortic valve replacement and the other does not. The combination of severe coronary artery disease and severe aortic stenosis (or incompetence) is usually an indication for surgery in symptomatic patients since the medical prognosis is ominous[19].

Unlike mitral valve disease, patients with aortic valve disease often do well for a long time, but their condition deteriorates rapidly once symptoms appear. Accentuated angina pectoris or angina at rest, syncope on effort, and accelerated dyspnoea or pulmonary oedema indicate a grave prognosis. Such patients are at risk for sudden death. The decision to operate must be made expeditiously in such patients.

Multivalvular disease

The combination of aortic and mitral disease is usually due to rheumatic fever. Bivalvular disease has a long course similar to that of isolated mitral valve disease. Indications for surgery are similar to those for isolated mitral or aortic valve disease.

Tricuspid valvular disease

This is usually overshadowed by coexistent severe rheumatic deformities of the mitral and aortic valves. Functional tricuspid incompetence is more common than organic disease of this valve, but the distinction can usually only be made at operation. Functional insufficiency is treated by annuloplasty rather than by valve replacement. Tricuspid valve replacement is nearly always performed in conjunction with replacement of left-sided heart valves.

Indications for heart valve replacement

The following are the indications for heart valve replacement for rheumatic valvular disease at Groote Schuur Hospital, Cape Town:

1. Aortic stenosis and/or aortic incompetence plus symptoms.
2. Mitral stenosis may undergo closed valvotomy if there are class III symptoms and the valve is suitable. The valve should be replaced if there are class III symptoms and the valve is not suitable for valvotomy e.g., if it is severely calcified.
3. Mitral incompetence with class III symptoms on medical treatment.
4. Asymptomatic patients with aortic incompetence and mitral incompetence may need valve replacement if there are signs of increasing left ventricular dilatation.

Most valve replacements at Groote Schuur Hospital are done because of rheumatic heart disease.

Miscellaneous diseases[20-23] necessitating valve replacement include, e.g., papillary muscle rupture; infective endocarditis; chordal rupture; aortic incompetence due to aortic diseases such as syphilitic aortitis, sinus of Valsalva aneurysm, aortic dissection, rheumatoid aortic incompetence; Marfan's syndrome; lupus valvulitis; Whipple's disease; ochronosis of the aortic valve; and endomyocardial fibrosis. Other reports deal with valve replacement in special groups of patients, e.g. children[24,25], the elderly[26] and patients with valve prostheses who need reoperation[27].

15

Congenital heart disease

Decisions regarding cardiac operations on children with congenital heart disease have to be handled individually by the physician in consultation with the parents[28]. The clearest indication for operation is a matter of life or death, e.g. a newborn child with transposition of the great arteries and an intact ventricular septum. Without operation there is a 90% mortality rate in a few months; with surgery the survival rate is 90% over the same period. Some cases of transposition with associated hypoplastic pulmonary valve and infundibulum may require use of a valved conduit to link the right ventricle to the distal pulmonary artery. This is usually done as part of a Rastelli operation[29].

Although stenosis and infective endocarditis are commonly appreciated complications of the congenitally bicuspid aortic valve, pure severe aortic regurgitation complicating this congenital malformation, unassociated with either stenosis or infection, can occur[30]. Severe mitral incompetence in symptomatic patients with ostium primum atrial septal defects may require very complex surgical techniques or mitral valve replacement (Figure 2.1). Attempts have been made to correct complete atrioventricular canal defects

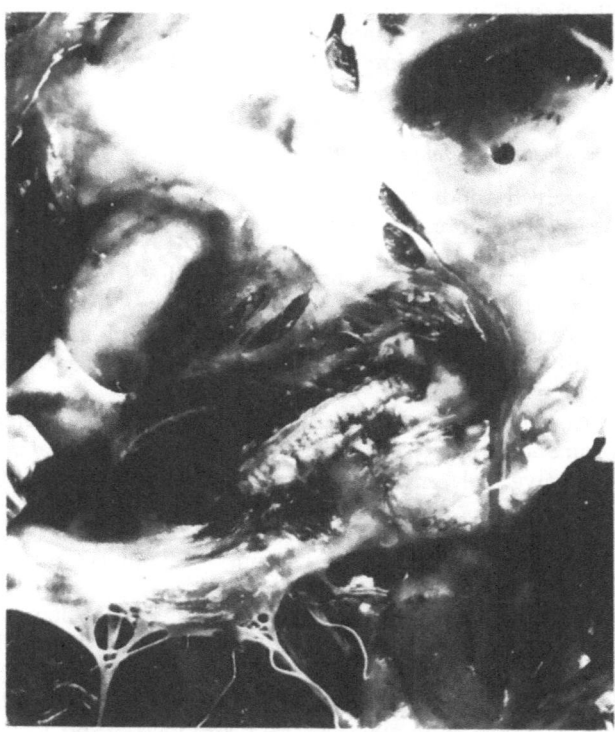

Figure 2.1 View into right atrium and right ventricle. Sewing ring of mitral valve prosthesis is visible through portion of ostium primum defect, which the surgeon had attempted to close by direct suture. Excessive tension caused the sutures to cut through the tissue

by closure of the defect and reconstruction of the atrioventricular valve. Prosthetic valve replacement can be avoided in the overwhelming majority of such patients. Some patients with persistent truncus arteriosus have required replacement of the truncal valve at the time of total correction.

Valve replacement is necessary in 10–15% of cases of congenital mitral valve malformation. However, valve replacement is associated with a higher morbidity and mortality compared to valve repairs. Schwarze and Bernhard[31] describe the special pathology of reconstructable or only prosthetically correctable congenital malformations of the mitral valve, including, e.g., the hammock valve (mitral arcade) and absent papillary muscles. Congenital mitral valve incompetence is usually treated by reconstructive surgery, and valve replacement is seldom indicated. Tricuspid valve replacement may be performed in patients with Ebstein's anomaly.

Patients with tricuspid atresia (and normal ventriculoarterial connections) usually need some form of systemic to pulmonary artery or cavopulmonary arterial anastomosis in the first few years of life to alleviate progressive hypoxia. In the Fontan procedure[32], the atrial septal defect is closed and the right atrium is anastomosed to the outlet chamber, either directly or by an external conduit. As the outlet chamber is expected to act as a ventricle, there is a theoretical advantage in inserting a valve between the right atrium and the outlet chamber. A Fontan-like surgical approach is also applicable to patients with tricuspid atresia, transposition of the great arteries and pulmonary stenosis.

An extracardiac valved conduit has been used to treat pulmonary atresia. The conduit is anastomosed to the distal main pulmonary artery or to its branches, and to a right ventriculotomy incision. Double-outlet left ventricle and double-outlet right ventricle have similar indications for operation: early repair or pulmonary artery banding in infants with high pulmonary blood flow, aortopulmonary shunt and subsequent repair using external valved conduit in patients with associated pulmonary or subpulmonary stenosis.

Transannular outflow tract patches may be used to overcome right ventricular outflow tract obstruction. If such patients have haemodynamically significant pulmonary insufficiency in association with residual pulmonary artery stenosis, pulmonary hypertension from other causes, or associated tricuspid regurgitation, a prosthetic valve can be implanted at the level of the annulus under the outflow patch, or a valved conduit may be used.

With regard to univentricular hearts, most centres have abandoned the approach of septation of such hearts plus use of a valved conduit to establish continuity between the newly created 'right' ventricle and the pulmonary artery. However, this technique may still be applied in the patient with single left ventricle, left-sided infundibular chamber supporting a discordantly connected and laevopositioned aorta, naturally occurring pulmonary outflow tract obstruction, or two functionally normal atrioventricular valves. The likelihood of damage to, and the need to replace, the abnormal atrioventricular valves, contributed to the high initial mortality of the procedure and to the postoperative morbidity.

MATCHING PROSTHESIS TO PATIENT

Consideration should be given to the unique concerns of any given patient before a particular prosthesis is chosen[33-36]. Roberts[33] discussed the choice of a substitute cardiac valve with reference to type, size and surgeon. He regarded the caged-disc prosthesis as the least desirable since it obstructs, it thromboses and disintegrates. The other three types of valve prostheses have more favourable characteristics. Because of its large size, the caged-ball prosthesis might be limited to patients with mainly regurgitant lesions. The tilting disc has favourable haemodynamics and is durable. Long-term anticoagulant therapy is necessary with all of the mechanical valves. The glutaraldehyde-treated porcine xenograft valve lacks the latter disadvantage, but its durability is suspect and it is unsuitable for use in young patients due to calcification.

Roberts[33] believes that if the valve replacement is performed in a large, well-equipped medical centre by an experienced surgical team, the operative result is more dependent on the type and size of substitute valve inserted than on the surgeon who inserts the valve.

Guidelines for the use of tissue valves (bioprostheses)

Chung[34] has proposed the following guidelines for use of tissue valves for heart valve replacement: (1) patients unable to have adequate control of anticoagulation; (2) patients with less than 10 years life expectancy, especially if the patient is older than 60 years of age; (3) women wanting to have children, or patients engaged in potentially traumatic activity. They should not be used in children or in patients receiving dialysis for renal failure. McClung et al.[35] state that although few anatomical complications have been described, the Ionescu–Shiley pericardial bioprosthesis may be more suitable for aortic valve replacement due to its greater flow capacity, whilst the porcine xenograft may be more suitable in the mitral position because of anatomical considerations.

Guidelines for the use of mechanical prosthetic valves

(1) Patients aged 35 years or younger. (2) Patients on renal dialysis or having disorders of calcium metabolism. (3) Patients needing long-term anticoagulation for other indications, e.g. atrial fibrillation or past thrombo-embolism.

ASSESSING THE AETIOLOGY OF EXCISED DISEASED HEART VALVES

About two-thirds of excised natural heart valves are submitted to the pathologist without the surgeon indicating the suspected aetiology of the valvular disease necessitating the operation[7]. The pathologist is able to make an aetiological diagnosis in only one-third of excised valves. This is not surprising since fibrous thickening, distortion or destruction of the normal architecture, and superimposition of thrombus, are non-specific findings, which may occur in both congenital and acquired valve lesions. The only feature identifying the acquired lesions histologically is the increased vascularity[10]. Since some rheumatic-type valves are very sparsely vascularized, even this histological feature is of dubious specificity[9]. In a personal series[7], review of the operation notes, in conjunction with the macroscopical description of the excised valve and the cuspal histology, enabled one to make an aetiological diagnosis in 81% of excised valves. The crucial information needed for improving the aetiopathological diagnosis is knowledge of the appearance of the intact valve.

The mitral valve is usually excised *in toto* and thus its macroscopical morphology may be interpreted by the pathologist. Few pathologists seem prepared to label severe mitral valve stenosis as a chronic rheumatic-type of deformity; usually only a description is given without any reference being made as to the likely aetiology. Although there are other rare causes of mitral stenosis, e.g. Whipple's disease, carcinoid syndrome, treatment with methysergide, Fabry's disease, Hurler–Schei syndrome and pseudoxanthoma elasticum, the presence of this lesion is pathognomonic of previous rheumatic fever.

In the case of the aortic valve it is important that the pathologist be given a guide as to the appearance of the valve at operation and/or the clinically suspected aetiology of the valvular disease, since the aortic valve is usually removed in fragments and it is often not possible for the pathologist to reconstruct the appearance of the intact valve. Davies[11] points out that it is not possible to report meaningfully on one cusp. Each report should note the number of cusps, their shape, the presence of fibrosis or calcification, and whether commissural fusion is present. This is usually easily recognizable, even in a surgically excised valve. Since infection[36] of the native heart valve at the time of heart valve replacement may predispose to infection of the prosthetic valve, it is important to alert the pathologist to this possibility, since antibiotics may mute the inflammatory response and appropriate stains for micro-organisms may not be performed. An additional problem is that a non-specific chronic valvulitis is a common finding in chronic rheumatic valvular disease.

INCIDENCE OF ASCHOFF BODIES IN SURGICALLY REMOVED CARDIAC TISSUE

The Aschoff body (nodule) in its granulomatous (proliferative) phase is the pathognomonic myocardial lesion of rheumatic fever[37]. Not everyone agrees on what constitutes a typical Aschoff body. Fassbender[38] stresses the perivascular situation of the classical Aschoff body and describes three evolutionary patterns of rheumatic carditis:

1. The 'exudative' variety of the rheumatic process may run a fulminating clinical course, especially in children, with death from heart failure within

3 weeks. Not a single Aschoff body may be present, only an interstitial fibrinous exudate with large numbers of neutrophiles and occasional lymphocytes. This form may represent a type of Arthus phenomenon.

2. The granulomatous (proliferative) form of rheumatic carditis (Colour Plate B) is the classical Aschoff body, the features of which will be described below. The Aschoff body passes through four phases: (a) exudative, (b) granulomatous (proliferative), (c) resolving and (d) healed phases. It is only the granulomatous phase which is diagnostic of rheumatic fever. This phase is noted 1 month or more after an acute attack of rheumatic fever and may persist in the tissue for 3–6 months or even longer after the symptoms of the acute attack have abated.

A small area of fibrinoid necrosis may be present at the centre of the nodule in the early granulomatous phase. It becomes surrounded and finally replaced by histiocytes, giant cells, lymphocytes, plasma cells and fibroblasts arranged in roughly parallel rows. The histiocytes (so-called Anitschkow 'myocytes') have a characteristic owl's-eye appearance of the nucleus due to a bar-like arrangement of the chromatin. These cells gives rise to giant cells (Aschoff cells) which are usually found towards the centre of the nodule.

3. The muscle-associated ('myoaggressive granuloma') spares the connective tissue, is usually not seen in association with typical Aschoff nodes and is found in the myocardium itself or in the loose subendothelial tissues in juxtaposition to necrotic myofibres. No fibrinoid is seen, only small fragments of necrotic muscle. Autoantibodies directed against cardiac muscle may cause the necrosis, which may be a late complication of long-continued rheumatic carditis. The granulomata produced experimentally in rabbit hearts by Murphy[39], who repeatedly injected the animals with killed group A streptococci, appear to be of a similar nature to the muscle-associated granuloma and are unlike the Aschoff body.

The records of the University of Cape Town Pathology Department list 116 out of 468 atrial appendages of patients with mitral valve stenosis (with or without mild incompetence) as containing Aschoff bodies (24.8%). These diagnoses had been made by several different pathologists, all of whom had ostensibly been looking for granulomatous (proliferative) phase Aschoff bodies. Table 2.3 summarizes my findings after reviewing the histology of these 116 patients.

I found that if strict criteria[37] were applied for granulomatous phase Aschoff bodies, then only 82 of the 116 patients had acceptable Aschoff bodies; this corresponds to 17.5% of the total group of 468 patients. The

Table 2.3 Review of 116 surgically removed atrial appendages (from patients with mitral stenosis) diagnosed by a variety of pathologists as containing Aschoff bodies

No. of patients	Granulomatous phase Aschoff bodies	Review negative for Aschoff bodies		
		Mononuclear cells	Non-specific granuloma	Organizing thrombus
116	82	25	4	5

Table 2.4 Incidence of Aschoff bodies in atrial appendages of patients operated upon for mitral valve disease

Authors	Year	Reference	Incidence (%)
Pinniger	1951	40	67
Waaler	1952	41	25
Decker et al.	1953	42	46
McKeown	1953	43	45
McNeely et al.	1953	44	46
Gil et al.	1955	45	75
Lannigan	1961	46	64
Ruebner and Boitnott	1961	47	41
Roberts and Virmani	1978	48	21
Silver	1983	49	40
Vijayanagar et al.	1983	50	2
Present series			18

commonest error was the labelling of focal collections of mononuclear cells (mainly lymphocytes) as Aschoff bodies. Four patients had muscle-associated granulomata of the type described by Fassbender[38] without typical Aschoff bodies. Organizing endocardial thrombi were misinterpreted as Aschoff bodies in five other patients.

The reported incidence of active Aschoff bodies in atrial appendages removed from patients with mitral stenosis varies from centre to centre (Table 2.4). While all record the incidence of 'Aschoff nodules', there are some differences in the histological criteria. Another factor is the variation from centre to centre of the types of patient selected for operation. The Cape Town incidence correlates best with the incidences of 25% reported by Waaler[41] and the 21% noted by Roberts and Virmani[48].

REFERENCES

1. John, S., Jairaj, P. S., Muralidharan, S., Bashi, V. V., Vinod, A., Krishnaswamy, S. and Sukumar, I. P. (1986). Aortic valve replacement in India. Early and long-term results. *J. Cardiovasc. Surg.*, **27**, 207
2. Krause, R. M. (1979). The influence of infection on the geography of heart disease. *Circulation*, **60**, 972
3. Besterman, E. (1970). The changing face of acute rheumatic fever. *Br. Heart J.*, **32**, 579
4. Silver, M. D. (1976). Recent advances in the knowledge of pathology of natural and artificial valves. In Kalmanson, D. (ed.) *The Mitral Valve: a Pluridisciplinary Approach*, pp. 51-63. (London: Edward Arnold)
5. Pomerance, A. and Davies, M. J. (1975). *The Pathology of the Heart*. (London: Blackwell Scientific Publications)
6. Roberts, W. C., Dangel, J. C. and Bulkley, B. H. (1973). Nonrheumatic valvular cardiac disease: a clinicopathologic survey of 27 different conditions causing valvular dysfunction. *Cardiovasc. Clin.*, **5**, 333
7. Rose, A. G. (1986). Etiology of acquired valvular heart disease in adults. A survey of 18,132 autopsies and 100 consecutive valve replacement operations. *Arch. Pathol. Lab. Med.*, **110**, 385
8. Editorial. (1984). Hartkwaal by kinders. *S. Afr. Med. J.*, **65**, 945
9. Roberts, W. C. (1973). Valvular, subvalvular and supravalvular aortic stenosis. Morphologic features. *Cardiovasc. Clin.*, **5**, 97
10. Falcone, M. W., Roberts, W. C., Morrow, A. G. and Perloff, J. K. (1971). Congenital aortic

stenosis resulting from a unicommissural valve. Clinical and anatomic features in twenty-one adult patients. *Circulation*, **44**, 272

11. Davies, M. J. (1980). *Pathology of Cardiac Valves*. (London: Butterworths)
12. Olsen, E. G. J. (1973). *The Pathology of the Heart*. (New York: Intercontinental Medical Book Corporation)
13. Rapaport, E. (1975). Natural history of aortic and mitral valve disease. *Am. J. Cardiol.*, **35**, 221
14. Edwards, J. E. (1979). Pathology of acquired valvular disease of the heart. *Sem. Roentgen.*, **14**, 96
15. Chizner, M. A., Pearle, D. L. and de Leon, A. C. Jr. (1980). The natural history of aortic stenosis in adults. *Am. Heart J.*, **49**, 419
16. Matloff, J. M. and Chaux, A. (1977). What is the current status of prosthetic cardiac valve replacement? *Cardiovasc. Clin.*, **8**, 279
17. Roberts, W. C. (1978). Substitute cardiac valves. Advantages and disadvantages of four commonly used ones. *Adv. Cardiol.*, **22**, 252
18. New York Heart Association (1973). *Nomenclature and criteria for the diagnosis of diseases of the heart and great vessels*, 7th edn. (New York: Little, Brown)
19. Ellis, L. B. (1971). Indications for surgery in patients with acquired valvular disease. *Cardiovasc. Clin.*, **3**, 61
20. Rostad, H., Hall, K. V. and Froysaker, T. (1979). Mitral insufficiency following myocardial infarction. *Scand. J. Thorac. Cardiovasc. Surg.*, **13**, 277
21. Shore, D. F., Wong, P. and Paneth, M. (1982). Valve repair versus replacement in the surgical management of ruptured chordae. A post-operative echocardiographic assessment of mitral valve function. *J. Cardiovasc. Surg.*, **23**, 378
22. Taguchi, K., Sasaki, N., Matsuura, Y. and Umera, R. (1969). Surgical correction of aneurysm of the sinus of Valsalva. A report of forty-five consecutive patients including eight with total replacement of the aortic valve. *Am. J. Cardiol.*, **23**, 180
23. Danielson, G. K., Titus, J. L. and DuShane, J. W. (1974). Successful treatment of aortic valve endocarditis and aortic root abscesses by insertion of prosthetic valve in ascending aorta and placement of bypass grafts to coronary arteries. *J. Thorac. Cardiovasc. Surg.*, **67**, 443
24. Van der Horst, R. L., le Roux, B. T., Rogers, N. M. A. and Gotsman, M. S. (1973). Mitral valve replacement in childhood. A report of 51 patients. *Am. Heart J.*, **85**, 624
25. Attie, F., Kuri, J., Zanoniani, C., Renteria, V., Buendia, A., Ovseyevitz, J., Lopez-Soriano, F., Garcia-Cornejo, M. and Martinez-Rios, M. A. (1981). Mitral valve replacement in children with rheumatic heart disease. *Circulation*, **64**, 812
26. Barnhorst, D. A., Giuliani, E. R., Pluth, J. R., Danielson, G. K., Wallace, R. B. and McGoon, D. C. (1974). Open-heart surgery in patients more than 65 years old. *Ann. Thorac. Surg.*, **18**, 81
27. Shemin, R. J., Guadiani, V. A., Conkle, D. M. and Morrow, A. G. (1979). Prosthetic aortic valves. Indications for and results of reoperation. *Arch. Surg.*, **114**, 63
28. Nadas, A. S. (1971). Indications for surgery in patients with congenital heart disease. *Cardiovasc. Clin.*, **3**, 51
29. Rastelli, G. C., McGoon, D. C. and Wallace, R. B. (1969). Anatomic correction of transposition of the great arteries with ventricular septal defect and subpulmonary stenosis. *J. Thorac. Cardiovasc. Surg.*, **58**, 545
30. Roberts, W. C., Morrow, A. G., McIntosh, C. L., Jones, M. and Epstein, S. E. (1981). Congenitally bicuspid aortic valve causing severe, pure aortic regurgitation without superimposed infective endocarditis. Analysis of 13 patients requiring aortic valve replacement. *Am. J. Cardiol.*, **47**, 206
31. Schwarze, E. W. and Bernhard, A. (1975). The pathological anatomy of surgically reconstructed or prosthetically correctable congenital valvular malformation of the mitral region. *Virchow's Arch. (Pathol. Anat.)*, **367**, 149
32. Fontan, F. and Baudet, E. (1971). Surgical repair of tricuspid atresia. *Thorax*, **26**, 240
33. Roberts, W. C. (1976). Choosing a substitute cardiac valve: type, size, surgeon. *Am. J. Cardiol.*, **38**, 633
34. Chung, G. K. (1982). The cardiac valve controversy: a point of view. *Hawaii Med. J.*, **41**, 56

35. McClung, J. A., Stein, J. H., Ambrose, J. A., Herman, H. V. and Reed, G. E. (1983). Prosthetic heart valves : A review. *Prog. Cardiovasc. Dis.*, **26**, 237

36. Leitersdorf, E., Friedman, G., Gozal, D., Appelbaum, A., Sacks, T. and Levij, I. (1982). Hypothesis : new concepts on the pathogenesis of early prosthetic valve endocarditis. *Med. Hypotheses*, **9**, 325

37. Aschoff, L. (1939). The rheumatic nodules in the heart. *Ann. Rheum. Dis.*, **1**, 161

38. Fassbender, H. G. (1975). *Pathology of Rheumatic Diseases*. (Berlin: Springer-Verlag)

39. Murphy, G. E. (1950). The induction of rheumatic-like cardiac lesions in rabbits by repeated focal infections with group A streptococci; comparison with cardiac lesions of serum disease. *J. Exp. Med.*, **91**, 485

40. Pinniger, J. L. (1951). The left auricular appendage in mitral stenosis. *St Thom. Hosp. Rep.*, **7**, 54

41. Waaler, E. (1952). Activity of the rheumatic auriculitis in chronic valvular disease. The distribution of rheumatic auriculitis. *Acta Pathol. Microbiol. Scand.*, **93**(Suppl.), 211

42. Decker, J. P., Hawn, C. van Z. and Robins, S. L. (1953). Rheumatic 'activity' as judged by the presence of Aschoff bodies in the auricular appendages of patients with mitral stenosis. I. Anatomic aspects. *Circulation*, **8**, 161

43. McKeown, E. F. (1953). The left auricular appendage in mitral stenosis. *Br. Heart J.*, **15**, 433

44. McNeely, V. F., Ellis, L. B. and Harken, D. E. (1953). Rheumatic 'activity' as judged by the presence of Aschoff bodies in auricular appendages of patients with mitral stenosis. II. Clinical aspects. *Circulation*, **8**, 337

45. Gil, J. R., Rodriguez, H. and Ibarra, J. J. (1955). Incidence of asymptomatic active rheumatic cardiac lesions in patients submitted to mitral commissurotomy and the effect of cortisone on these lesions. *Am. Heart J.*, **50**, 912

46. Lannigan, R. (1961). Sub-clinical rheumatic carditis. *Br. Heart J.* **23**, 35

47. Ruebner, B. H. and Boitnott, J. K. (1961). The frequency of Aschoff bodies in atrial appendages of patients with mitral stenosis. Relationship to age, atrial thrombosis, and season. *Circulation*, **23**, 550

48. Roberts, W. C. and Virmani, R. (1978). Aschoff bodies at necropsy in valvular heart disease. Evidence from an analysis of 543 patients over 14 years of age that rheumatic heart disease, at least anatomically, is a disease of the mitral valve. *Circulation*, **57**, 803

49. Silver, M. D. (1983). *Cardiovascular Pathology*. (New York: Churchill Livingstone).

50. Vijayanagar, R., Bognolo, D., Eckstein, P., Jeffery, D., Toole, J., Natarajan, P. and Willard, E. (1983). Surgical treatment of mitral valve disease: pathologic findings and atrial dysrhythmia. *South. Med. J.*, **76**, 703

3

Design, Classification and Identification of Prosthetic Heart Valves: Gross Examination of the Heart containing a Prosthesis, Analysis of Removed Prostheses

DESIGN CRITERIA FOR PROSTHETIC HEART VALVES[1-3]

For satisfactory long-term function in man, a prosthetic heart valve must fulfil numerous design criteria:

1. It must be chemically inert and compatible with human tissues. There should be no toxic, allergenic or carcinogenic effects. There should be no host reaction deleterious to the prosthesis.
2. The valve should cause little trauma to the formed elements of the blood.
3. It must have a low thrombogenicity. In third world countries a lack of need for anticoagulants is an advantage, as too, is a low price.
4. It should be durable over many years of function (i.e. outlast the lifespan of the patient), bearing in mind that such a prosthesis has to open and close about 100 000 times a day. A single-block construction (i.e. no welds) is preferable.
5. The prosthesis should present minimal obstruction to forward blood flow when open; it should open and close quickly in response to changes in pressure gradients; it should also be relatively competent in the closed position.
6. Fixation in a physiological position must be technically feasible, safe, and secure over many years.
7. The valve should not be noisy, and it should not require the patient to modify his lifestyle appreciably[4].
8. The valve should be resistant to infection.

Many heart valve prostheses, some of which are no longer in use, have been aimed at achieving these objectives[5-10]. Silver and Wilson[11] illustrate some of the recent prostheses. Figures 3.1 to 3.3 summarize the process of heart valve development, the designs of currently used major categories of

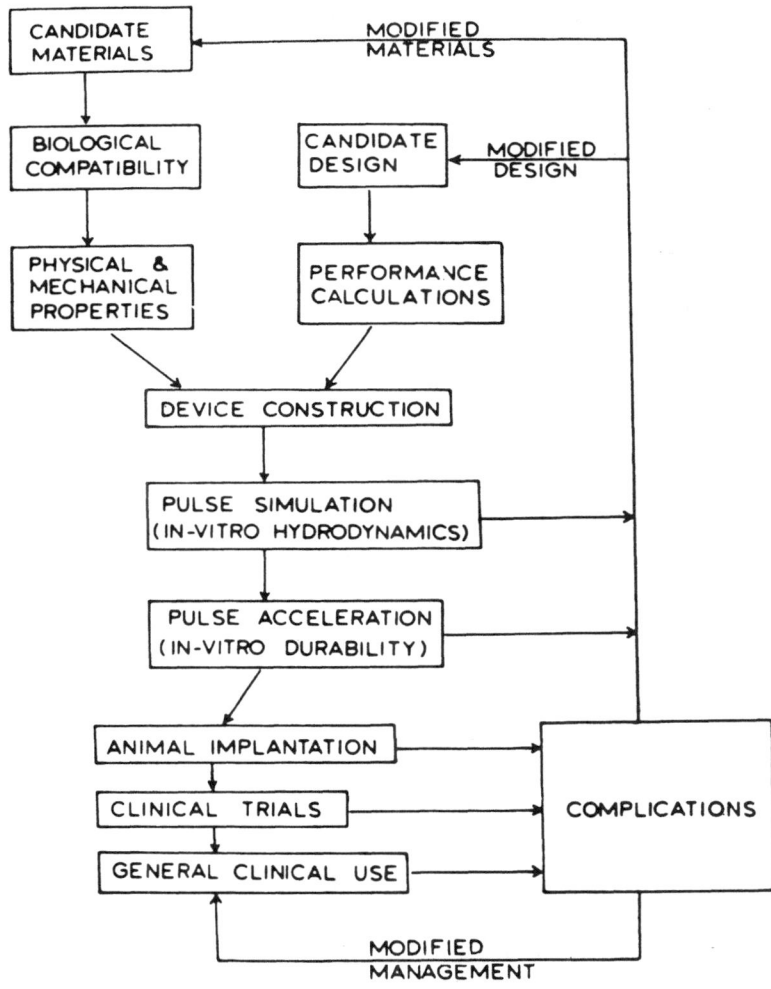

Figure 3.1 Flow chart of heart valve development process. (Schoen, F. J., Titus, J. L. and Lawrie, G. M. (1982) Bioengineering aspects of heart valve replacement. *Ann. Biomed. Eng.,* **10**, 97-128; by permission)

prostheses and the sequential popularity of various valves. There are prominent regional differences in the utilization of the various prostheses. Table 3.1 gives a classification of the various types of prosthetic heart valves previously and currently available, and lists most of the prostheses falling into each

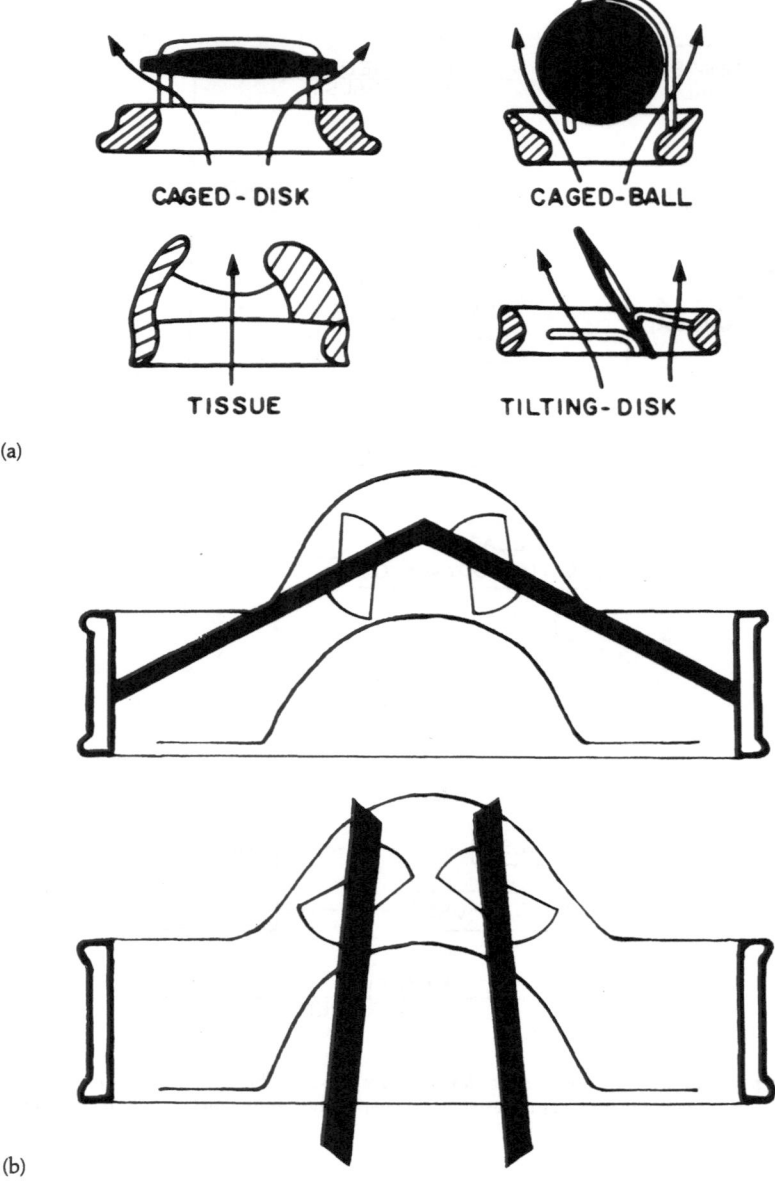

(a)

(b)

Figure 3.2 Designs and flow patterns of major categories of presently used prosthetic heart valves. (a) Caged-ball, caged-disc, tilting-disc, and bioprosthesis (tissue valve). (Schoen, F. J., Titus, J. L., Lawrie, G. M. (1982). Bioengineering aspects of heart valve replacement. *Ann. Biomed. Eng.*, **10**, 97–128; by permission). (b) Bileaflet tilting-disc valve in opened and closed positions

category. The reasons for the decline in use of certain types of heart valves are listed in Table 3.2.

IDENTIFICATION OF PROSTHETIC HEART VALVES

Several articles outline the morphological[4-7] and radiological[8,9] criteria for the identification of prosthetic heart valves. Identification is rendered difficult due to the continuing introduction of new prosthetic heart valves. There is an increasing recognition of prosthesis-related complications. The pathologist performing an autopsy on such patients should be aware of the types of prostheses used in the region and, if available, the operation notes should provide useful information in this regard.

Firstly (Figures 3.4 and 3.5, and Table 3.2), one has to decide if the valve in question is a mechanical prosthesis (made of artificial materials) or a xenograft prosthesis (made of biological tissue). With regard to mechanical prostheses, there are high-profile valves which have a ball (Figure 3.4) as the mobile portion (Starr–Edwards, Smeloff–Cutter, DeBakey–Surgitool,

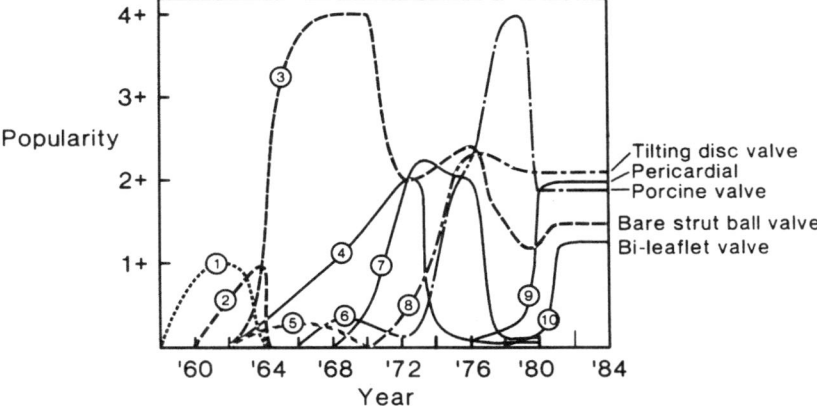

Figure 3.3 Popularity of prosthetic heart valves plotted against time. *Line 1*, short-lived technique of debridement of the calcified valve antedated valve replacement. *Line 2*, beginning at 1960, represents the Teflon cloth valve, either single cusps or a trileaflet type. *Line 3*, which reaches the highest point on the graph, is the bare-strut ball-valve prosthesis, the archetype of which is the Starr–Edwards 1260 valve; it declined in popularity after 1970 due to competition from several new approaches. *Line 4*, the homograft valve, which declined steeply in popularity in the early 1970s. *Line 5*, non-tilting, disc-type valve. *Line 6*, heterograft porcine valve, first of limited popularity because of the inadequacy of formaldehyde fixation, but by late 1970s its glutaraldehyde-preserved form had gained exceptional popularity. Latterly it has declined in popularity due to increasing concern about durability. *Line 7*, cloth-covered ball-valve design; this has disappeared from use. *Line 8*, tilting-disc valve, the archetype being the Bjork–Shiley valve, which has enjoyed rather steady increase in popularity. *Line 9*, bovine pericardial bioprosthesis, the archetype being the Ionescu–Shiley valve, which has gained in popularity due to its haemodynamic advantage. *Line 10*, the bileaflet all-synthetic valve (St Jude) has enjoyed increasing acceptance. (McGoon, D. C. (1982) Long-term effects of prosthetic materials. *Am. J. Cardiol.*, **50**, 621–629; by permission)

Table 3.1 Classification of the various types of prosthetic heart valves

A. Mechanical prostheses

1. *Caged-ball valves*
   - (i) Starr–Edwards ball valve
   - (ii) Smeloff–Cutter (now Smeloff–Sutter) valve
   - (iii) Harken valve
   - (iv) Magovern–Cromie valve
   - (v) Braunwald–Cutter valve
   - (vi) DeBakey–Surgitool valve

2. *Caged-disc valves*
   - (i) Hufnagel–Conrad valve
   - (ii) Cross–Jones valve
   - (iii) Kay–Suzuki valve
   - (iv) Harken–Cromie valve
   - (v) Kay–Shiley valve
   - (vi) Beall valve
   - (vii) Starr–Edwards disc valve
   - (viii) Cooley–Cutter valve
   - (ix) University of Stellenbosch valve
   - (x) Alvarez valve

3. *Hinged-leaflet valve*
   Gott–Daggett hinged-leaflet valve

4. *Tethered plunger valve*
   University of Cape Town valve

5. *Cageless, central-flow, low-profile, tilting disc valves*
   - (i) Pierce valve
   - (ii) Wada–Cutter valve
   - (iii) Bjork–Shiley valve
   - (iv) Lillehei–Kaster valve
   - (v) Lillehei–Medical valve
   - (vi) Hammersmith valve
   - (vii) Hall–Kaster (Medtronic-Hall) valve
   - (viii). Omniscience valve
   - (ix) Omnicarbon valve

6. *Bileaflet (bivalve) prostheses*
   - (i) Kalke–Lillehei valve
   - (ii) St Jude Medical valve
   - (iii) Duromedics valve

B. Tissue valves

1. *Homograft aortic valves*
   - (i) Fresh homograft aortic valve
   - (ii) Sterilized homograft aortic valve

2. *Xenograft aortic valves*
   - (i) Unfixed xenograft valves
   - (ii) Formaldehyde-treated valve
   - (iii) Glutaraldehyde-treated valves
      - (a) Carpentier valve
      - (b) Hancock valve
      - (c) Carpentier–Edwards valve
      - (d) Angell–Shiley valve
      - (e) Low-profile bioprosthesis
      - (f) Xenomedica bioprosthesis
      - (g) Tascon bioprosthesis

Table 3.1 *Continued*

3. *Autologous fascia lata valve*

4. *Dura mater homograft valve*

5. *Bovine pericardial xenograft valves*
   (i) Ionescu–Shiley bioprosthesis
   (ii) Carpentier–Edwards bioprosthesis
   (iii) Mitroflow Medical bioprosthesis
   (iv) Meadox–Gabbay bioprosthesis
   (v) Bicuspid mitral bioprosthesis
   (vi) Hancock bioprosthesis

6. *Polymeric trileaflet valve prosthesis*
   Abiomed heart valve prosthesis

C. Valve-containing conduits
   1. Pulmonary artery and valve substitutes
   2. Left ventricle-to-aorta bypass
   3. Replacement of ascending aorta and aortic valve

Braunwald–Cutter, Magovern–Cromie, Harken, and Surgitool 200 prostheses) and low-profile valves, which have a mobile disc (Figure 3.5). The latter include the following prostheses: Lillehei–Kaster, Wada–Cutter, Bjork–Shiley, Cooley–Cutter, Kay–Suzuki, Harken, Starr–Edwards model 6520, Cross–Jones, Beall model 103, Beall–Surgitool model 105, and the Kay–Shiley (T series, K series, MGCD series and TGCD series) prostheses.

Next the number of struts should be examined. With the low-profile valves it is important to note whether the struts have an acute angle to the base ring plane (Lillehei–Kaster), emerge into the valve orifice (Wada–Cutter, Bjork–Shiley), or arise at right angles to the base ring plane (Cooley–Cutter, Kay–Suzuki, Starr–Edwards models 6500 and 6520 disc valves, Harken disc valve, Cross–Jones, Beall model 103, Beall–Surgitool model 105, and Kay–Shiley (series T, K, MGCD, TGCD prostheses).

Note whether the cage is single (Starr–Edwards) or double (Smeloff–Cutter) and whether the cage is open (Braunwald–Cutter, Magovern–Cromie, and Starr–Edwards models 2300, 2310, 6300, 6310). In the latter Starr–Edwards models the cloth covering the struts obscures the opening, which is easily identified only by radiography. The Magovern–Cromie valve has a large cage opening, whereas the above-listed Starr–Edwards models have a small cage opening. The other models of the Starr–Edwards prostheses have a closed cage. Other distinguishing features[4-7] include the strut–ring junction, the shape of the base ring edge, the site at which the poppet seats (e.g. near its equator or otherwise), and the radiolucency of the ball or disc occluder.

Radiography of a prosthesis may help to identify the type of heart valve prosthesis (Table 3.3 and Figures 3.6–3.17); this is of particular value with bioprostheses. Whereas radiography of the Hancock porcine aortic valve prosthesis, like that of the Hancock pericardial heart valve, reveals only a narrow wire-like base ring, the Carpentier–Edwards bioprosthesis has a radiolucent base ring and only the serpentine-like wire stent is radiopaque (Figure 3.7). Updating an earlier report[8], Mehlman[9] has recently reviewed

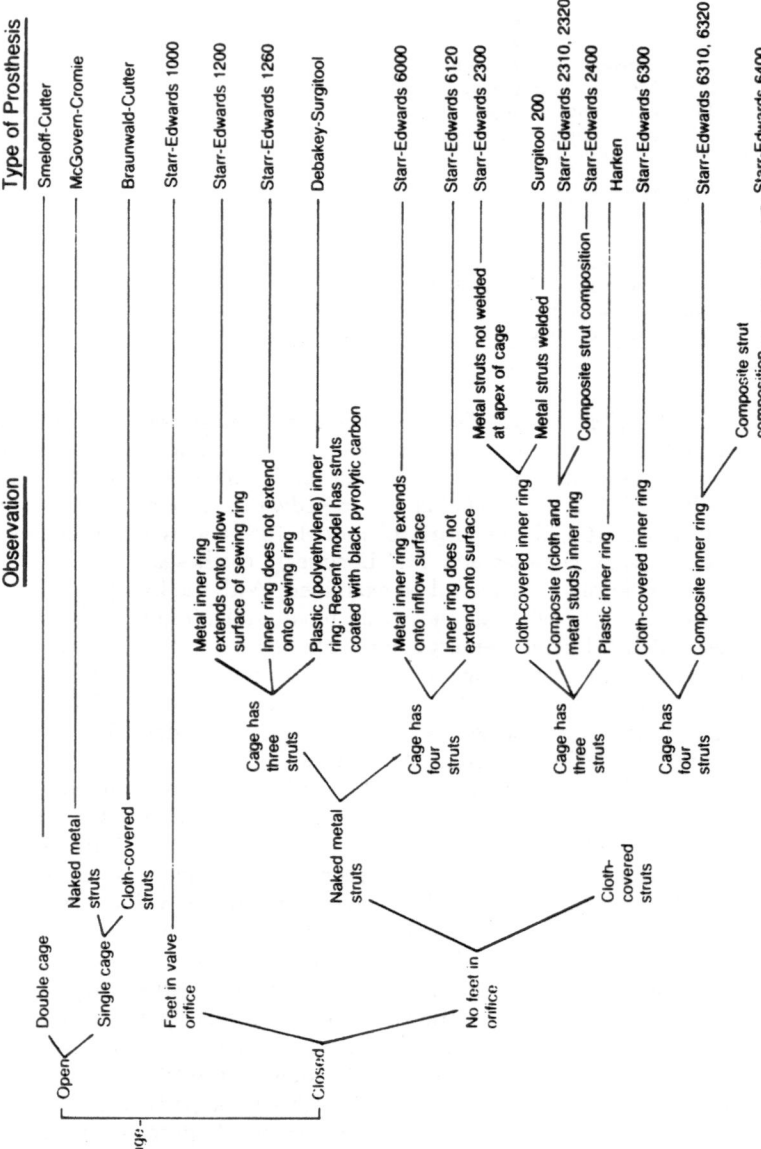

Figure 3.4 Key to identify ball-valve prostheses. (Modified after ref. 5; copyright 1975 by American Medical Association)

Table 3.2 The 'rise and fall' of replacement valves

	Reason for	
Type of valve	Introduction	Decline in use
Cloth cusp	Hydrodynamic*	Failure in durability
Central disc	Hydrodynamic*	Failure in durability
Bare strut ball	Hydrodynamic*	(Thrombogenicity)
Homograft	Less thrombogenic	Failure in durability
Tilting disc	Hydrodynamic	(Failure in 'durability'†)
		(Thrombogenicity)
Heterograft	Less thrombogenic	(Failure in durability)
Cloth-covered ball valve	Less thrombogenic	Failure in durability
		Not less thrombogenic
Pericardial	Hydrodynamic	(?Failure in durability)
Bileaflet	Hydrodynamic	?

* Compared with previously unreplaceable diseased valve
( ) Valves which remain popular, but which would be even more successful
were it not for the limitation given
† 'Durability' in this usage refers to thrombotic immobilization of the disc

(McGoon, D. C. (1982). Long-term effects of prosthetic materials. *Am. J. Cardiol.*, **50**, 621–629; by permission.)

Table 3.3 Radiographic identification of xenograft heart valve prostheses

Prosthesis	Special features	Base ring
Angell–Shiley	All parts radiolucent	Radiolucent
Carpentier–Edwards	Radiopaque, serpiginous wire stent	Radiolucent
Hancock	Radiolucent stent	Radiopaque
Ionescu–Shiley	Flat, mono-unit base ring and stent with perforations	Radiopaque

the radiographic features of ten of the newer valvular prostheses marketed since 1978.

Although superficially similar to the radiographic silhouette of the Carpentier–Edwards bioprosthesis, in the Carpentier–Edwards SupraAnnular (SAV) bioprosthesis the change of shape of the wireform as it shifts from base ring to stent is more gradual, giving the wire a gently curving instead of a right-angle appearance (Figure 3.8). In the Carpentier–Edwards pericardial valve prosthesis (Figure 3.9) the base ring is marked radiographically by a flattened circular ring with three holes. The flattened ring does not extend into the stent as is the case with the Ionescu–Shiley bioprosthesis. In addition, a narrow wireform outlines each of the three stent posts and the base ring.

The base ring and stent of the Hancock II porcine xenograft valve are radiolucent (Figure 3.11). Three tiny circular rings mark the distal external aspects of the three supporting posts. In the case of the Ionescu–Shiley bioprosthesis the base ring and stent form a single radiopaque structure, which appears flattened with many perforations in both (Figure 3.7). By contrast the Ionescu–Shiley low-profile pericardial xenograft (Figure 3.12) has a base ring consisting of three narrow wireform arcs, each length being

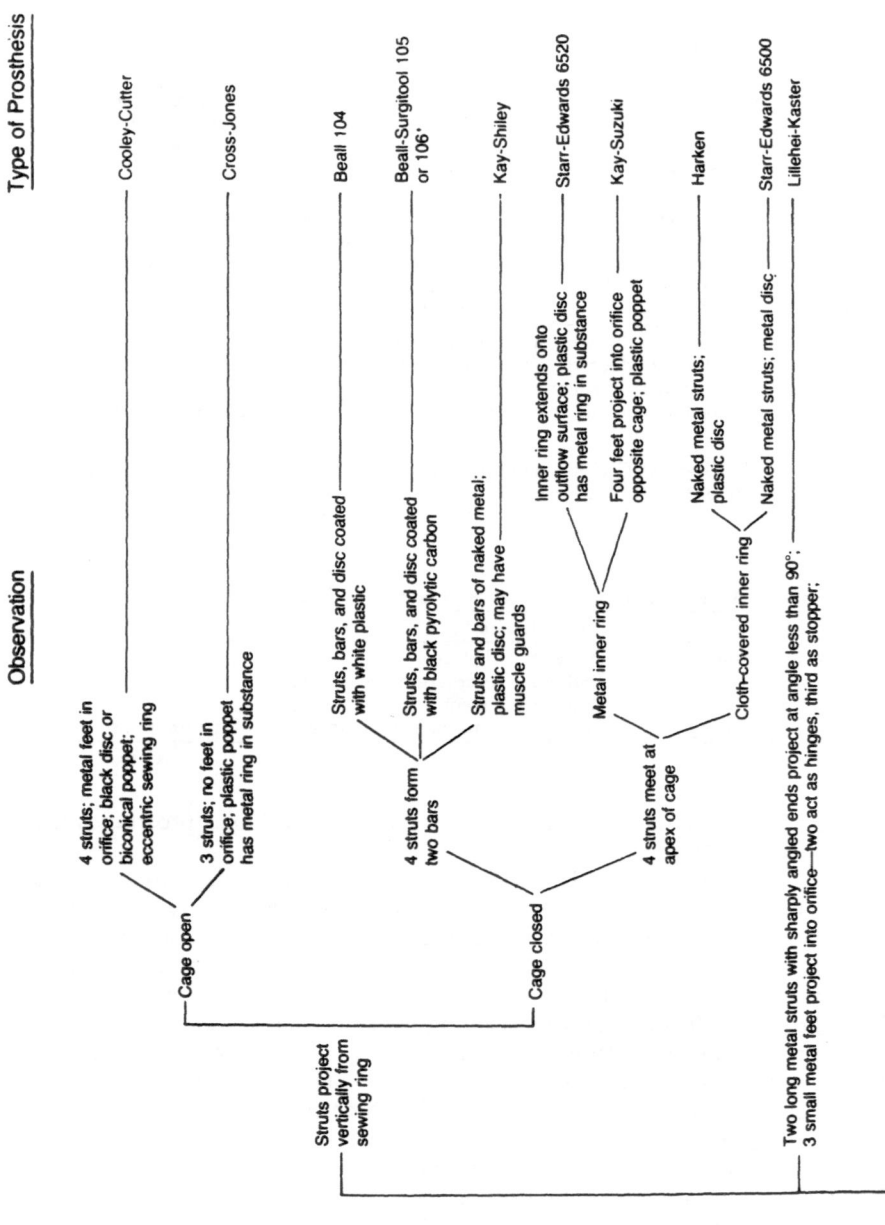

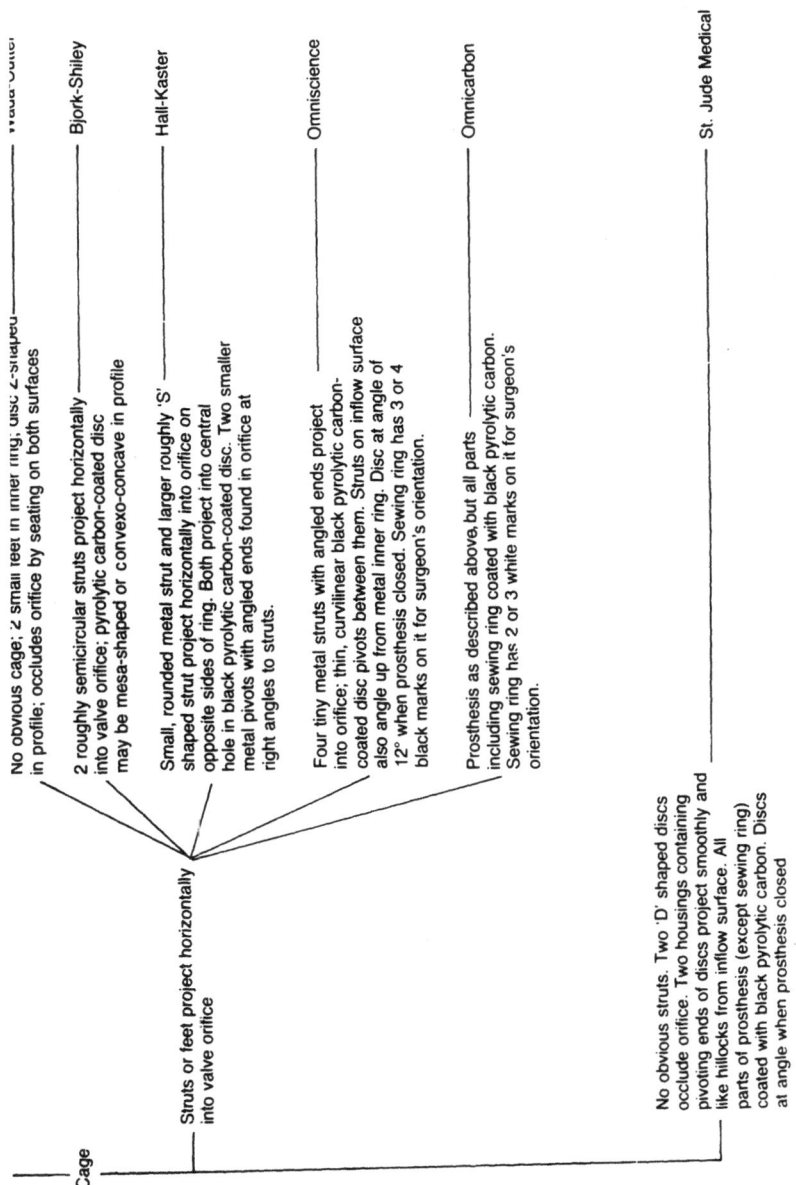

Figure 3.5 Key to identify disc valve prostheses. (Modified after ref. 5; copyright 1975 by American Medical Association)

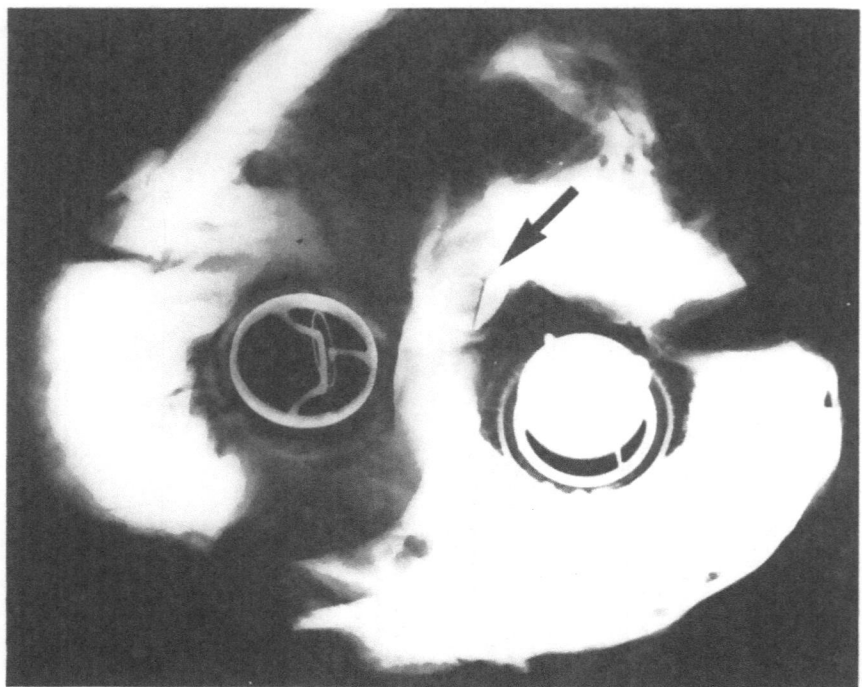

Figure 3.6 Postmortem radiograph of heart containing three different mechanical valve prostheses: Bjork–Shiley monostrut valve in tricuspid position (left), St Jude Medical aortic valve (arrow), and Starr–Edwards mitral valve prosthesis (right)

approximately one-third of the circumference of the base ring. Adjoining arcs are separated by small radiolucent areas. The stent posts are radiolucent.

The Starr–Edwards caged-ball prosthesis has a readily recognizable appearance (Figure 3.13). The St Jude Medical valve (Figure 3.14), which has two leaflets that open to right-angles to the base ring, is radiolucent. When viewed on edge the discs may be weakly radiopaque. The discs are more clearly seen on a radiograph of the explanted prosthesis (Figure 3.15). The Bjork–Shiley heart valve prosthesis with the convexo-concave disc has the same X-ray appearance as the Bjork–Shiley valve with the straight disc (Figure 3.16) and incorporated disc marker. Emerging from the base ring towards its centre are two eccentrically located U-shaped structures of unequal size. The Bjork–Shiley integral monostrut cardiac valve prosthesis (Figures 3.6 and 3.17) has only one U-shaped structure. Perpendicular to the flattened portion of the U is a short straight projection with a very small hook or bulge on its end. The radiolucent disc also has a radiopaque circular disc marker.

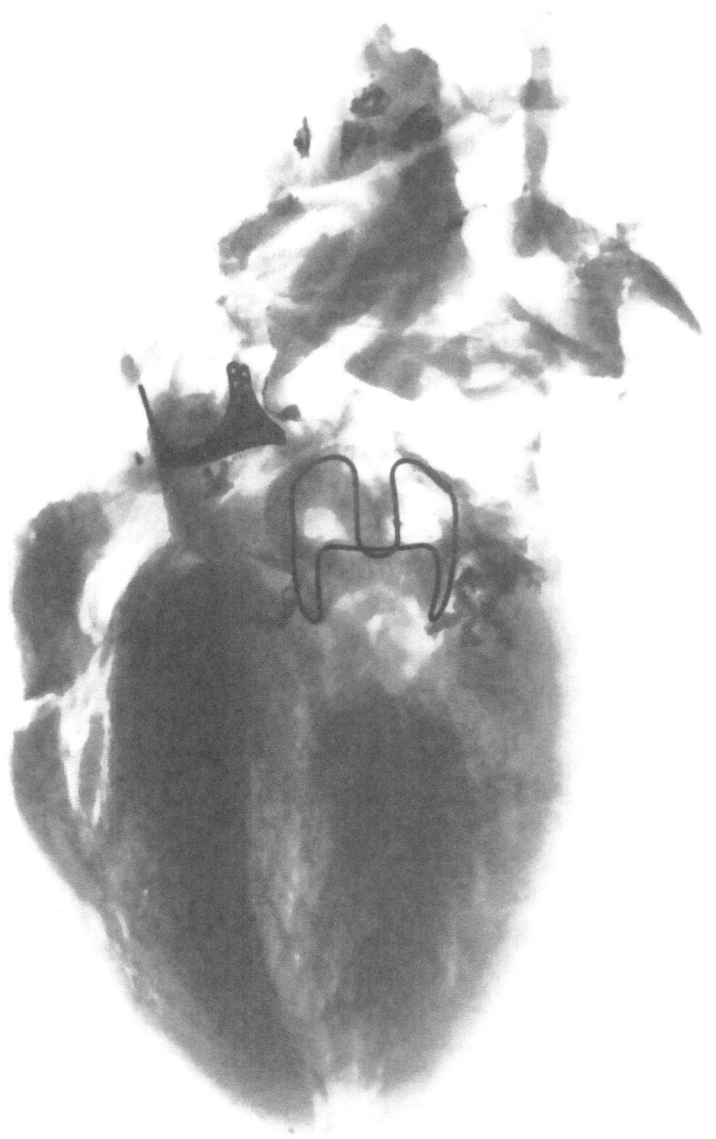

Figure 3.7 Postmortem radiograph of heart containing an Ionescu–Shiley aortic standard pericardial xenograft bioprosthesis (rigid titanium stent) and a Carpentier–Edwards mitral (model 6625) bioprosthesis (wireform stent)

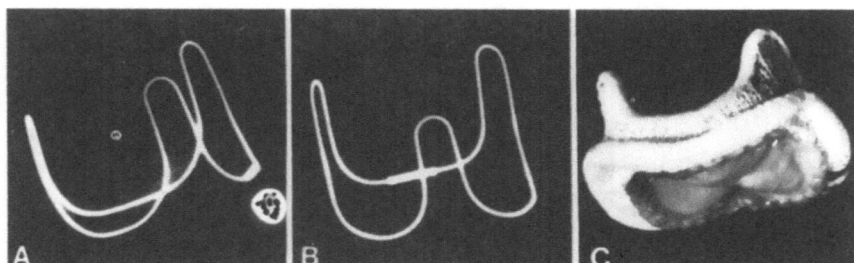

Figure 3.8 Carpentier–Edwards SupraAnnular (SAV) bioprosthesis (aortic position: **A**, PA radiograph; **B** and **C**, LL radiograph and photograph). One continuous narrow wireform outlines each of the three stents and that portion of the base ring between the stents. Although superficially similar to the radiographic silhouettes of the Carpentier–Edwards bioprosthesis (see Figure 3.7), in the SupraAnnular model the change of shape of the wireform as it shifts from base ring to stent is more gradual, giving the wire a gently curving appearance rather than a right-angle appearance. (From ref. 9; by permission of the American Heart Association, Inc.)

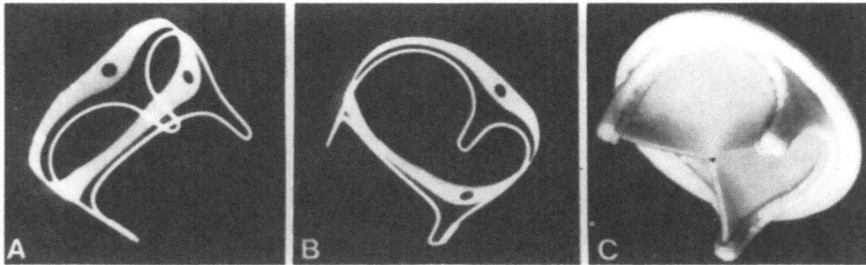

Figure 3.9 Carpentier–Edwards pericardial bioprosthesis (mitral position: **A**, PA radiograph; **B** and **C**, LL radiograph and photograph). The base ring is marked by a flattened circular ring with three holes. The flattened ring does not extend into the stents as is seen in the Ionescu–Shiley xenograft. In addition, a narrow wireform outlines each of the three stents and the base ring between the stents. The wire curves gently between stent and base ring, similar to the Carpentier–Edwards SupraAnnular bioprosthesis (From ref. 9; by permission of the American Heart Association, Inc.)

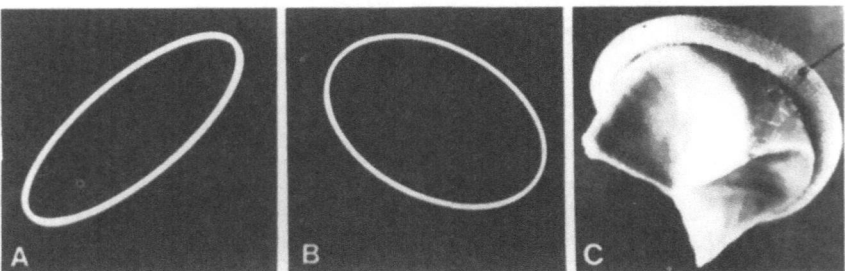

Figure 3.10 Hancock pericardial heart valve (mitral position: **A**, PA radiograph; **B** and **C** LL radiograph and photograph). The base ring has a narrow, circular, wirelike form. The remainder of the valve is radiolucent. The radiographic silhouette is similar to that of the Hancock porcine xenograft. (From ref. 9; by permission of the American Heart Association, Inc.)

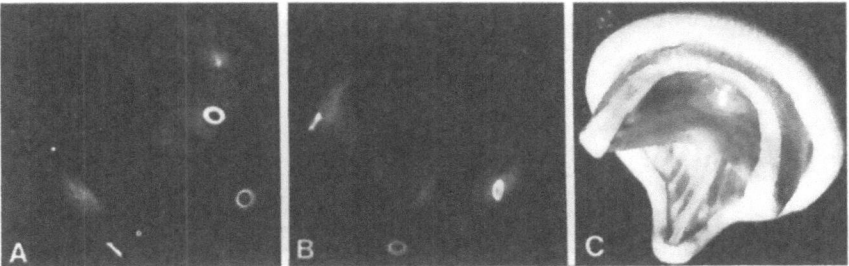

Figure 3.11 Hancock II porcine xenograft (mitral position: **A**, PA radiograph; **B** and **C**, LL radiograph and photograph). The base ring and stents are radiolucent. Three tiny rings mark the distal external aspects of the three stents. (From ref. 9; by permission of the American Heart Association, Inc.)

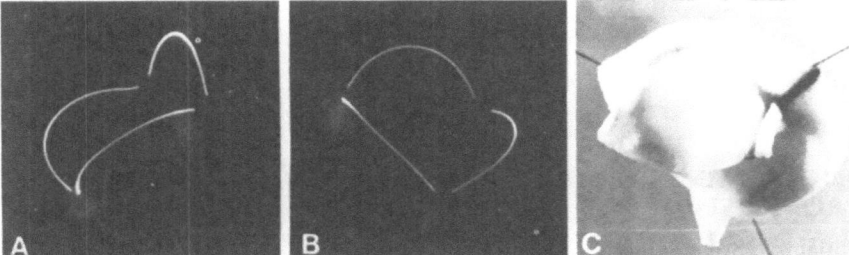

Figure 3.12 Ionescu–Shiley low-profile pericardial xenograft (mitral position: **A**, PA radiograph; **B** and **C**, LL radiograph and photograph). The base ring consists of three narrow wireform arcs, each length approximately one-third the circumference of the base ring. Adjoining arcs are separated by small radiolucent areas. The stents are radiolucent. (From ref. 9; by permission of the American Heart Association, Inc.)

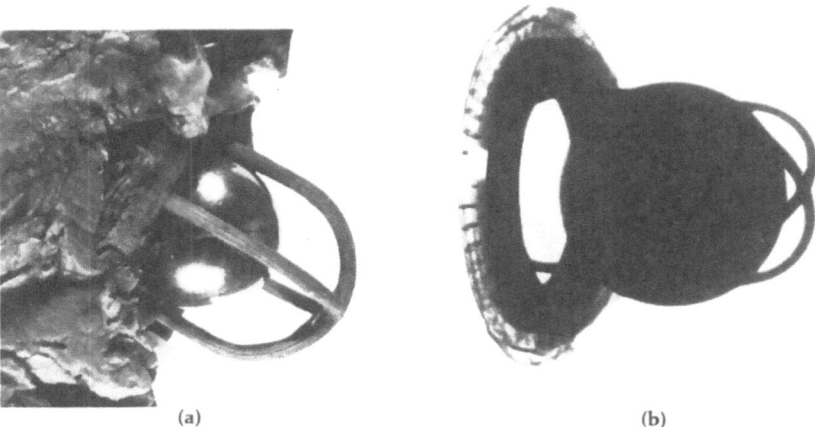

(a) (b)

Figure 3.13 (a) Starr–Edwards caged-ball valve (model 6320) with cloth covering the struts, which diverge slightly towards the apex. Poppet material is a Stellite alloy ball. (b) Radiographic features are a high-profile, closed cage composed of four struts. The base ring is smooth and the ball is radiopaque

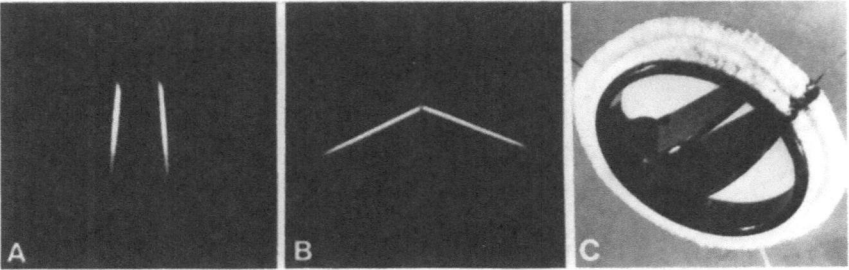

Figure 3.14 St Jude Medical cardiac valve (mitral position: **A**, oblique radiograph demonstrating both discs on edge in the open position; **B**, oblique radiograph demonstrating both discs on edge in the closed position; **C**, LL photograph). On routine chest radiographs the St Jude Medical valve is likely to be radiolucent. When viewed on edge the discs are radiopaque. The base ring is radiolucent. (From ref. 9; by permission of the American Heart Association, Inc.)

GROSS EXAMINATION OF A HEART CONTAINING A VALVE PROSTHESIS

Patients may come to autopsy with valvular prostheses replacing their mitral and/or aortic and/or tricuspid valves. The pulmonary valve is seldom directly replaced, but its function may be replaced by a valved conduit linking the right ventricle to the pulmonary artery. Any of the standard techniques for opening and examining the heart may be used[10,11] with adaptations being made for the fact that the valve ring cannot be cut across where a prosthesis is present. Adequate exposure of both aspects of the prosthetic valve can be obtained by opening the chamber or great vessel on either side of the prosthesis right down to the sewing ring. This should only be done after

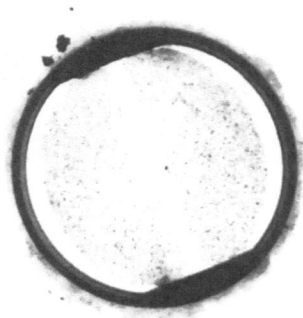

Figure 3.15 Low-density radiograph of explanted St Jude Medical prosthesis shows some details of base ring and both discs

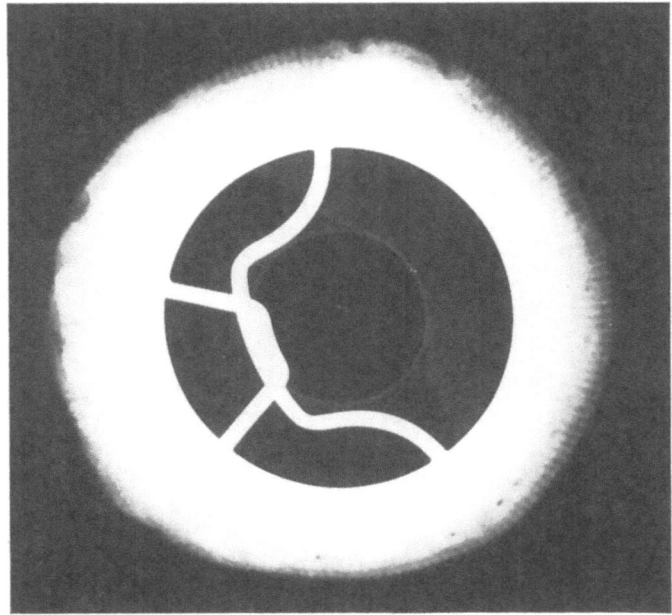

Figure 3.16 Radiograph of explanted Bjork–Shiley mitral tilting standard disc valve with radiolucent disc

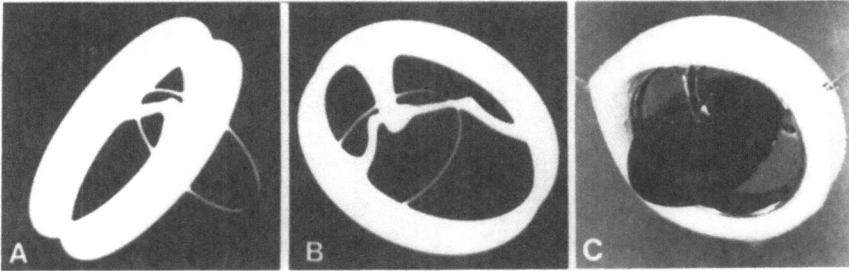

Figure 3.17 Bjork–Shiley integral monostrut cardiac valve prosthesis (mitral position: **A**, PA radiograph; **B** and **C**, LL radiograph and photograph). The radiographic silhouette is similar to that of the Bjork–Shiley convexoconcave and straight disc valves. The flattened base ring is circled by a groove. Emerging from the base ring towards its centre is a wide U-shaped structure. Perpendicular to the flattened portion of the U is a short straight projection with a very small hook or bulge on its end. The radiolucent disc contains a narrow circular radiopaque disc marker which is seen from any projection. (From ref. 9; by permission of the American Heart Association, Inc.)

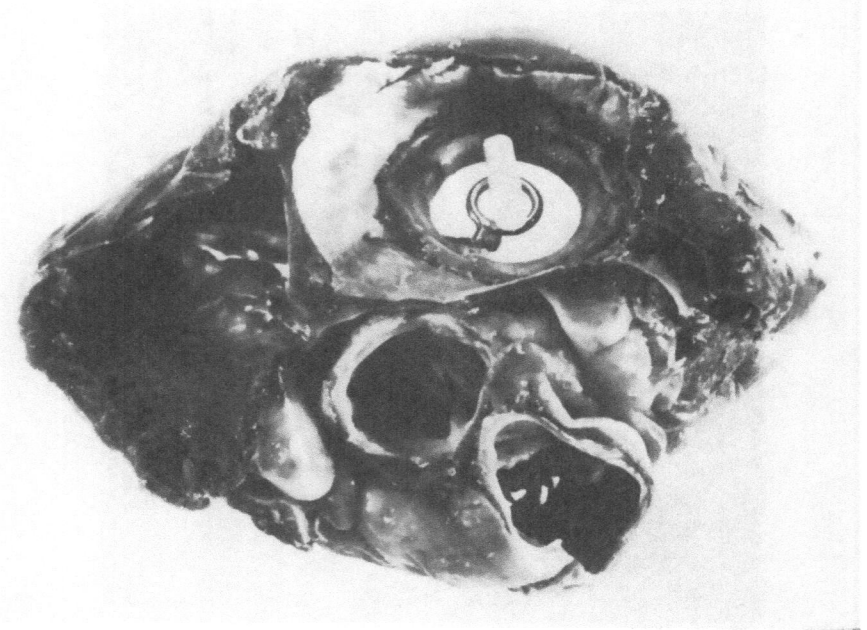

(a)

(b)

Figure 3.18 Slice of heart base containing the valves. Mitral valve has been replaced by a University of Cape Town lenticular prosthesis. (a) Trimming down of atria and great arteries allows heart valves and prosthesis to be easily inspected. (b) Transection of ventricles close to atrioventricular valves exposes mitral prosthesis and tricuspid valve for close inspection

careful circumferential probing of the host—prosthesis junction for paravalvular leaks.

A convenient way to expose the implanted valves is to transversely section the ventricles about 1 cm below the lower edge of the atrioventricular prosthesis. The atria may be similarly sectioned just above the atrioventricular prosthesis and the aorta is transected just above the level of the coronary ostia. The pulmonary artery is transected separately just above the pulmonary valve, since this valve lies at a higher level than the aortic valve. The latter method provides one with the base of the heart containing the prostheses, which can be easily photographed *in situ* (Figure 3.18). Having been fully examined *in situ*, the prosthesis may be removed by cutting through the securing interrupted sutures.

Aortic valve prosthesis

If the aortic valve has been replaced, one should examine the external appearance of the aortotomy wound and check for the presence of coronary bypass vein grafts or tube grafts. The ascending aorta should be opened longitudinally on both sides down to the aortic valve ring, taking care to avoid the coronary ostia, or the aortic root may be transected as described above. The internal aspect of the aortotomy wound should be assessed for the stage of healing and for the presence of infection or aneurysm. After checking for paravalvular leaks, thrombi or vegetations, host tissue overgrowth, freedom of bobbin movement or impingement on cardiac structure (see checklist below), note whether any portion of the prosthesis is obstructing a coronary ostium. This applies particularly to bioprostheses, which have broad stents. Occasionally a sewing ring may partially obstruct an ostium.

Look for evidence of disproportion between the relative sizes of the aortic root and the prosthesis; this should be done prior to fixation of the specimen. If a bulky Starr—Edwards prosthesis is placed in a too small aortic root, ball movement may be limited by its impingement against the aortic wall. For photography of the prosthesis it is often necessary to excise the aorta a few millimetres above the aortic ring.

The inferior aspect of the aortic valvular prosthesis is available for inspection once the left ventricle has been opened and cleared of clots. Cut the chordal attachments of the mitral valve's anterior leaflet and fold the leaflet posteriorly for better exposure of the inferior aspect of the aortic prosthesis. Even better exposure is obtained by cutting the anterior mitral leaflet free from its attachment to the posterior aortic cusp.

Mitral valve prosthesis

The outflow and inflow aspects of the prosthesis are examined from the left ventricular and left atrial aspects respectively (see checklist below for points to be noted). In early postoperative deaths one should examine the atriotomy suture lines; massive thrombosis on the inner aspect of the wound may predispose to spread of thrombus on to the prosthesis. If a bulky (high-profile) prosthesis (e.g. a Starr–Edwards valve) has been inserted, one should watch out for prosthetic-induced subaortic obstruction. This is especially prone to occur if the left ventricle is not dilated and there is a short posterior wall, which favours angulation of the prosthesis into the left ventricular outflow tract.

Tricuspid valve prosthesis

Similar principles to those noted above, and in the checklist below, apply to examination of a prosthesis in the tricuspid position.

Valve prosthesis within a conduit

When opening the chest at autopsy in such patients it is important to note whether the sternum is unduly compressing an anteriorly placed valved conduit. (Some degree of compression occurs in all cases and is one of the reasons for using a valved rather than a non-valved conduit.) The steel ring of the prosthesis may compress one of the major epicardial coronary arteries. Note the size and adequacy of the proximal and distal anastomoses, the size of the more distal pulmonary artery to which the conduit has been anastomosed, as well as the angle of each anastomosis. Kinking of the graft, layering of the interior of the graft by thrombus or thrombotic occlusion of the graft may also occur. Intraconduit obstruction by pannus formation is another possibility.

CHECKLIST FOR EXAMINING A HEART CONTAINING A PROSTHETIC VALVE

1. Consider the possibility of a future publication or coroner's inquest – photograph unusual features before you mar the specimen by cutting it. Fresh specimens may be photographed in colour, but prior fixation in formaldehyde (for even just a few hours) to remove highlights is preferable for black and white photography.
2. Open heart chambers and/or great vessels down to sewing ring of prosthesis after probing for paraprosthetic leaks.
3. Note the number, sites, types and model of prostheses present; look for ring abscesses or defects in the valve ring due to surgical trauma (haematoma/aneurysm); watch out for prosthesis–patient mismatch, impingement of bobbin on cardiac structure.
4. Note the degree of patency of the coronary ostia; the position of the prosthetic sewing ring and stents are important in this regard. Post-cannulation ostial stenosis is rarely encountered. The circumflex branch of the left coronary artery may be at risk to sewing ring sutures during mitral valve replacement. Immediate division of the left coronary artery into its two major branches has caused problems in the past by leading to

cannulation perfusion of only one of the branches during aortic valve replacement. Cannulation may lead to dissection too. Transverse sectioning of the coronary arteries at 4 mm intervals should be performed, the degree of narrowing noted and the appropriate histological samples taken.

5. Note the severity and distribution of endocardial sclerosis in the ventricles. Possible aetiological factors include turbulent blood flow due to the prosthesis, direct trauma by the prosthesis, chamber dilatation and scarring following excision of papillary muscles. Sometimes the cause is unknown.

6. Rupture of the left ventricle may occur at the level of the mitral valve ring (due to sutures, excessive excision of ring tissue or a too-large prosthesis), or at the site of papillary muscle excision or at midventricular level (due to the effects of a bulky prosthesis, scissors or cardiotomy ischaemia). Small coronary arterial branches may be damaged by the rupture too.

7. Record the heart weight after clots have been removed. The ventricles should be sectioned transversely at multiple levels between their apices and bases in order to gauge the macroscopical appearance of the myocardium (fresh or healed regional infarction, subendocardial haemorrhagic infarction, subendocardial fibrosis). Sections for histology should be taken from the left ventricle (anterior, lateral and inferior walls), septum and right ventricle, as well as the papillary muscles, atria and coronary arteries.

EXAMINATION OF REMOVED PROSTHETIC VALVES

The pathologist should be adept at examining valve prostheses, which have either been surgically removed or have been excised from the heart at autopsy to facilitate their closer examination. Optimal examination of the prosthesis often aids in patient management, helps to provide a sound rationale for patient–prosthesis matching and serves to assist the bioengineer in developing an improved valve[12].

1. Note the type and make of the prosthesis; expect to encounter prostheses which may no longer be in production. Several reports[3–9,13] plus data contained in the present chapter should enable one to identify most valve prostheses.

2. Examine the prosthesis macroscopically from the inflow and outflow aspects for thrombi (culture infected vegetations); assess the mobility of the bobbin/leaflets, and look for variance and cloth/metal wear, host tissue overgrowth or incorporation of prosthesis into the endomyocardium. It is useful to photograph the prosthesis.

3. Radiography (e.g. in a Faxitron apparatus) is very useful for aiding the identification of the type of bioprosthesis and allows one to accurately gauge the severity of bioprosthetic calcification.

4. Histology should be performed on bioprosthetic cusps, on tissue covering the sewing ring and on neighbouring anatomical structures, e.g. the aorta. Stains for phosphate (the von Kossa method) or calcium (alizarin red) are

useful. In the case of mechanical valves only thrombi or tissue covering the sewing ring can be examined microscopically.

5. Transmission electron microscopy may be used to assess the degree of preservation of the collagen in bioprosthetic cusps, and scanning electron microscopy gives information on the cuspal surface.

6. Removal of cloth covering mechanical prostheses may reveal unsuspected metal fractures, e.g. at weld points.

7. More specialized examinations may be indicated in certain cases, e.g. biochemical quantification of calcium, phosphorus and osteocalcins[14].

REFERENCES

1. Byrne, J. P., Behrendt, D. M., Kirsh, M. M. and Orringer, M. B. (1977). Replacement of heart valves by prosthetic devices. In Joachim, H. L. (ed.) *Pathobiology Annual*, Vol. 7, pp. 83–114. (New York: Appleton-Century-Crofts)
2. Angell, W. W., Angell, J. D. and Kosek, J. C. (1978). Clinical and experimental comparisons establishing the glutaraldehyde treated xenograft as the standard for tissue heart valve replacement. In Ionescu, M. I. (ed.) *Tissue Heart Valves*. pp. 89–126. (London: Butterworths)
3. Lefrak, E. A. and Starr, A. (1979). *Cardiac Valve Prostheses*. (New York: Appleton-Century-Crofts)
4. Chun, P. K. and Nelson, W. P. (1977). Common cardiac prosthetic valves. *J. Am. Med. Assoc.*, **238**, 401
5. Silver, M. D., Datta, B. N. and Bowes, V. F. (1975). A key to identify heart valve prostheses. *Arch. Pathol.*, **99**, 132
6. Wallace, R. B. (1966). Prosthetic valves: available types. In Brest, A. N. (ed.) *Heart Substitutes: Mechanical and Transplants*. p. 18. (Springfield, Illinois: Charles C. Thomas Publisher)
7. Silver, M. D. and Wilson, G. W. (1983). Pathology of cardiovascular prostheses including coronary artery bypass and other vascular grafts. In Silver, M. D. (ed.) *Cardiovascular Pathology*. Vol. 2, p. 1225. (New York: Churchill Livingstone)
8. Mehlman, D. J. and Resnekov, L. A. (1978). A guide to the radiographic identification of prosthetic heart valves. *Circulation*, **57**, 613
9. Mehlman, D. J. (1984). A guide to the radiological identification of prosthetic heart valves: an addendum. *Circulation*, **69**, 102
10. Layman, T. E. and Edwards, J. E. (1966). A method for dissection of the heart and major pulmonary vessels. *Arch. Pathol.*, **82**, 314
11. Silver, M. M. (1983). Gross examination of the heart. In Silver, M. D. (ed.) *Cardiovascular Pathology*. pp.1-30. (New York: Churchill Livingstone)
12. Schoen, F. J. and Hobson, C. E. (1985). Anatomic analysis of removed prosthetic heart valves: causes of failure of 33 mechanical valves and 58 bioprostheses, 1980–1983. *Human Pathol.*, **16**, 549
13. Morse, D. and Steiner, R. M. (1985). Cardiac valve identification atlas and guide. In Morse, D., Steiner, R. M. and Fernandez, J. (eds.) *Guide to Prosthetic Cardiac Valves*. pp. 257-346. (New York: Springer-Verlag)
14. Levy, R. J., Zenker, J. A. and Bernhard, W. F. (1983). Porcine bioprosthetic valve calcification in bovine left ventricle-aorta shunts: studies of the deposition of vitamin K-dependent proteins. *Ann. Thorac. Surg.*, **36**, 187

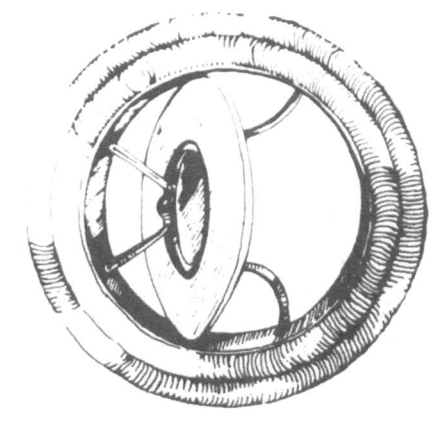

MECHANICAL VALVES

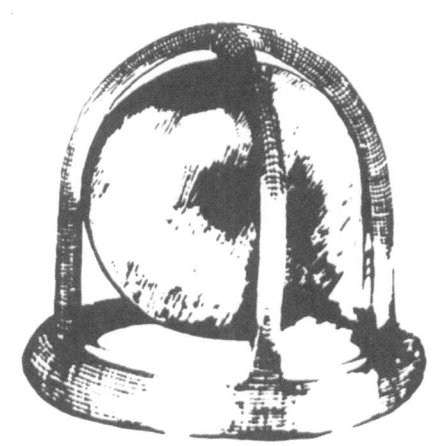

4
Caged-ball Valves

STARR–EDWARDS PROSTHESIS

The basic design of the Starr–Edwards ball valve prosthesis (Colour Plates G and H) has remained virtually unchanged since its introduction in 1960, although numerous modifications have been made (Table 4.1). The initial Starr–Edwards prostheses (model 1000 aortic, 6000 mitral) had a Stellite-21 cage (Figures 4.1 and 4.2), a compression-moulded Silastic (silicone rubber) poppet and a knitted Teflon (polytetrafluoroethylene) sewing ring. Stellite is an alloy composed of cobalt, chromium, molybdenum and nickel. Model 1000 had three feet in the orifice and a lot of metal on the inflow surface.

Many modifications have been made in the design of the Starr–Edwards valve between the initial design and the current reversion to use of an early

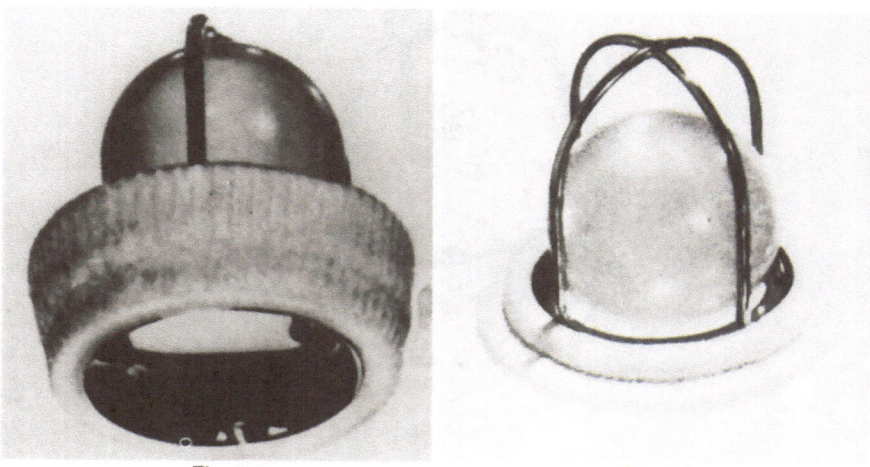

Fig. 4.1 Fig. 4.2

Figure 4.1 Starr–Edwards model 1000 aortic caged ball-valve has three Stellite struts, three feet in the orifice, significant metal on the inflow surface, a radiolucent Silastic ball and a cloth sewing ring (Picture courtesy of American Edwards Laboratories)
Figure 4.2 Starr–Edwards model 6000 mitral valve prosthesis has four Stellite struts joined at the apex, significant metal on the inflow surface, a radiolucent poppet and a cloth sewing ring (Picture courtesy of American Edwards Laboratories)

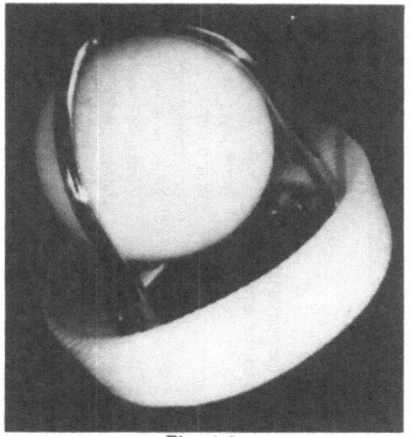

Fig. 4.3

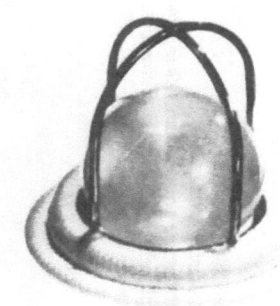

Fig. 4.4

Figure 4.3 Starr–Edwards model 1200 aortic valve prosthesis (presently available). It has three Stellite struts, a shortened cage, a silicone rubber poppet containing 2% (by weight) barium sulphate and a knitted cloth sewing ring. Poppets of the early valves had no barium sulphate and were thus radiolucent (Picture courtesy of American Edwards Laboratories)
Figure 4.4 Starr–Edwards model 6120 mitral valve prosthesis (presently available). The prosthesis has four Stellite struts joined at the apex, cloth extends into the inflow orifice and there is a seamless sewing ring. Initially there was a radiolucent poppet, now it is radiopaque due to contained barium sulphate (Picture courtesy of American Edwards Laboratories)

valve design. The design was changed in 1965 (Figures 4.3 and 4.4). In the model 1200 aortic there were no feet in the orifice, the cage was shortened and some poppets contained barium sulphate. In the 6120 mitral valve and 1260 aortic valve cloth extended into the inflow orifice. This reduced thromboembolism and a modified curing technique greatly diminished deterioration of the Silastic ball[1]. This early design has been the most successful, and is still in use at the present time. In order to encourage endothelialization and so further reduce thrombosis, the entire cage was cloth-covered in the models 2300 aortic and 6300 mitral valves (Figures 4.5 and 4.6) which were introduced in 1967. However, the cloth covering led to a smaller orifice size as well as tissue ingrowth, which was excessive in some patients.

The 2310–2320 aortic and the 6310–6320 mitral prostheses had protective metal studs on the inner aspect of the valve ring. The studs (Colour Plate G) protruded through the cloth covering and were intended to protect the latter from the hollow Stellite-21 metal ball which was introduced in 1967. The change of the ball structure from Silastic to Stellite-21 was made in order to abolish the problem of ball variance. These prostheses had a larger orifice size and there was less risk of tissue ingrowth. Due to strut cloth wear the struts were lined by tracks made of Stellite-21 in the models 2400 aortic and 6400 mitral prostheses introduced in 1972.

Table 4.1 Details of different models of Starr–Edwards ball valve prosthesis

Model	Cage/struts	Sewing ring components		Ball occluder (poppet)	Difference from previous model
		Outer ring	Inner ring		
Mitral prostheses					
Non-cloth-covered					
Pre-6000	Lucite	Teflon cloth	Lucite	Solid Silastic; seats proximal to its equator	
6000	Closed cage Four Stellite struts joined at apex	Knitted Teflon	Exposed metal inflow aspect	Ditto (some with barium sulphate)	Main problem: Thrombosis
Extended cloth prosthesis					
6120	Closed cage; no feet in orifice. Stellite 21; four naked struts	Teflon + polypropylene cloth	Cloth-covered inflow surface	Ditto	Cloth covers inflow aspect of ring Main problem: Thrombosis
Cloth-covered					
6300	Closed cage; four cloth-covered Stellite struts not joined at the apex. Perforations in metal ring	Teflon cloth	Teflon cloth	Hollow Stellite	Totally cloth-covered valve; metal ball. Main problem: Cloth wear on ring, poor haemodynamics
6310	Ditto	Ditto	Composite seat; Dacron cloth and studs	Ditto (poppet seats close to the equator)	Studs in orifice
6320	Ditto; struts diverge slightly towards apex	Ditto	Ditto	Ditto	Inner layer of Teflon and outer polypropylene. Main problem: Cloth wear on struts.
6400	Ditto plus composite struts (metal liners and polypropylene cloth) which do not diverge towards the apex.	Teflon and polypropylene	Ditto	Solid Silastic	Metal tracks on inside of struts. Main problem: Encourage neo-intima.
Beaded	Stellite 21 with metal beads on non-contact areas.			Ditto	Metal beads on non-contact areas. Silastic ball

(continued)

Non-cloth-covered Pre-1000					
1000	Three or four stellite struts Stellite 21 cage; three struts joined at apex. Three feet in orifice	Teflon and polypropylene Ditto	Stellite 21 Ditto	Radiolucent Ditto	Three struts; foam in sewing ring. Barium sulphate in some poppets *Main problem:* Ball variance
1200	Ditto; tapered support at each strut junction Shortened cage.	Ditto	Ditto	Ditto	No feet in orifice Spherical seat made convex. Barium sulphate in some poppets. Modified curing technique
1260	Ditto	Ditto	Ditto Reduced metal on inflow surface	Solid Silastic	Scalloped outflow metal ring. All poppets contained barium sulphate *Main problem:* Thrombosis
2300	Three cloth-covered struts	Seamless cloth	Cloth-covered orifice	Hollow Stellite	Totally Teflon-covered orifice, double layers of Dacron (later Teflon) on struts *Main problems:* Poor haemodynamics and cloth wear.
2310	Two models: first had low clearance and second intermediate clearance between ball and cage. A perforated metal ring. Three thin struts joined at apex after December 1969. Struts more divergent at apex.	Teflon and polypropylene	Composite seat; Dacron cloth and studs	Ditto	Struts covered by inner Teflon and outer polypropylene. *Main problem:* Sticking ball in open position.

Table 4.1 *(continued)*

Model	Cage/struts	Sewing ring components			Difference from previous model
		Outer ring	*Inner ring*	*Ball occluder (poppet)*	
2320	Struts covered by inner Teflon and outer polypropylene.	Ditto	Ditto	Ditto	*Main problem:* Strut cloth wear
2400	Three cloth covered struts with metal track on inside of each strut	Compressible	Ditto	Ditto	Stellite tracks inside struts.
Beaded metal	Same as mitral prosthesis (see above)				

Lucite = methyl methacrylate
Stellite = alloy of cobalt, chromium, molybdenum and nickel
Teflon† = polytetrafluoroethylene
Dacron† = polyester
Silastic* = silicone rubber
*Dowcorning
†Dupont

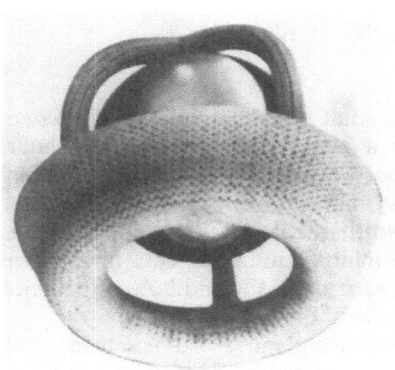 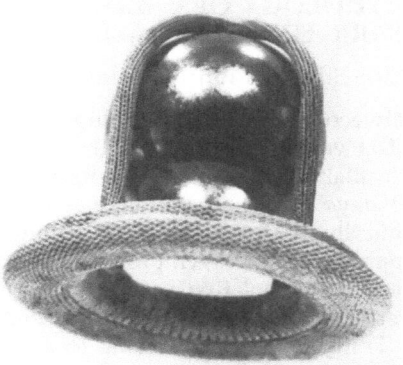

Fig. 4.5 Fig. 4.6

Figure 4.5 Starr–Edwards model 2300 aortic valve prosthesis had three cloth-covered struts, a cloth-covered orifice, a hollow Stellite poppet and a seamless cloth sewing ring (Picture courtesy of American Edwards Laboratories)
Figure 4.6 Starr–Edwards model 6300 mitral valve prosthesis had four cloth-covered struts, a cloth-covered orifice, a hollow Stellite poppet and a seamless sewing ring

The periods of usage of the various Starr–Edwards prosthetic heart valves are as follows:

Aortic prostheses
Model No. and approximate years used

Pre-1000	1961–64
1000	1964–66
1200	1966–present
1260	1968–present
2300	1967–68
2310	1968–70
2320	1970–76
2400	1972–81

Mitral prostheses
Model No. and approximate years used

Pre-6000	1960–64
6000	1964–65
6120	1966–present
6300	1967–68
6310	1968–70
6320	1970–76
6400	1972–81
6500	1968–70
6520	1970–76

PATHOLOGY OF CARDIAC VALVE REPLACEMENT WITH THE STARR–EDWARDS BALL VALVE PROSTHESIS

Starr–Edwards mitral valve prosthesis

Between January 1970 and June 1976, 332 adult patients underwent isolated mitral valve replacement with a Starr–Edwards prosthesis at Groote Schuur Hospital[2]. The operative, in-hospital, or postoperative mortality rate within 30 days of the operation was 8.0%. Thromboembolism was encountered clinically in 15 late survivors, among whom there was fatal embolism in five, transient embolic symptoms in four and minor embolic effects in another four. The cumulative survival rate at 5–6 years was 64%, and 50% of patients were clinically free of significant embolism events[3].

Thirty-four patients came to autopsy following mitral valve replacement with a Starr–Edwards prosthetic valve. Fifteen patients died 30 days or less after operation (group 1) and 19 died later (group 2). The mean age of the patients was 35.1 years (S.D. = 15.2). There were 13 males and 21 females. The mean period of postoperative survival in group 1 was 10 days (S.D. = 9) and that for group 2 was 37.9 months (S.D. = 35.6). Most of the valves implanted were model Nos. 6320 or 6400 Starr–Edwards valves. The principal causes of death in these patients are given in Table 4.2

In the early postoperative period the commonest reason for death was 'unknown cause' (?arrhythmia), followed by myocardial failure and thromboembolism. Seventy-five per cent of the late deaths were related to thrombus deposition on the prosthesis (Figure 4.7). The most frequent sites of thrombus deposition on the 18 Starr–Edwards mitral prostheses bearing thrombi were the inflow aspect of the sewing ring and the inner aspect of the cage.

Table 4.2 Principal causes of death (one per patient) in 34 patients with Starr–Edwards mitral valve prostheses

Group 1	
Unknown	5
Myocardial failure	4
Systemic thromboembolism	3
Unrelated to cardiac operation	2
Incorrect preoperative diagnosis	1
Group 2	
Systemic thromboembolism	11
Thrombosed prosthesis (cloth wear)	3 (2)
Myocardial failure	2
Unrelated to cardiac operation	2
Infected prosthesis	1

Starr–Edwards aortic valve prosthesis

Only seven patients with isolated Starr–Edwards aortic valve prostheses were autopsied. Their mean age was 46 years (S.D. = 10.1) with a range of 34–62 years. The mean postoperative survival period was 482.4 days (S.D. = 935),

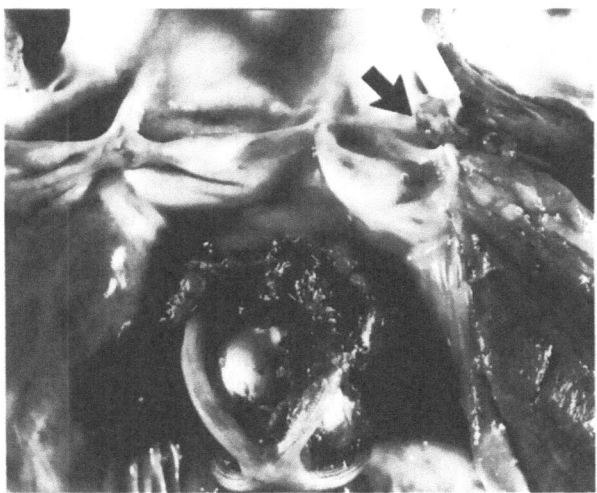

Figure 4.7 Thrombus deposition on strut and base ring of Starr–Edwards mitral valve prosthesis. Thromboembolus (arrow) occludes origin of left coronary artery

with a range from 0 to 2520 days. Six patients received model 2400 Starr–Edwards aortic valve prostheses and one received a model 2320 prosthesis. Principal causes of death are given in Table 4.3.

Three patients who had two valves replaced by Starr–Edwards valves died of pneumonia, heart failure and uncorrected associated valvular heart disease.

Table 4.3 Principal causes of death (one per patient) in seven patients with Starr–Edwards aortic valve prostheses

Group 1	
Bypass accident-induced cerebral anoxia	1
Ruptured aortotomy wound (medionecrosis)	1
Prosthetic disproportion	1
Group 2	
Infected prosthesis	3
Thrombosed prosthesis	1

PRINCIPAL CAUSES OF DEATH IN 44 PATIENTS WITH STARR–EDWARDS PROSTHESES

The principal causes of death in the 44 patients with Starrr–Edwards valvular prostheses were as follows: (a) error in preoperative diagnosis, 1; (b) error in operative technique, 2; (c) problems inherent in the prosthetic valve, 23; (d)

postoperative complications, 9; (e) unrelated to the valve replacement operation, 4; and (f) unknown causes, 5.

COMMENT

Starr et al.[4] reported a 10-year follow-up of 290 patients with isolated mitral valve replacement with non-cloth- and cloth-covered Starr–Edwards prostheses. The 10-year projection of the percentage of patients alive and free of emboli (disregarding transient ischaemic attacks) for the model 6310–6320 (50%) was similar to that actually observed for the model 6120 (46%). Salomon et al.[5] reported that thromboemboli were more common with the Starr–Edwards valve than with aortic allografts or porcine xenograft valves. Fraser and Waddell[6] found a statistically significant lower incidence of emboli in patients with aortic prostheses who were on 'well-controlled' anticoagulants. Lewis et al.[7] found that thromboembolism was a major problem after aortic valve replacement. Herr et al.[8] encountered fatal prosthetic infection in five of 266 patients who had Starr–Edwards valves implanted over a 4-year period.

Roberts and Morrow[9] reported on 98 autopsied patients with Starr–Edwards valves. In the 65 early deaths (less than 1 month postoperatively) major causes of death included mechanical interference with functioning of the prostheses in 22 patients, uncontrolled bleeding (22 patients), and acute myocardial infarction (16 patients). Less frequent early fatal complications were associated uncorrected valvular disease, pulmonary complications, arrhythmia, and infection. Causes of the 33 late deaths included prosthetic valve infection (in five patients), congestive heart failure (eight patients) sometimes due to prosthetic thrombosis, and sudden unexpected death.

Prosthetic valve thrombi were found at autopsy in 27 of their 33 patients. Other complications included intimal thickening of the aortic root and proximal portions of the major coronary arteries, traumatic intravascular haemolysis, and ball variance. The latter problem is reviewed by Laforet[10], who states that 29 of 1400 Starr–Edwards valves returned to Edwards Laboratories Inc. for examination showed ball variance of some degree. This consisted of change in colour, mass, hardness, shape or surface appearance. The ball of the prosthesis sometimes increased in size so that it became stuck in the open position. Ball variance has not been encountered at Groote Schuur Hospital since only Starr–Edwards prostheses with metal (Stellite) balls have been used. Ball fracture may lead to systemic embolism, and Gobel et al.[11] reported a patient with fatal coronary arterial embolism resulting from this complication.

Cloth wear (Figure 4.8 and Colour Plate G), which may be a significant problem, was seen in five out of 47 Starr–Edwards prosthetic valves implanted in 44 patients at Groote Schuur Hospital. All five were model 6310-6320 mitral prostheses in which wearing away of the metal studs had led to subsequent cloth wear. Bonchek and Starr[12] reported cloth wear in 10 patients with Starr–Edwards valves and expressed the hope that the newer model 2400 aortic and 6400 mitral composite track valves would overcome this

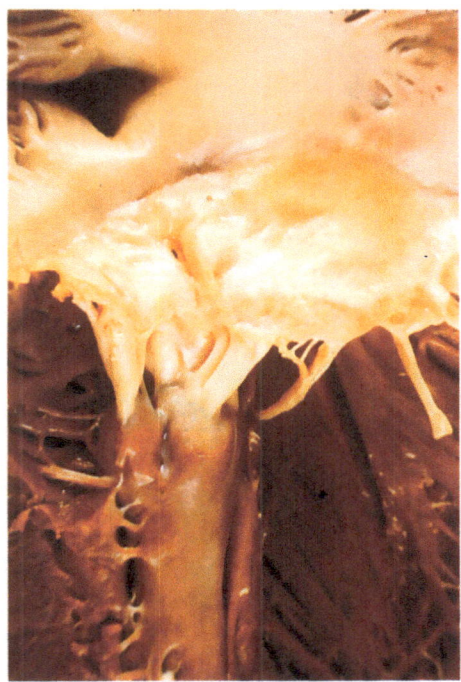

Plate A Severe post-rheumatic mitral stenosis and incompetence

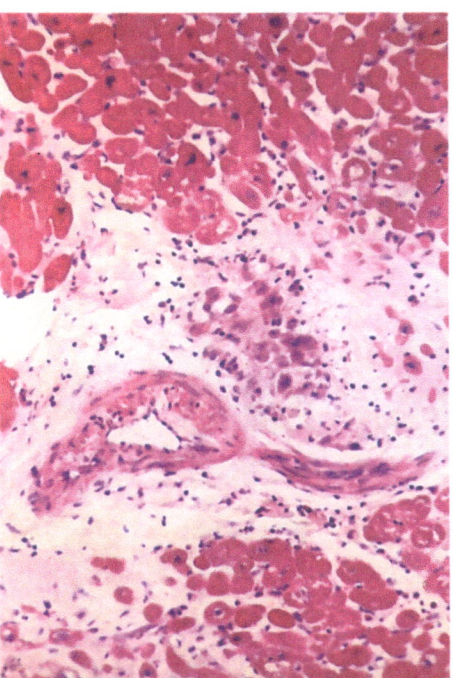

Plate B Proliferative phase Aschoff body alongside intra-myocardial coronary artery

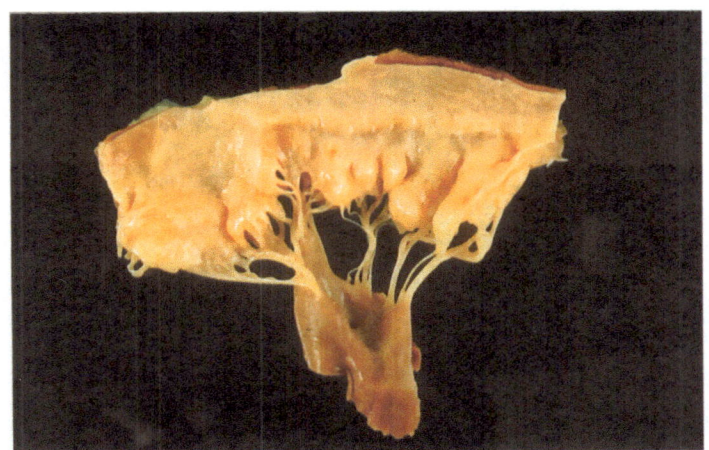

Plate C Floppy mitral valve with prominent hooding of posterior leaflet

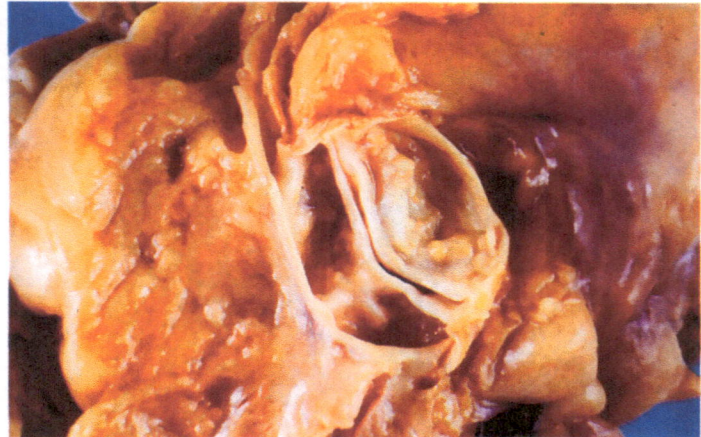

Plate D   Calcified, stenotic, congenitally bicuspid aortic valve

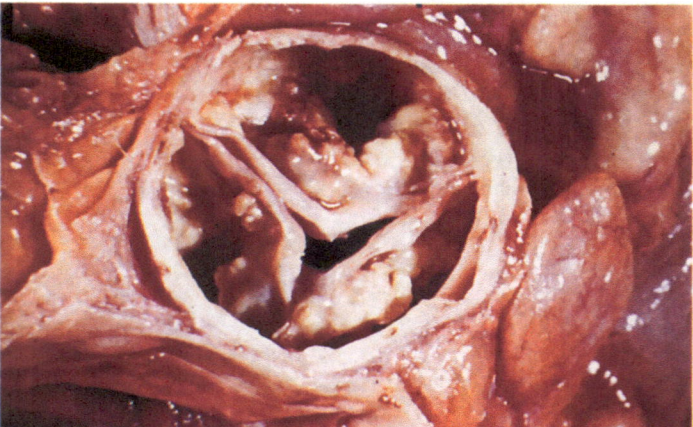

Plate E   Senile calcific tricuspid aortic stenosis (aortic nodular sclerosis)

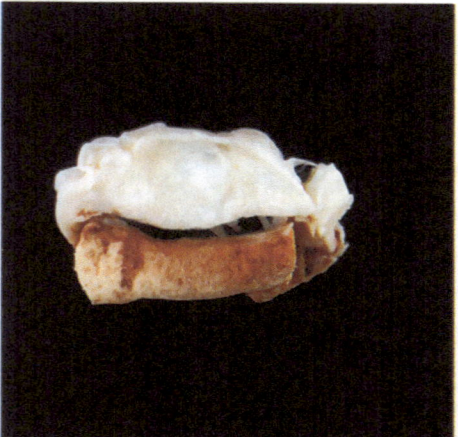

Plate F   Ivalon sponge prosthesis used to bolster deficient posterior mitral valve leaflet has become calcified

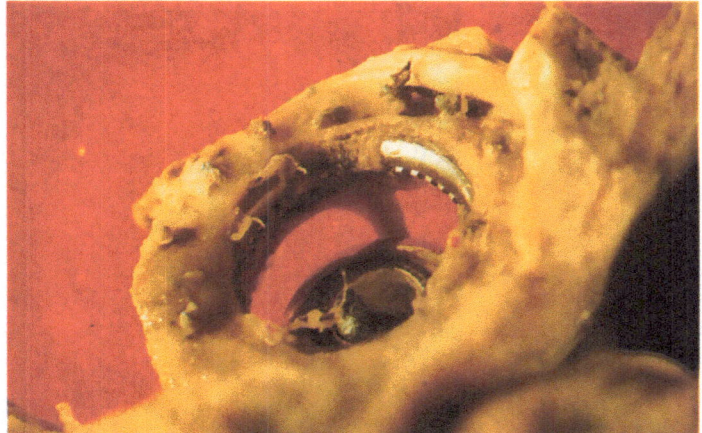

Plate G   Removal of abdundant thrombus from this Starr–Edwards model 6310 mitral prosthesis revealed cloth wear and loss over much of the base ring due to wear of the protective studs on the contact zone of the ring

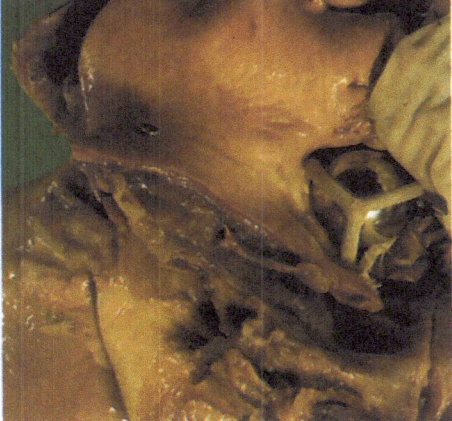

Plate H   Despite being widened with a patch, the narrow aortic root still impinges on the ball of the Starr–Edwards prosthesis

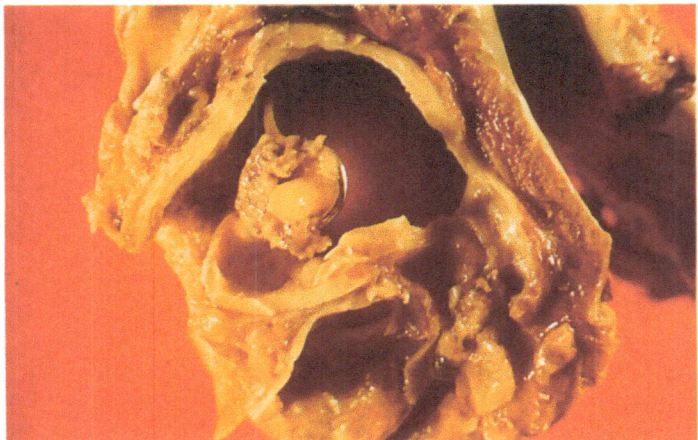

Plate I   Non-infected thrombus covers most of the upper retaining ring of a UCT aortic valve prosthesis. A thromboembolus occludes the left main coronary artery

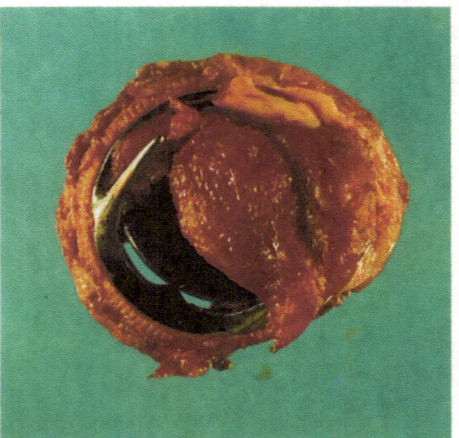

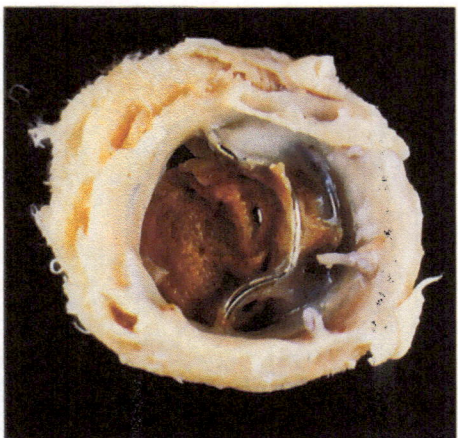

Plate J   Bjork–Shiley prosthetic disc is immobilized by an overgrowth of host tissue following organization of thrombus. Residual unorganized thrombus is seen on the undersurface of the disc. Immobilization favours further thrombosis on the valve

Plate K   Massive thrombosis in lesser orifice has led to total immobilization of this Lillehei–Kaster mitral valve prosthesis

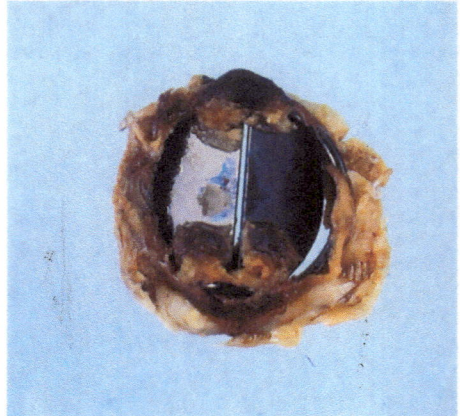

Plate L   Limited thrombosis at the two hinge sites has immobilized the two discs of this St Jude Medical prosthesis

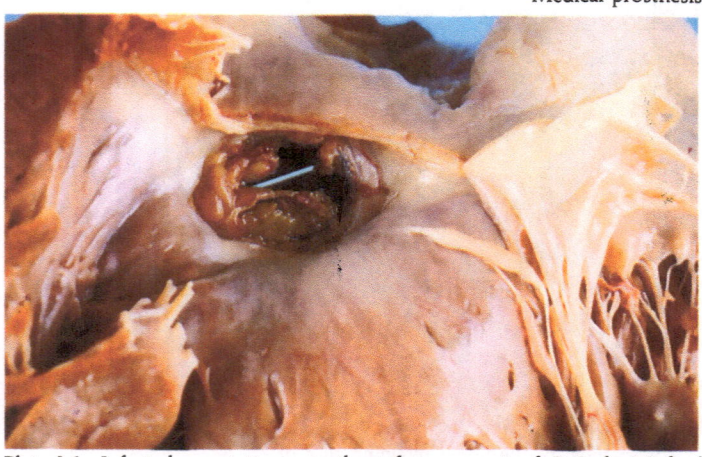

Plate M   Infected vegetations on the inferior aspect of St Jude Medical aortic valve prosthesis reduce the effective orifice of the valve

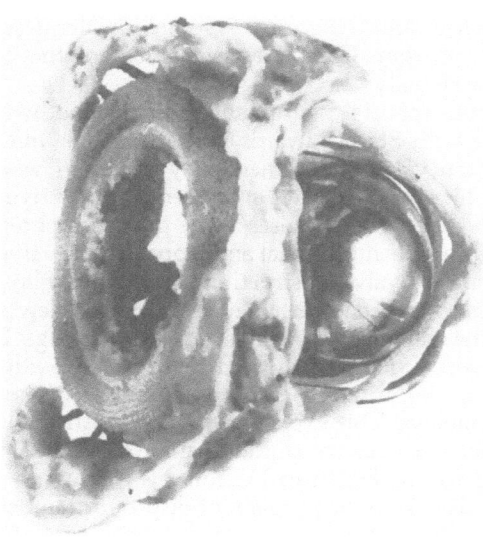

Figure 4.8 Severe wear of cloth covering of struts and base ring of explanted Starr–Edwards model 6300 mitral valve prosthesis

problem. Shah *et al.*[13] suggest that the following clinical findings should arouse suspicion of cloth wear: (a) recurrent transient cerebral ischaemic attacks or other systemic emboli despite adequate anticoagulation; (b) systemic arterial embolization more than 4 years after valve replacement with cloth-covered prostheses; (c) increase in loudness of the prosthetic valve clicks on auscultation, particularly with a metallic pitch; (d) persistent severe haemolytic anaemia with or without regurgitation across the prosthesis; and (e) incomplete seating of the poppet on the valve orifice seen on cinefluorography or intravalvular regurgitation seen on angiography.

The true incidence of cloth wear in general, and of clinically significant cloth wear in particular, is unknown. Twelve of 18 patients with cloth-covered aortic valves (models 2310-2320) who were reoperated upon for a variety of reasons showed cloth wear[14]. Four of these 12 patients were reoperated upon for haemolytic anaemia and all four had strut cloth wear. Significant cloth wear was present in 1% of the patients of Isom *et al.*[15]. Shah *et al.*[13] observed an overall incidence of 2.5% (aortic valve prostheses 3.3% and mitral valve 1.2%). Teflon fibre embolism resulting from cloth wear has been observed at autopsy[16]. Sudden death due to fatal coronary arterial obstruction due to Starr–Edwards aortic valve cloth wear has also been reported[17]. The composite strut valves do not develop strut cloth wear, but the metal studs that protrude through the sewing ring cloth may wear away and lead to cloth wear[18].

Ringel *et al.*[19] reported a unique form of structural failure of a Starr–Edwards aortic track valve. Fractures of the three struts and their liners had occurred above their insertion into the valve ring. At operation the ball was found in the aortic root and the cage was lodged in the descending aorta at the level of the diaphragm. Complete detachment of the entire prosthesis may also occur occasionally[20].

There are numerous reports[4,9,21,22] detailing the haemodynamic and clinical findings in patients with Starr–Edwards prostheses. The inference has often been made that mitral valve replacement may cause left ventricular outflow tract obstruction. This was confirmed in a recent comparative haemodynamic study with various types of prostheses[23]; the greatest degree of obstruction occurs with the high-profile mechanical and bioprosthetic valves. Other papers address the problems of valve obstruction due to thrombosis[24], infection[25], mitral valve remnants[26] and encroachment by pannus[27]. Few reports[28–32] give detailed data on the valvular or general autopsy findings in patients with Starr–Edwards valves. Vasconez[33] showed that the Starr–Edwards prosthesis with a Teflon sewing ring is held in place predominantly by sutures, and host tissue ingrowth is minimal. This explains why paraprosthetic leakage has been common. These authors welcomed the change of the sewing ring of the Starr–Edwards valve from Teflon to Dacron.

Seningen *et al.*[34] discussed the problem of disproportion between the bulky Starr–Edwards prosthesis and a too narrow aortic root (Colour Plate H), which may lead to prosthetic aortic stenosis and death due to too low a cardiac output. Prosthetic stenosis was observed in one of my patients with a tricuspid prosthesis in which a strut had become fused to the ventricular wall by fibrous tissue, probably due to organized thrombus (Figure 4.9). Scanty thrombus within the cage may limit free motion of the ball (Figure 4.10).

In 1983, Starr[35] reviewed ball-valve prostheses from a perspective of 22 years. He suggests that the Starr–Edwards mitral Silastic ball-valve, which

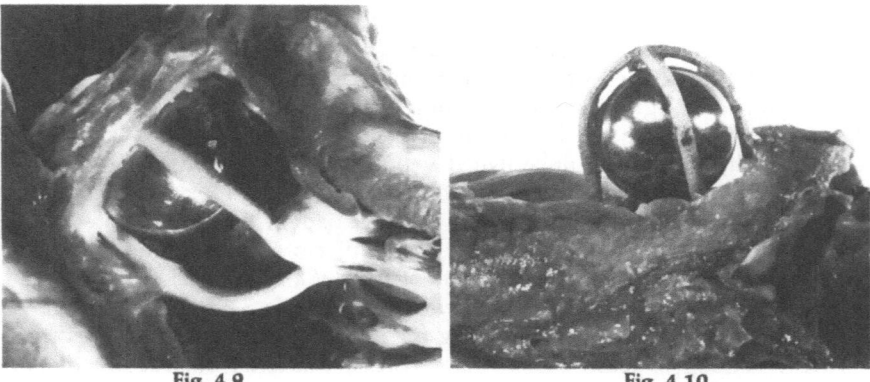

Fig. 4.9   Fig. 4.10

Figure 4.9   Disproportion between the bulky Starr–Edwards tricuspid valve prosthesis and a mildly dilated right ventricle has led to incorporation of part of the cage into the right ventricular free wall
Figure 4.10   Scanty thrombus on the inner aspect of the struts is limiting movement of the ball, which is stuck in an open position

has been in use for 17 years, is the valve of choice except in very elderly patients and those in whom anticoagulant therapy poses a big risk. He also concluded that there are no major differences in the incidence of thromboembolism between currently available tissue valves and the ball-valve during the same time frame (from 1973 onwards). He also claims that the St Jude Medical valve has a thromboembolism-free rate comparable to that of the Starr–Edwards Silastic ball-valve. Regarding thrombotic stenosis in aortic valve replacement, he cited evidence to show that the Bjork–Shiley valve was 97% free of this complication at 5 years, whereas the Starr–Edwards ball-valve was 99.5% free. In a recent study[36], *in vitro* velocity, shear stress, and pressure drop measurements were made under steady-flow conditions and used to interpret some of the failure modes of the Starr–Edwards prosthesis as observed at autopsy. Comparison of the valve model used today with the same model used in the late 1960s shows greatly improved results, especially with regard to thromboembolism[37]. Current model Starr–Edwards valves compare favourably with other valves introduced since 1970. Long-term complications are primarily thromboembolism, endocarditis, haemolysis and anticoagulation-related complications[38].

SMELOFF–SUTTER (previously SMELOFF–CUTTER) VALVE

This full-orifice (non-overlapping) caged-ball prosthesis (Figure 4.11 and Table 4.4) was developed during the early 1960s by Drs Smeloff, Cartwright, Davey and Kaufman[39–41]. The prosthesis is machined from a single piece of pure titanium. The orifice and struts are bare metal. The two cages each have three struts, which are not continuous across the ring. The full orifice design aims

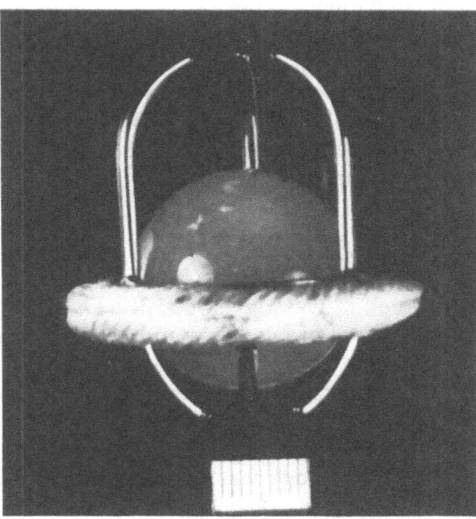

Figure 4.11 Smeloff–Sutter (previously Smeloff–Cutter) valve prosthesis has been available from 1966 to the present. Note the distinctive double cage arrangement (Picture courtesy of Dr M. D. Silver)

to reduce thromboembolism by a washing effect produced by regurgitation of blood around the ball. The one cage is shorter than the other. In the mitral position the silicone rubber poppet occupies less of the left ventricular cavity than is the case with the Starr—Edwards prosthesis, because the poppet rests partially in the left atrium in systole. Thus, if the left ventricle is small, there is less chance of the valve causing left ventricular outflow tract obstruction. The full-orifice design allows a larger prosthetic orifice than is possible with a conventional ball valve. The sewing ring consists of Teflon.

There is a narrow clearance between the ball and the cages. Design-related complications include ball variance (swelling due to lipid absorption, which was corrected by altering the curing process). Rarely the tip of a metal strut (open-ended cages) penetrated the endocardium or became entangled in a papillary muscle remnant[42]. Unfortunately, cardiac catheterization studies failed to show the improved haemodynamics expected of the full-orifice prosthesis[43]. Thromboembolic rates were similar to those of other non-cloth-covered prostheses. Thrombotic stenosis was rarer than with disc valves. A fibrous subvalvular pannus caused prosthetic mitral stenosis in 16 of 376 patients with this prosthesis[44]. This finding prompted Smeloff et al. to consider altering the design of their prosthesis. Harlan et al.[45] reported on the performance of the Smeloff aortic valve beyond 10 years, and concluded that it has excellent long-term durability and a low thromboembolic rate in anticoagulated patients.

HARKEN VALVE

Dr D. Harken and co-workers successfully implanted a caged-ball prosthesis in the aortic root of human patients in the early 1960s with an initial operative mortality rate of 71%[46,47]. The early Harken valve incorporated both inner and outer cages with a total of eight struts. The outer cage aimed to prevent the aortic wall from interfering with poppet movement[48]. The modern model of the Harken caged-ball prosthesis (Table 4.4) has a hollow Stellite ball enclosed by three cloth-covered struts. A polyethylene inner ring seats the poppet proximal to its equator.

MAGOVERN—CROMIE VALVE

This sutureless heart valve[48–50] was developed by Dr G. Magovern of the University of Pittsburgh School of Medicine and Mr H. Cromie, a machinist. The manufacturing company is Coratomic (previously Surgitool, then Medical Engineering Corporation). The initial Magovern—Cromie valve had a stainless steel closed cage surrounding a silicone rubber ball. The base ring of the valve incorporated curved metal pins (Figure 4.12) which were turned outward and through the aorta when the cage was rotated horizontally with a special instrument. Due to a tendency for thrombus to accumulate at the apex of the cage of this prototype valve, all subsequent valves (Table 4.4) were made with an open-ended cage (Figure 4.13). Model A1 introduced in 1963 had 24 pins attached to an upper metal plate, and the lower rim had 24 additional

Table 4.4 Details of other ball valve prostheses (excluding Starr–Edwards prostheses)

Valve	Used clinically from	Cage/struts	Sewing ring	Ball occluder (poppet)	Major problems
Harken	1960	Early: inner and outer cages with eight struts Later: three cloth-covered struts with plastic lining inside ring. Closed cage	Ivalon sponge	Hollow Stellite seats proximal to its equator	Thromboembolism
Magovern–Cromie	1962	Titanium open cage. Automatic fixation mechanism	No sewing ring; models A1, A2, A3 up to 1968. Dacron on sides and part of base from 1968 (model A4)	Silicone rubber with barium sulphate	Paravalvular leaks; thromboembolism
Smeloff–Sutter	1964	Titanium bare strutted open-ended double cage	Convex metal inner ring.	Radiolucent silicone rubber	Thromboembolism. Ball variance. Cage attached to ventricular septum
Braunwald–Cutter	1968	Single, open cage, Dacron cloth-covered struts	Polypropylene cloth over orifice	Radiolucent silicone rubber	Thromboembolism, variance, haemolysis, apical cloth wear, paravalvular leaks
De Bakey–Surgitool	1969	Closed cage, no feet in orifice, three bare titanium struts (recently coated with pyrolytic carbon)	Plastic (polyethylene) inner ring. Serrated metal ring	Radiolucent poppet (recently pyrolite ball)	Strut wear

59

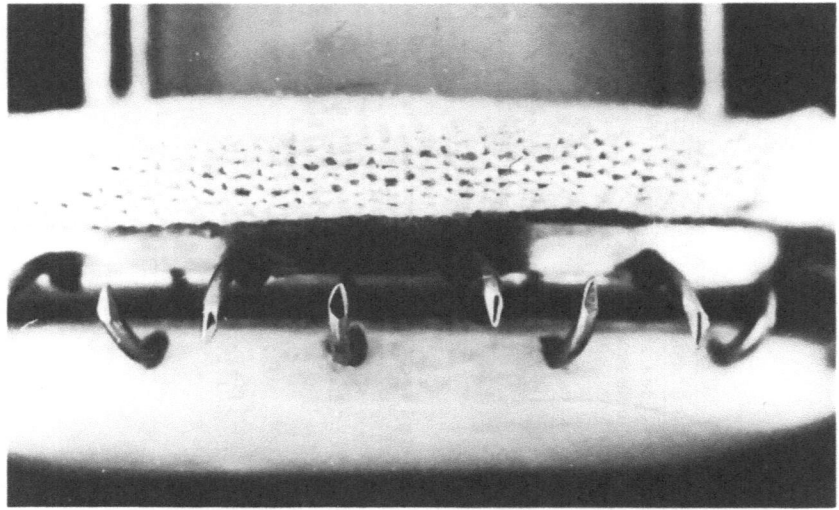

Figure 4.12 Base ring of Magovern–Cromie aortic valve prosthesis incorporates curved hooks, which allow rapid fixation of the prosthesis in the aortic annulus. (Picture courtesy of Dr M. D. Silver)

interdigitating pins. Model A2 of 1964 had a silicone rubber flange over the outflow aspect of the ring to limit paraprosthetic leaks and the radiopaque poppet contained barium sulphate. Model A3, which was introduced in 1965 to overcome the problem of thromboembolism, had Teflon partially covering its inflow surface. Model A4 of 1968 had Dacron covering most of the base and bare struts. In this model only the aortic valve used the sutureless technique and the mitral prosthesis was abandoned. The establishment of safe techniques for cardiopulmonary bypass and myocardial protection rendered the rapidly implantable sutureless Magovern–Cromie valve redundant.

BRAUNWALD–CUTTER VALVE

Since host tissue covers fabric leaflet valves[51], Braunwald reasoned that covering mechanical prostheses with porous cloth would combine the advantages of both devices. Several non-cloth-covered (Starr–Edwards, Cross–Jones, Kay–Shiley) prostheses had their struts covered by loosely knit polypropylene and the metal ring was clothed with stretch-knit Dacron[52]. Experiments with these modified prostheses showed that:

1. The fabric covering the metal increases thrombogenicity of the prosthesis, but the more adherent thrombus gets covered by endothelial cells, thereby producing a non-thrombogenic autologous surface.
2. The thrombus which forms is seldom more than twice as thick as the underlying cloth. Anticoagulation leads to a thinner thrombus-tissue layer.

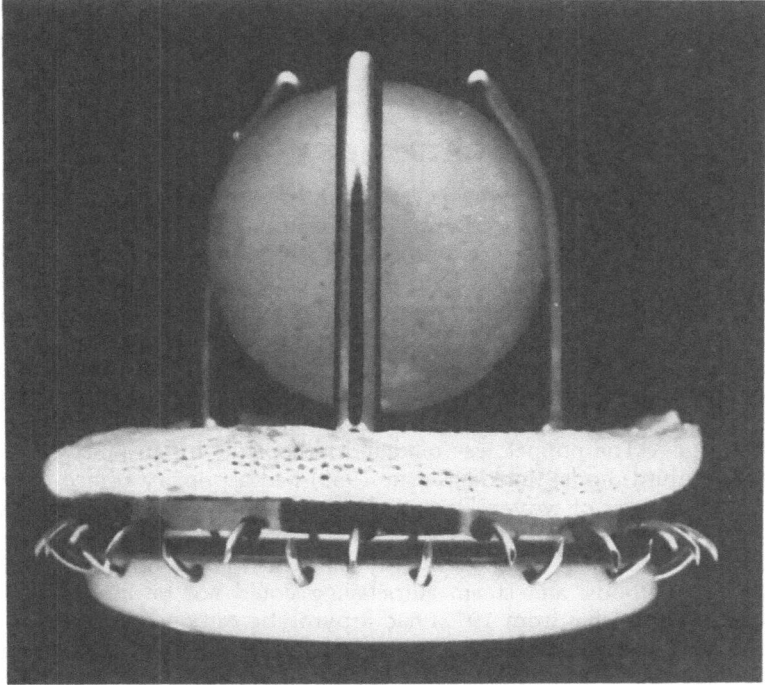

Figure 4.13 Magovern–Cromie caged-ball aortic valve prosthesis has an open-ended titanium cage and a silicone rubber poppet; since 1964 the poppet has been rendered radiopaque by barium sulphate. (Picture courtesy of Dr M. D. Silver)

3. A coarse fibre weave in the cloth favours a uniform fibroblast infiltration of the thrombotic layer resulting in better adherence.
4. The cloth covering the struts had an abrasive action which led to wear of soft poppets (e.g. those made from silicone rubber), whereas hard poppets (made of Stellite) resulted instead in wear of the cloth.

In 1967 Braunwald and co-workers started clinically to use standard, non-cloth-covered Starr–Edwards prostheses, which they had completely covered with cloth. Thromboembolism was rare, but the platelet–fibrin layer developed slowly in humans (unlike the experimental results in calves) and the human neo-intima was thin and delicate. In addition the cloth covering the ring rendered the smaller prostheses stenotic[52]. In order to overcome the latter difficulty, Cutter Laboratories produced a totally cloth-covered prosthetic heart valve. The Braunwald–Cutter caged-ball valve[53] had a titanium frame with an open-ended cage (Table 4.4). The ring was covered by polypropylene mesh and the struts with knitted Dacron. The mild-cure silicone rubber poppet was similar to that used in 1966 in the Smeloff–Cutter valve.

Late morphology of Braunwald–Cutter valve prostheses[54] includes severe cloth and poppet wear, escape of the poppet, retraction of cloth covering the distal portions of the struts and trivial calcific deposits deep in the tissue coating.

DEBAKEY–SURGITOOL AORTIC VALVE

The aim of this prosthesis, which was designed by Dr M. E. DeBakey and associates of Baylor College of Medicine, Houston, Texas and Mr H. Cromie of Surgitool, Inc., was to devise a prosthesis which would not suffer the ball variance that was encountered with the early model Starr–Edwards aortic valves. Several different models were manufactured in the evolution of this prosthesis. The first DeBakey–Surgitool valve had a titanium poppet and the struts plus the ring were covered with Dacron velour. This totally cloth-covered design was unsuccessful due to severe haemolysis. The second model (Table 4.4) had a pyrolytic carbon–silicone alloy coated ball with a bare titanium cage[55]. The poppet was rendered radiopaque by an inner tungsten screen. The third model (introduced in 1969) had a primary orifice covered with a double layer of woven Dacron. Severe haemolysis prohibited its use. The fourth model introduced in 1971 was characterized by a base ring made of ultra-high molecular weight polyethylene which could only be sterilized by gaseous methods, and steam autoclaving could not be used. The fifth valve design (available from 1972) had a pyrolytic carbon base ring[48].

There have been very few reports published of results using the DeBakey–Surgitool valve[56,57]. Embolism had a similar incidence to other non-cloth-covered prostheses. Wear and/or fracture of the struts occurred due to the combination of an extremely hard pyrolytic carbon ball and a soft titanium cage. Design alterations in the mid-1960s by Cutter Laboratories virtually eliminated ball variance with silicone rubber poppets[48]. The long-term durability of such poppets has still to be proved.

DEBAKEY–SURGITOOL MITRAL VALVE

Although this prosthesis has been used at Baylor College by DeBakey and co-workers for several years, it has not been made available for general use. Like the Beall–Surgitool valve it has a pyrolytic carbon disc and Dacron velour covers the orifice. The struts cross on the DeBakey valve, unlike the parallel arrangement of the Beall valve.

REFERENCES

1. Starr Edwards cardiac valve prostheses (statistical data sheet). (1972). (Santa Ana, California: Edwards Laboratories)
2. Forman, R., Beck, W. and Barnard, C. N. (1978). Results after mitral valve replacement with cloth-covered Starr–Edwards prostheses (Models 6300, 6310/6320 and 6400). Br. Heart J., 40, 612
3. Rose, A. G. (1984). Pathology of Heart Valve Replacement by Valvular Prostheses. MD thesis, University of Cape Town
4. Starr, A., Grunkemeier, G., Lambert, L., Okies, J. E. and Thomas, D. (1976). Mitral valve

replacement. A 10-year follow-up of non-cloth-covered vs. cloth-covered caged-ball prostheses. *Circulation*, **54**, (Suppl. 3), III-47

5. Salomon, N., Stinson, E. B., Griepp, R. B. and Shumway, N. E. (1976). Mitral valve replacement: long-term evaluation of prosthesis-related mortality and morbidity. *Circulation*, **56**, (Suppl. 2), II-94
6. Fraser, R. S. and Waddell, J.(1967). Systemic embolization after aortic valve replacement. *J. Thorac. Cardiovasc. Surg.*, **54**, 81
7. Lewis, R. P., Herr, R. H., Starr, A. and Griswold, H. E. (1966). Aortic valve replacement with the Starr–Edwards ball-valve prosthesis. *Am. Heart J.*, **71**, 549
8. Herr, R., Starr, A., McCord, C. W. and Wood, J. A. (1965). Special problems following valve replacement. Embolus, leak, infection, red cell damage. *Ann. Thorac. Surg.*, **1**, 403
9. Roberts, W. C. and Morrow, A. G. (1967). Anatomic studies of hearts containing caged-ball prosthetic valves. *Johns Hopkins Med. J.*, **121**, 271
10. Laforet, E. G. (1967). Death due to swelling of ball component of aortic ball-valve prosthesis. *N. Engl. J. Med.*, **276**, 1025
11. Gobel, F. L., Hawkins, H. M., Hanson, R. and Wang, Y. (1968). Acute myocardial infarction secondary to thromboembolism from a fractured prosthetic aortic valve. *Circulation*, **38**, 672
12. Bonchek, L. I. and Starr, A. (1975). Ball valve prostheses: current appraisal of late results. *Am. J. Cardiol.*, **35**, 843
13. Shah, A., Dolgin, M., Tice, D. A. and Trehan, N. (1978). Complications due to cloth wear in cloth-covered Starr–Edwards aortic and mitral valve prostheses — and their management. *Am. Heart J.*, **96**, 407
14. Starr, A., Bonchek, L. I., Anderson, R. P., Wood, J. A. and Chapman, R. D. (1975). Late complications of aortic valve replacement with cloth-covered composite-seat prostheses. *Ann. Thorac. Surg.*, **19**, 289
15. Isom, O. W., Spencer, F. C., Glassman, E., Teiko, P., Boyd, A. D., Cunningham, J. N. and Reed, G. E. (1977). Long term results in 1375 patients undergoing valve replacement with the Starr–Edwards cloth-covered steel ball prosthesis. *Ann. Surg.*, **186**, 310
16. Niles, N. R. (1970). Teflon embolism from Starr–Edwards valves. *J. Thorac. Cardiovasc. Surg.*, **59**, 794
17. Maronas, J. M., Such, M. and Sanchez, P. (1982). Fatal coronary obstruction due to cloth-wear of a cloth-covered Starr–Edwards aortic valve prosthesis. *Chest*, **82**, 645
18. Warnes, C. A., McIntosh, C. L. and Roberts, W. C. (1983). Wear of the metallic studs on the composite seat of the 2320 Starr–Edwards aortic valve and its clinical consequences. *Am. J. Cardiol.*, **52**, 1062
19. Ringel, R. E., Moulton, A. L., Burns, J. E., Brenner, J. I. and Berman, M. A. (1983). Structural failure of a Starr–Edwards aortic track valve. *Texas Heart Inst. J.*, **10**, 81
20. Bruhlmann, W. F., Neftel, K. A. and Tartini, R. (1982). Misleading supine chest x-ray in complete detachment of a Starr–Edwards prosthetic aortic valve. *Europ. J. Radiol.*, **4**, 317
21. Aris, A., Fast, A. J., Tector, A. J., Flemma, R. J. and Lepley, D. (1974). A comparative study of ball and disc prostheses in mitral valve replacement. *J. Thorac. Cardiovasc. Surg.*, **68**, 335
22. Miller, D. C., Oyer, P. E., Stinson, E. B., Reitz, B. A., Jamieson, S. W., Baumgartner, W. A., Mitchell, R. S. and Shumway, N. E. (1983). Ten to fifteen year reassessment of the performance characteristics of the Starr–Edwards model 6120 mitral valve prosthesis. *J. Thorac. Cardiovasc. Surg.*, **85**, 1
23. Jett, G. K., Jett M. D., Barnhart, G. R., van Rijk-Swikker, G. L., Jones, M. and Clark, R. E. (1986). Left ventricular outflow tract obstruction with mitral valve replacement in small ventricular cavities. *Ann. Thorac. Surg.*, **41**, 70
24. Bache, R. J., From, A. H., Castaneda, A. R., Jorgensen, C. R. and Wang, Y. (1972). Late thrombotic obstruction of Starr–Edwards tricuspid valve prosthesis. *Chest*, **61**, 613
25. Schelbert, H. R. and Muller, O. F. (1972). Detection of fungal vegetations involving a Starr–Edwards mitral prosthesis by means of ultrasound. *Vasc. Surg.*, **6**, 20
26. Bisarya, R. K., Englebrecht, W., Burr, L. H. and Allen, P. (1974). Obstruction of a mitral ball-valve prosthesis by adhesions from an intact mural leaflet complex. *J. Thorac. Cardiovasc. Surg.*, **68**, 116
27. Mond, H. G., Clarebrough, J. K. and Dowling, J. T. (1972). Entrapment of the metal ball in series 6310 and 2310 Starr–Edwards prosthetic valves. *J. Thorac. Cardiovasc. Surg.*, **64**, 186

28. Roberts, W. C., Bulkley, B. H. and Morrow, A. G., (1973). Pathologic anatomy of cardiac valve replacement: a study of 224 necropsy patients. *Prog. Cardiovasc. Dis.*, **15**, 539

29. Joassin, A. and Edwards, J. E. (1973). Causes of death within 30 days of mitral valvular replacement. Analysis of 93 cases. *Cardiovasc. Clin.*, **5**, 169

30. Joassin, A. and Edwards, J. E. (1973). Late causes of death after mitral valve replacement: analysis of 36 cases. *J. Thorac. Cardiovasc. Surg.*, **65**, 255

31. Schoen, F. J., Titus, J. L. and Lawrie, G. M. (1983). Autopsy-determined causes of death after cardiac valve replacement. *J. Am. Med. Assoc.*, **249**, 899

32. Niles, N. R. and Sandilands, J. R. (1969). Pathology of heart valve replacement surgery: autopsies of 62 patients with Starr–Edwards prostheses. *Dis. Chest.*, **56**, 373

33. Vasconez, L. O., Shanklin, D. R. and Wheat, M. W. (1968). Healing around the Starr–Edwards aortic valve prosthesis in patients. *Ann. Thorac. Surg.*, **6**, 25

34. Seningen, R. P., Bulkley, B. H. and Roberts, W. C. (1974). Prosthetic aortic stenosis. A method to prevent its occurrence by measurement of aortic size from preoperative aortogram. *Circulation*, **49**, 921

35. Starr, A. (1983). Ball valve prostheses : A perspective after 22 years. In DeBakey, M. E. (ed.) *Advances in Cardiac Valves: Clinical Perspectives.* p. 1 (New York: Yorke Medical Books)

36. Yoganathan, A. P., Reamer, H. H. and Corcoran, W. H. (1981). The Starr–Edwards aortic ball valve: flow characteristics, thrombus formation, and tissue overgrowth. *Artif. Organs*, **5**, 6

37. Starr, A. (1985). The Starr–Edwards valve. *J. Am. Coll. Cardiol.*, **6**, 899

38. Best, J. F., Hassanein, K. M., Pugh, D. M. and Dunn, M. (1986). Starr–Edwards aortic prosthesis: a 20-year retrospective study. *Am. Heart J.*, **111**, 136

39. Cartwright, R. S., Palich, W. E. and Ford, W. B. (1962). Combined replacement of aortic and mitral valves: an original transatrial approach to the aortic valve. *J. Am. Med. Assoc.*, **130**, 86

40. Cartwright, R. S., Giacobine, J. W., Ratan, R. S., Ford, W. B. and Palich, W. E. (1963). Combined aortic and mitral valve replacement. *J. Thorac. Cardiovasc. Surg.*, **45**, 35

41. Cartwright, R. S., Smeloff, E. A. and Davey, T. B. (1964). Development of a titanium double-caged ball valve. *Trans. Am. Soc. Artif. Intern. Organs*, **10**, 231

42. Kalke, B., Korns, M. E., Goott, B., Lillehei, C. W. and Edwards, J. E. (1969). Engagement of ventricular myocardium by open-cage atrioventricular valvular prosthesis. *J. Thorac. Cardiovasc. Surg.*, **58**, 92

43. Frater, R. W. M., Wexler, H. R. and Yellin, E. (1969). The *in vivo* comparison of hemodynamic function of ball, disc, and eccentric monocusp artificial mitral valves. In Brewer, L. A. III (ed.) *Prosthetic Heart Valves.* p. 262. (Springfield, Illinois: Charles C. Thomas)

44. Smeloff, E. A., Davey, T. B., Riemenschneider, T. A., Epstein, M. L., Janos, G. and Marshall, R. (1982). Modification of the Smeloff mitral prosthesis. *Am. J. Surg.*, **144**, 158

45. Harlan, B. J., Smeloff, E. A., Miller, G. E., Kelly, P. B., Junod, F. L., Ross, K. A. and Shankar, K. G. (1986). Performance of the Smeloff aortic valve beyond 10 years. *J. Thorac. Cardiovasc. Surg.*, **91**, 86

46. Harken, D. E., Soroff, H. S. and Taylor, W. J. (1960). Partial and complete prostheses in aortic insufficiency. *J. Thorac. Cardiovasc. Surg.*, **40**, 744

47. Harken, D. E., Soroff, H. S. and Taylor, W. J. (1961). Aortic valve replacement. In Merendino, K. A. (ed.) *Prosthetic Valves for Cardiac Surgery.* p. 508. (Springfield, Illinois: Charles C. Thomas)

48. Lefrak, E. A. and Starr, A. (1979). *Cardiac Valve Prostheses.* (New York: Appleton-Century-Crofts)

49. Magovern, G. J. and Cromie, H. W. (1963). Sutureless prosthetic heart valves. *J. Thorac. Cardiovasc. Surg.*, **46**, 726

50. Magovern, G. J., Kent, E. M., Cromie, H. W., Cushing, W. B. and Scott, S. (1964). Sutureless aortic and mitral valves: clinical results and operative technique on sixty patients. *J. Thorac. Cardiovasc. Surg.*, **48**, 346

51. Braunwald, N. S. and Morrow, A. G. (1965). A late evaluation of flexible teflon prosthesis utilized for total aortic valve replacement. *J. Thorac. Cardiovasc. Surg.*, **49**, 485

52. Braunwald, N. S. and Morrow, A. G. (1968). Tissue ingrowth and the rigid heart valve:

review of clinical and experimental experience during the past year. *J. Thorac. Cardiovasc. Surg.*, **56**, 307

53. Braunwald, N. S., Tatooles, C., Turina, M. and Detmer, D. (1971). New developments in the design of fabric-covered prosthetic heart valves. *J. Thorac. Cardiovasc. Surg.*, **62**, 673

54. Schoen, F. J., Goodenough, S. H., Ionescu, M. I. and Braunwald, N. S. (1984). Implications of late morphology of Braunwald-Cutter mitral heart valve prostheses. *J. Thorac. Cardiovasc. Surg.*, **88**, 208

55. Bokros, J. C. and Akins, R. J. (1971). Applications of pyrolytic carbon in artificial heart valves: a status report. *Proc. 4th Buhl International Conf. on Materials.* (Pittsburgh, Pennsylvania: Carnegie Press, Carnegie—Mellon University)

56. Scott, S. M., Sethi, G. K., Bridgman, L. H. *et al.* (1976). Experience with the DeBakey—Surgitool aortic prosthetic valve. *Ann. Thorac. Surg.*, **21**, 483

57. Paton, B. C. and Pine, M. D. (1976). Aortic valve replacement with the DeBakey valve. *J. Thorac. Cardiovasc. Surg.*, **72**, 652

5
Caged-disc, Hinged-leaflet and Tethered Plunger Valves

The caged-ball design gained worldwide acceptance following early successes with mitral valve replacement in 1960[1,2]. Initially there was concern that caged-ball valves may produce subaortic outflow tract obstruction, resulting in a low cardiac output, or that ventricular fibrillation might result from the cage impinging on the septum. Pathological specimens occasionally supported this contention[3,4]. Concern regarding the suitability of caged-ball valves for mitral valve replacement in patients with small left ventricles led to the development of low-profile prostheses, which have a shorter (lower profile) cage than the ball valve. The reduced weight of a lens valve lowers the inertial force necessary to start the lens through its range of motion and the prosthesis is also quieter.

CAGED-DISC VALVES

Hufnagel–Conrad valve

This polypropylene and silicone-rubber caged-disc prosthesis was developed by Drs Hufnagel and Conrad at the Georgetown University Hospital[5]. Various shapes of disc were evaluated, but this valve and its numerous modifications were not satisfactory in a blood medium. Its use was soon abandoned due to problems of wear and thrombosis.

Cross–Jones valve

The Cross–Jones prosthesis[6], manufactured by Pemco Inc. between 1967 and 1974, had an open-ended cage composed of three struts. The radiolucent silicone-rubber disc contained a radiopaque titanium ring, which also served to strengthen the disc. The cage was also made of titanium. No feet projected into the valve orifice. Significant complications included thrombosis, thromboembolism, cocking of the disc, retrograde dislodgement[7] and disc variance.

Kay–Suzuki valve

The valve (Figure 5.1) designed by Drs E. B. Kay and A. Suzuki[4] and manufactured from 1964 by Valve Research, had a closed-ended high cage with four struts. Four short, open base feet projected into the orifice opposite the cage. The valve had a narrow double-ring valve base (metal inner ring) and a radiolucent poppet. Major problems were thromboembolism and disc variance. The valve has been discontinued.

Harken–Cromie valve

The Harken P2 low-profile prosthetic mitral valve (manufactured by Surgitek–Surgitool from 1967) had a closed cage composed of four thin, crossing struts and a radiopaque poppet[8]. Thromboemboli, fluttering of the disc due to uncorrected aortic regurgitation[9] and disc wear/variance were recognized complications. Production of the valve has ceased.

Kay–Shiley valve[10,11]

The type I Kay–Shiley valve had four struts which projected vertically from the Stellite sewing ring to form two parallel bars made of bare metal (Stellite). The closed cage held a radiolucent silicone rubber disc. This valve was used for mitral and tricuspid valve replacements[12,13]. The type II valve had knitted Teflon cloth extending on to the orificial metal to reduce thromboembolism[14]. The type III valve had a muscle guard projecting from the ring to prevent the disc from engaging the adjacent myocardium. This modification nullifies the theoretical advantage of the low-profile valve, namely that it avoids contact with the myocardium[15]. The addition of a second guard gave rise to the type IV valve, which also substituted Delrin for silicone rubber as the

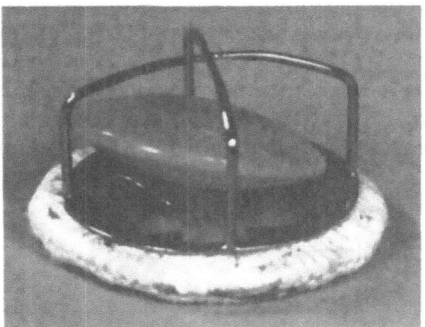
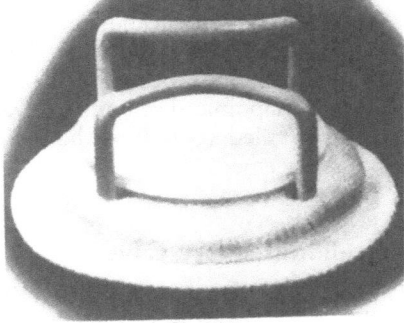

Fig. 5.1   Fig. 5.2

Figure 5.1 Kay–Zuzuki disc valve has a cage with four struts and four feet project into the orifice. (Picture courtesy Dr M. D. Silver)
Figure 5.2 Beall model 103 caged-disc mitral valve prosthesis

disc material[16].

Since low profile prostheses should produce less obstruction of the tertiary orifice (the space between the poppet and the aortic wall), Bjork implanted the Kay–Shiley valve in the aortic position in 60 consecutive patients. Postoperatively the average systolic gradient was disappointing[17]. Major complications encountered with the Kay–Shiley prosthesis included thromboembolism, sudden death, grooving and disc wear, restenosis with tissue ingrowth, perivalvular leaks, disc cocking and disc variance[18]. According to Lefrak and Starr[1] the established vulnerability of the Kay–Shiley prosthesis to catastrophic malfunction is typical of disc prostheses; a small amount of thrombus may critically interfere with disc mobility, rendering it stenotic and susceptible to a vicious cycle of rapidly progressive thrombosis. Deaths from low cardiac output dsyndrome or arrhythmias continue to occur despite the use of low-profile valves.

Beall valve

Dr A. Beall and Coratomic (initially Surgitek/Surgitool Inc., then Medical Engineering Corporation) produced a partially cloth-covered, low-profile valve (Figure 5.2) from 1974 to the present. The disc was made of extruded Teflon, and solid Teflon covered the titanium struts[19]. Due to premature disc wear[20,21] the disc was changed to a thicker, compression-moulded Teflon disc in Model 103. Due to poor haemodynamic responses during exercise[22], the small-sized model 104 Beall prosthesis had enlarged primary and secondary orificial areas.

Later it became apparent that wear of the disc edge was still a significant problem[23]. Disc wear manifested clinically as increased haemolysis and mitral incompetence or stenosis. Model 105, introduced in 1971, no longer had a Teflon disc and there was no Teflon on the struts. A pyrolytic carbon–silicone alloy coated the new graphite disc and the titanium wire struts. However, strut fracture[24] due to cracking of the brittle carbon alloy was a serious problem in model 105. Strut fracture, which is related to metal fatigue, tends to occur at the base and may be concealed by the cloth covering. Careful handling of the valve is recommended prior to implantation.

In model 106 the thickness of the strut wire was increased and its packaging and sterilization was improved[1]. The greater degree of haemolysis associated with the Beall–Surgitool valve is probably related to the valve's combination of an overlapping disc with a Dacron velour cloth-covered orifice. The prosthesis failed to reduce the incidence of thromboembolism after mitral valve replacement.

Starr–Edwards disc valve

The first Starr–Edwards disc valve (Figure 5.3) had a poppet made of hollow Stellite 21 and the cage was made from the same metal alloy[25]. The heat-tempered poppet was made harder than the cage legs to prevent edge wear, and the latter were also thick enough to withstand wear. The sewing ring was made of Teflon cloth. While the problem of disc edge wear was eliminated by this valve model, it later became evident that thromboembolism, poor hydraulic function and thrombotic entrapment of the disc were significant problems[1,26]. The model 6520 Starr–Edwards disc prosthesis (Figure 5.4) had a disc made from Hifax (ultrahigh molecular weight polyethylene), which contained a radiopaque titanium ring. The hydraulics were improved by enlarged primary and secondary orifices. The same closed cage design of Stellite 21 as the previous design was used in this new model.

Up until 1979 Edwards Laboratories had not been notified of a single case of disc wear, strut fracture, or poppet embolization with either the 6500 or 6520 models. In common with other disc valves it shares a haemodynamic effect inferior to caged-ball or tilting disc valves, and a tendency to disc immobilization by thrombus or endocardium. It also has a similar embolic rate to other non-cloth-covered valves[1].

Cooley–Cutter valve

Dr D. Liotta of Texas produced an eccentrically hinged disc valve, which closed too slowly and allowed an unacceptable amount of incompetence[27]. This was followed by the Cooley–Liotta–Cromie prosthesis, which was a modification of the Starr–Edwards valve. It had a titanium ball and Dacron velour completely covered the ring and the struts[28]. Its use was discontinued due to cloth wear and haemolysis. The Cooley–Bloodwell–Cutter prosthesis introduced in 1966 had a silicone rubber disc and bare titanium cage legs. The orifice of the valve was covered with Dacron cloth. Thromboembolism[29] and disc wear soon led to its use being discontinued.

The *Cooley–Cutter valve*[30], made available between 1971 and 1978 by Cutter Biomedical Corporation, had a double cage made of titanium struts

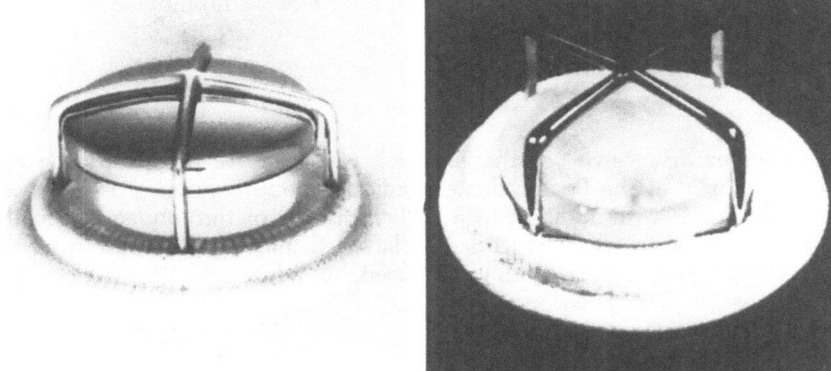

Fig. 5.3   Fig. 5.4

Figure 5.3   Starr–Edwards model 6500 caged-disc prosthesis with hollow Stellite disc which was available between 1968 and 1970
Figure 5.4   Starr–Edwards model 6520 caged-disc prosthesis which was available between 1970 and 1976. The disc contained a titanium ring to provide visibility on X-ray

(all machined from a single piece of titanium). The radiolucent poppet consisted of pyrolite with a tungsten insert. It had a peripheral, self-washing regurgitant stream in the closed position and the knitted Teflon sewing ring was eccentric in order to reduce the danger of poppet entrapment by mural endocardium. Initially there was a mitral prosthesis only. In 1973 an aortic prosthesis with a biconical occluder was introduced, and the mitral poppet was fashioned in this way too.

Like the DeBakey–Surgitool and the Lillehei–Kaster prostheses, the Cooley–Cutter valve has a hard pyrolytic carbon poppet and relatively soft titanium struts. Titanium strut wear has been reported with the DeBakey–Surgitool valve and the Cooley–Cutter valve may have the potential for similar wear. Strut fracture of the Cooley–Cutter prosthesis has been reported[31]. Thrombosis and thromboembolism have also been noted[18].

University of Stellenbosch valve

The University of Stellenbosch mitral valve prosthesis was developed by Dr P. M. Barnard and colleagues at the University of Stellenbosch, South Africa. The Silastic (silicone rubber) disc was enclosed in an open-ended, stainless steel cage having four bare metal struts. The original disc incorporated a stainless steel ring which was later changed for a perforated nylon plate. Electron beam-welding was used to hold the components together. The sewing ring of the prosthesis was covered with Dacron velour.

Following on testing of the valve in baboons, clinical use of the prosthesis started in July 1967[32]. In 1970 Barnard *et al.*[33] reported their clinical experience with 25 patients in whom the valve had been implanted. Thirty per cent of patients showed early thromboembolism (none fatal) and 9% had late embolism. In contrast to other reports, the cloth covering (Dacron velour) on the University of Stellenbosch mitral valve prosthesis did not reduce the incidence of early embolism. Due to the high rate of thromboembolism, the valve is no longer used.

Alvarez valve

The Alvarez disc valve prosthesis, which was made of polypropylene and was developed at the Postgraduate Medical School, London, was first used clinically in 1964. In addition to a high incidence of thromboembolism the valve was liable to wear, which led to late detachment of the disc from the valve ring. The prosthesis is no longer used, but a few patients have survived as long as 18 years postoperatively[34].

HINGED-LEAFLET VALVE

Gott–Daggett valve

In the mid-1960s Dr V. L. Gott and colleagues devised a hinged-leaflet, low-profile valve[35,36]. The Gott–Daggett valve (Figure 5.5) manufactured by

Daggett had a central cross strut with multiple prongs projecting from the inner aspect of the ring. The radiolucent hinged leaflet was composed of Dacron-reinforced silicone rubber; metal pins anchored the leaflet to the valve housing. Major problems included thromboembolism and haemolysis. Extended survival after mitral valve replacement with a Gott–Daggett prosthesis has been reported[37].

TETHERED-PLUNGER VALVE

University of Cape Town (UCT) valve

This tethered-plunger prosthesis (available from 1961 to the early 1970s) had (mitral: flat lenticular) and (aortic: cone shaped) Silastic poppets[38,39]. The initial UCT mitral valve prosthesis (Figures 5.6–5.8) had a lenticular disc suspended from a T-piece, which lay within a ring at the end of a suspension arm. In the mitral prosthesis the restraining mechanism was sited within the atrium, overcoming the most important disadvantage of the ball-valve. The suspension arm was anchored to a larger steel ring, which formed the valve seat. This seat ring was initially bare (Figure 5.6) but later it was covered with Ivalon, and subsequently with Teflon, which also acted as a sewing ring. A variety of lenticular-shaped poppets was used. The UCT (lancer) aortic valve (Figure 5.9 and Colour Plate I) had two rings and two suspension arms to hold the I-pieces of the double cone-shaped poppet[38]. Problems with thrombosis and thromboembolism (Figures 5.10 and 5.11) led to the use of the UCT prosthesis being discontinued.

The clinical, haemodynamic[40–45], and pathological findings[46] in patients with UCT prostheses have been previously reported. Ninety-eight patients with UCT prostheses were autopsied at the UCT Medical School, Cape Town. The bobbin of the early model UCT valves showed variance due to accumulation of lipid. This change was prevented by altering the curing technique, but bobbin wear (see Figure 5.12) still occurred.

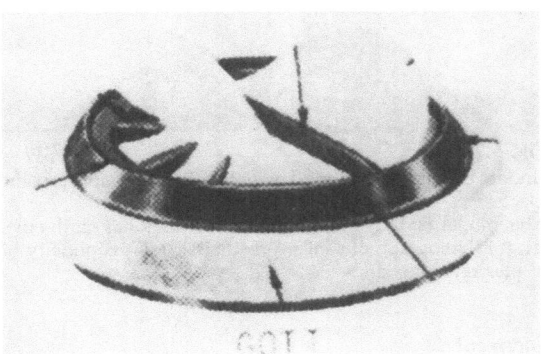

Figure 5.5 Gott–Daggett hinged bileaflet valve prosthesis with central cross strut and prongs projecting inwards from base ring

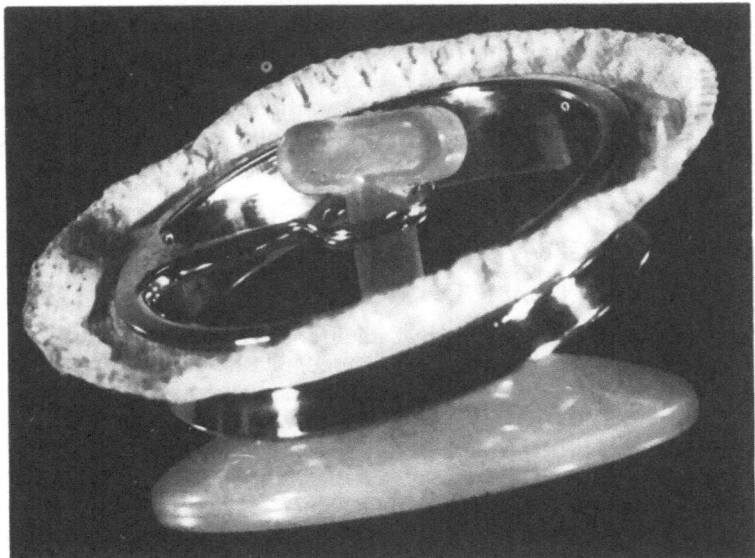

Fig. 5.6

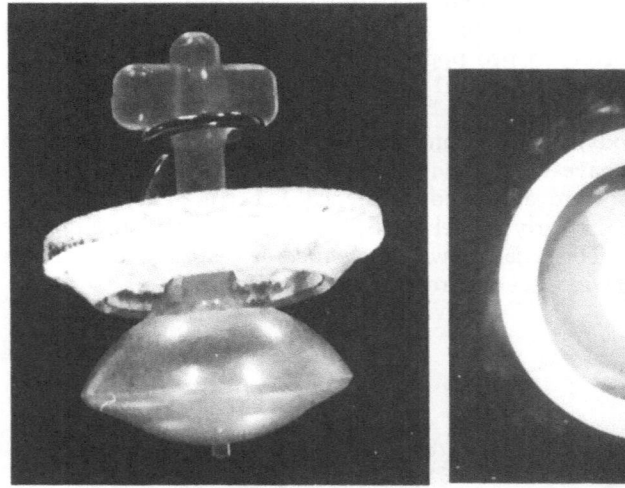

Fig. 5.7(a)   Fig. 5.7(b)

Figure 5.6   Early model University of Cape Town (UCT) mitral valve prosthesis has abundant metal on inflow aspect
Figure 5.7   (a) Later model of UCT mitral valve prosthesis has cloth-covered sewing ring and a thicker poppet. (b) Radiograph of similar prosthesis shows continuity between base ring and suspension arm plus retaining ring

Aortic valve replacement

Forty-one patients had UCT valves inserted. Their principal causes of death are given in Table 5.1 and the sites of thrombus deposition in relation to the

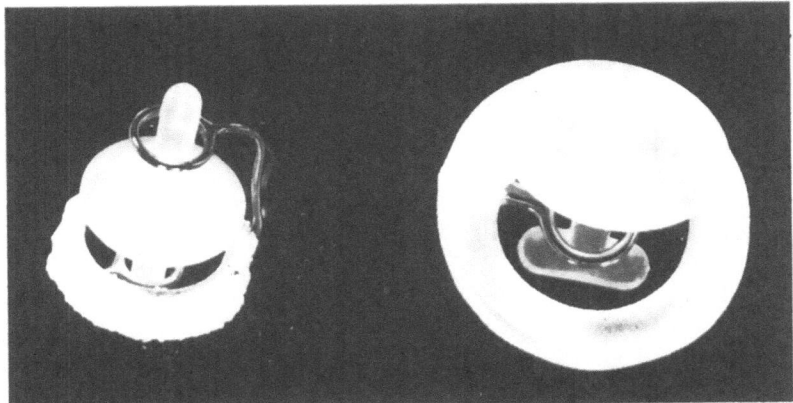

Fig. 5.8

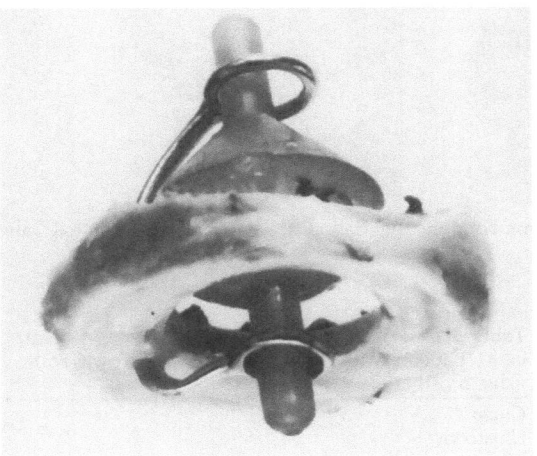

Fig. 5.9

Figure 5.8 UCT aortic valve prosthesis *(left)* and UCT mitral valve prosthesis *(right)* – the latter has a narrow profile disc
Figure 5.9 Explanted UCT aortic valve prosthesis shows evidence of wear of the lower edge of the bobbin

prosthesis are given in Table 5.2. There were 34 men and 7 women, with a mean age of 44.5 years (range 16–66 years). Postoperative survival ranged from 7 hours to 141 months. Twenty patients died 30 days or less after operation (group 1) and 21 patients died more than 30 days after surgery (group 2).

Mitral valve replacement

Thirty-six patients had isolated mitral valve replacement. Twelve patients (group 1) died less than 1 month postoperatively. Their mean age was 49

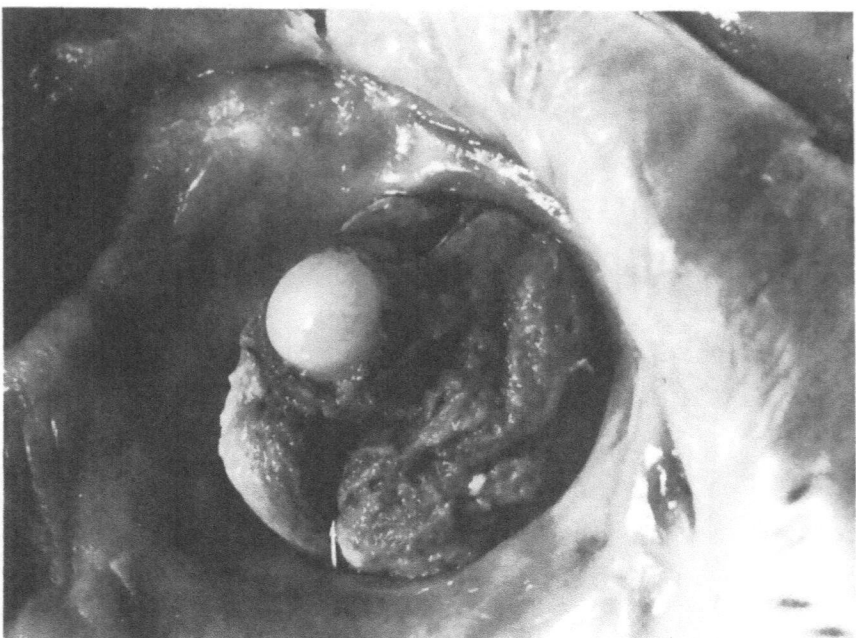

Figure 5.10 Thrombotic immobilization of late model UCT mitral valve prosthesis, (left atrial view)

Table 5.1 Principal causes of death (one per patient) in 41 patients with University of Cape Town aortic valve prosthesis

Group 1	
Unknown	7
Myocardial failure	7
Infected prosthesis (see Figure 5.13)	3
Myocardial perfusion error	1
Pneumonia	1
Ruptured aortotomy wound	1
Group 2	
Thromboembolism	6
Myocardial failure	3
Infected prosthesis	3
Unknown	3
Anticoagulant excess, bleeding	1
Air embolism	3
Aortic rupture (medionecrosis)	1
Detached prosthesis	1

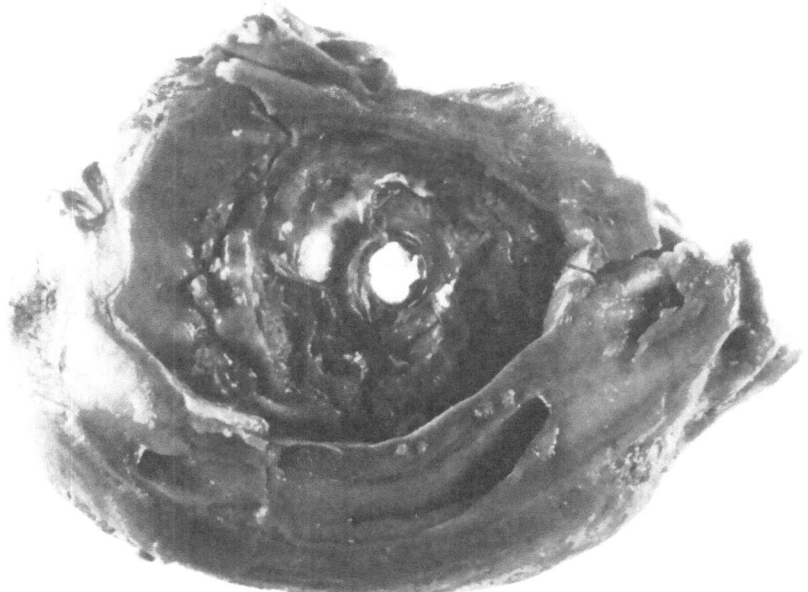

Fig. 5.11

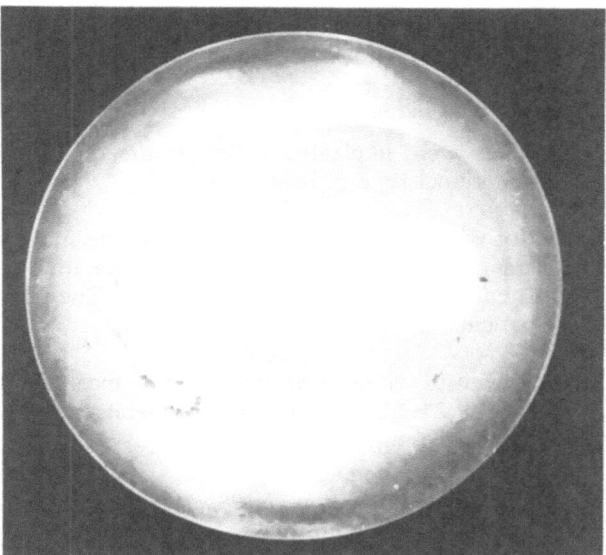

Fig. 5.12

Figure 5.11   Left ventricular view of thrombosed UCT mitral valve prosthesis after removal of bobbin
Figure 5.12   Removed bobbin of UCT mitral valve prosthesis shows evidence of severe wear of the disc's closing aspect

Table 5.2 Sites of thrombus deposition upon UCT aortic
and mitral valvular prostheses

	Aortic	Mitral
No. patients with UCT valves	41	36
No. UCT valves with thrombi	13 (32%)	12 (33%)
Sewing ring		
Inflow aspect	2 (5%)	6 (17%)
Outflow aspect	7 (17%)	1 (3%)
Both aspects	6 (15%)	2 (6%)
Metal guides for bobbin	5 (12%)	2 (6%)
Bobbin	3 (7%)	3 (8%)

years (SD = 9) with a range of 28–60 years. Seven patients were females
and the mean postoperative survival was 7.2 days (SD = 8.5) with a range
of a few hours to 21 days. Twenty-four patients who survived more than 30
days postoperatively (group 2) had a mean age of 49 years (SD = 14) and
a mean postoperative survival of 951 days (SD = 1314). The principal causes
of death of patients with UCT mitral valves are listed in Table 5.3.

Tricuspid valve replacement

Two patients underwent tricuspid valve replacement: one for Ebstein's disease
and the other for rheumatic valvular disease. One patient died of arrhythmia
and the other of septicaemia. The UCT prostheses appeared normal at
necropsy.

Multiple UCT prostheses in the same heart

Forty-one UCT valves were implanted in the hearts of 19 patients who
received no other additional type of heart valve.
Group 1
These six patients (of whom four were females) had a mean age of 30 years
(SD = 12) with a range of 16–44 years. Mean postoperative survival was
5.3 days (SD = 11) with a range of 8 hours to 27 days. The principal causes
of death in these patients are indicated in Table 5.4.
Group 2
These 13 patients (seven of whom were males) had a mean age of 36 years
(SD = 8) with a range of 21–52 years. Mean postoperative survival was 895
days (SD = 1066) and the range was 42–3285 days.

*Summary of the principal causes of death in the 98 patients with University of Cape
Town Prostheses*

The following groups of principal causes of death were encountered: (a)
due to an error in preoperative diagnosis, 1; (b) due to an error in operative
technique, 10 (10%); due to problems inherent in the cardiac valve prosthesis,
42 (43%); (c) postoperative complications, 22 (23%); (d) unrelated to the valve
replacement operation, 4 (4%); and unknown causes, 19 (19%).

Table 5.3 Principal causes of death in 36 patients with UCT mitral valve prosthesis

Group 1	
Unknown	4
Cerebral thromboembolism	3
Air embolism	2
Prosthetic disproportion	1
Sutures in coronary artery	1
Infected prosthesis	1
Group 2	
Thromboembolism	9
Infected prosthesis	4
Thrombosed prosthesis	3
Myocardial failure	2
Unknown	2
Anticoagulant excess, bleeding	1
Prosthetic dehiscence	1
Unrelated to cardiac surgery	1
Catheterization accident	1

Table 5.4 Principal causes of death in 19 patients with multiple UCT valvular prostheses

Group 1	
Myocardial failure	2
Air embolism	1
Dissecting aneurysm	1
Unrecognized associated valve disease	1
Unknown	1
Group 2	
Infection	5
Myocardial failure	3
Unrelated to operation (catheterization)	1
Thromboembolism	1
Thrombosed mitral and tricuspid prostheses	1
Anticoagulant excess, bleeding	1
Unknown	1

Comment

The UCT prosthesis was unsatisfactory since 43% of the deaths were due to prosthesis-related problems. In group 1 patients with aortic valve replacement the commonest principal cause of death was unknown causes (? arrhythmia) followed by myocardial failure. Due to poor patient selection in those early days in which the UCT prosthesis was used, there was a high incidence of myocardial failure. In modern times many of these patients would have either been operated upon earlier in the course of their disease, or they would have been refused surgery because of severe myocardial dysfunction. Less than adequate myocardial protection during cardiopulmonary bypass may also have played a role in the high incidence of myocardial failure postoperatively, since these operations were performed prior to the institution of cardioplegic myocardial protection.

The group 2 patients with isolated aortic valve replacement had thromboembolism, myocardial failure, infection and death due to unknown causes as the commonest reasons for demise. Although thrombus deposition was slightly less common on the UCT aortic valve compared to the UCT mitral prosthesis, thromboembolism was still an important complication with the UCT aortic prosthesis. Two patients in group 2 died of the late effects of operative air embolism.

In patients with a UCT mitral prosthesis the most important causes (in order) of early postoperative death (group 1) were unknown causes, thromboembolism and operative air embolism. Late deaths (group 2) were most often due to systemic thromboembolism, infection of the prosthesis or massive thrombotic occlusion of the prosthesis. Myocardial failure probably favoured the development of the latter complication in some instances. The high frequency of thrombosis on the UCT prosthesis was matched by numerous organ infarcts in these patients. The high thromboembolism rate stopped clinical usage of the UCT prosthesis.

REFERENCES

1. Lefrak, E. A. and Starr, A. (1979). *Cardiac Valve Prostheses.* (New York: Appleton-Century-Crofts)
2. Starr, A. and Edwards, M. L. (1961). Mitral replacement: Clinical experience with a ball-valve prosthesis. *Ann. Surg.*, **154**, 726
3. Roberts, W. C. and Morrow, A. G. (1967). Anatomic studies of hearts containing caged-ball prosthetic valves. *Johns Hopkins Med. J.*, **121**, 271
4. Kay, E. B., Suzuki, A., Demaney, M. and Zimmerman, H. A. (1966). Comparison of ball and disc valves for mitral valve replacement. *Am. J. Cardiol.*, **18**, 504
5. Hufnagel, C. A. and Conrad, P. W. (1965). Comparative study of some prosthetic valves for aortic and mitral replacement. *Surgery*, **57**, 205
6. Cross, F. S. and Jones, R. D. (1966). A caged-lens prosthesis for replacement of the aortic and mitral valves. *Ann. Thorac. Surg.*, **2**, 499
7. Schachner, A., Vidner, B. and Levy, M. J. (1979). Retrograde dislodgement of a Cross–Jones mitral valve occluder. *Scand. J. Thorac. Cardiovasc. Surg.*, **13**, 263
8. Harken, D. E., Matloff, J. M., Zuckerman, W. and Chaux, A. (1968). A new mitral valve. *J. Thorac. Cardiovasc. Surg.*, **55**, 369
9. Winsberg, F., Gabor, G., Hernberg, J. and Weiss, B. (1970). Fluttering of the mitral valve in aortic insufficiency. *Circulation*, **41**, 225
10. Kay, J. H., Kawashima, Y., Kagawa, Y., Tsuji, H. K. and Redington, J. V. (1966). Experimental mitral valve replacement with a new disc valve. *Ann. Thorac. Surg.*, **2**, 485
11. Kay, J. H., Tsuji, H. K., Redington, J. V., Kawashima, Y., Kagawa, Y., Yamada, T. and Caponegro, P. (1967). Clinical use of a new mitral disc valve. *Calif. Med.*, **106**, 165
12. Kitamura, S., Johnson, J. L., Redington, J. V., Mendez, A., Zubiate, P. and Kay, J. H. (1967). Surgery for Ebstein's anomaly. *Ann. Thorac. Surg.*, **11**, 320
13. Kay, J. H., Tsuji, H. K., Redington, J. V., Yamada, T., Kagawa, Y. and Kawashima, Y. (1967). The surgical treatment of Ebstein's malformation with right ventricular aneurysmorrhaphy and replacement of the tricuspid valve with a disc valve. *Dis. Chest*, **51**, 537
14. Kay, J. H., Tsuji, H. K. and Redington, J. V. (1969). Experiences with the Kay–Shiley disc valve. In Brewer, L. A. III (ed.) *Prosthetic Heart Valves.* p. 609. (Springfield, Illinois: Charles C. Thomas)
15. McGoon, D. C. (1972). The status of prosthetic cardiac valves. In Ionescu, M. I., Ross, D. N. and Wooler, G. H. (eds): *Biological Tissue for Heart Valve Replacement.* p. 3. (London: Butterworths)

16. Mori, T., Kitamura, S., Verruno, E., Kenaan, G. and Kay, J. H. (1974). Tricuspid valve replacement. *J. Thorac. Cardiovasc. Surg.*, **68**, 30
17. Bjork, V. O., Olin, C. and Anstrom, H. (1969). Results of aortic valve replacement with the Kay–Shiley disc valve. *Scand. J. Thorac. Cardiovasc. Surg.*, **3**, 39
18. Chun, P. K. C. and Nelson, W. P. (1977). Common cardiac prosthetic valves. *J. Am. Med. Assoc.*, **238**, 401
19. Beall, A. C. Jr, Bloodwell, R. D., Liotta, D., Cooley, D. A. and DeBakey, M. E. (1968). Elimination of sewing ring-metal seat interface in mitral valve prostheses. *Circulation*, **37-38**, (Suppl. II), 184
20. Beall, A. C., Jr., Bloodwell, R. D. and Abergast, N. R. (1969). Mitral valve replacement with Dacron-covered prosthesis to prevent thromboembolism : clinical experience in 202 cases. In Brewer, L. A. III (ed.) *Prosthetic Heart Valves*. p. 319. (Springfield, Illinois: Charles C. Thomas)
21. Robinson, M. J., Hildner, F. J. and Greenberg, J. J. (1971). Disc variance of Beall mitral valve. *Ann. Thorac. Surg.*, **11**, 11
22. Reid, J. A., Stevens, T. W., Sigwart, U., Fulweber, R. C. and Alexander, J. K. (1972). Hemodynamic evaluation of the Beall mitral valve prosthesis. *Circulation*, **45-46**, (Suppl. I), 1
23. Montoya, A., Sullivan, H. J. and Pifarre, R. (1976). Disc variance: a potentially lethal complication of the Beall valve prosthesis. *J. Thorac. Cardiovasc. Surg.*, **71**, 904
24. Gold, H. and Hertz, L. (1974). Death caused by fracture of Beall mitral valve prosthesis: report of a case. *Am. J. Cardiol.*, **34**, 371
25. Starr–Edwards mitral prosthesis, model 6500: *Technical Information*. Edwards Laboratories, Inc., Santa Ana, California, August 1968
26. Stross, J. K., Willis, P. W. III and Kahn, D. R. (1971). Diagnostic features of malfunction of disc mitral valve prostheses. *J. Am. Med. Assoc.*, **217**, 305
27. Klain, M., Leitz, K. H. and Kolff, W. J. (1969). Comparative testing of artificial heart valves in a mock circulation. In Brewer, L. A. III (ed.) *Prosthetic Heart Valves*. p. 114. (Springfield, Illinois: Charles C. Thomas)
28. Cooley, D. A., Liotta, D. and Cromie, H. W. (1967). Aortic valve prosthesis incorporating lightweight titanium ball, Dacron velour-covered cage and seat. *Trans. Am. Soc. Artif. Intern. Organs*, **13**, 93
29. Messmer, B. J., Okies, J. E., Hallman, G. L. and Cooley, D. A. (1972). Early and late thromboembolic complications after mitral valve replacement: a comparative study of various prostheses. *J. Cardiovasc. Surg.*, **13**, 281
30. Cooley, D. A., Okies, J. E., Wukasch, D. C., Sandiford, F. M. and Hallman, G. L. (1973). Ten-year experience with cardiac valve replacement: results with a new mitral prosthesis. *Ann. Surg.*, **177**, 818
31. Ansbro, J., Clark, R. and Gerbode, F. (1976). Successful surgical correction of an embolized prosthetic valve poppet. *J. Thorac. Cardiovasc. Surg.*, **72**, 652
32. Barnard, P. M. and Heydenrych, J. J. (1969). Mitral valve replacement in the baboon (Papio ursinus) and the human with the University of Stellenbosch mitral valve prosthesis. *Thorax*, **24**, 18
33. Barnard, P. M., Heydenrych, J. J. and De Wet Lubbe, J. J. (1970). Clinical experience with the University of Stellenbosch mitral valve prosthesis. *S. Afr. Med. J.*, **44**, 1377
34. Gibbs, J. L., Davies, G. A., Schofield, A., Wharton, G. A., Watson, D. A. and Gerlis, L. M. (1985). Mechanism of late failure of the Alvarez disc valve prosthesis. *Br. Heart J.*, **53**, 510
35. Gott, V. L., Daggett, R. L., Whiffen, J. D., Koepke, D. E., Rowe, G. G. and Young, W. P. (1964). A hinged-leaflet valve for total replacement of the human aortic valve. *J. Thorac. Cardiovasc. Surg.*, **48**, 713
36. Young, W. P., Gott, V. L. and Rowe, G. G. (1965). Open-heart surgery for mitral valve disease, with special reference to a new prosthetic valve. *J. Thorac. Cardiovasc. Surg.*, **50**, 827
37. Milano, A., Bortolotti, U., Mazzucco, A. and Gallucci, V. (1984). Extended survival after mitral valve replacement with a Gott–Daggett prosthesis. *Am. J. Cardiol.*, **54**, 1147
38. Barnard, C. N., Goosen, C. C., Holmgren, L. V. and Schrire, V. (1962). Prosthetic replacement of the mitral valve. *Lancet*, **2**, 1087
39. Barnard, C. N., Schrire, V., Frater, R. W. M. and Goosen, C. C. (1965). Further experiences with the UCT mitral, tricuspid and aortic prostheses. *Surgery*, **57**, 211

40. Barnard, C. N., Schrire, V. and Goosen, C. C. (1962). Total aortic valve replacement. *Lancet*, **2**, 856
41. Barnard, C. N., Gooosen, C. C., Holmgren, L. V. and Schrire, V. (1962). Prosthetic replacement of the mitral valve. *Lancet*, **2**, 1087
42. Beck, W., Barnard, C. N. and Schrire, V. (1966). The hemodynamics of the University of Cape Town aortic prosthetic valve. *Circulation*, **33**, 517
43. Schrire, V., Beck, W., Hewitson, R. P. and Barnard, C. N. (1967). Aortic valve replacement with the University of Cape Town lenticular prosthesis. A follow-up evaluation. *Am. J. Cardiol.*, **20**, 796
44. Schrire, V. and Barnard, C. N. (1970). Immediate and long-term results of mitral valve replacement with University of Cape Town mitral valve prosthesis. *Br. Heart J.*, **32**, 245
45. Schrire, V., Beck, W., Hewitson, R. P. and Barnard, C. N. (1970). Immediate and long-term results of aortic valve replacement with University of Cape Town aortic valve prosthesis. *Br. Heart J.*, **32**, 255
46. Rose, A. G. (1977). Pathology of aortic valve replacement. *S. Afr. Med. J.*, **52**, 551

6
Cageless, Central-flow, Low-profile, Tilting-disc Valves

PIERCE VALVE

This was the earliest tilting-disc prosthesis devised[1]. The sewing ring was cloth-covered and the plastic inner portion of the ring retained the ends of the spindle of the tilting disc. Laminar flow occurred through the larger orifice and the lesser orifice had a turbulent flow pattern. A small amount of thrombus or granulation tissue could seriously interfere with valve function.

WADA–CUTTER VALVE

This cageless valve (Figure 6.1), developed by Dr J. Wada of Sapporo, Japan, in conjunction with Cutter Biomedical Corporation, was available between 1967 and 1972. Two small feet, which project into the valve orifice, act as a

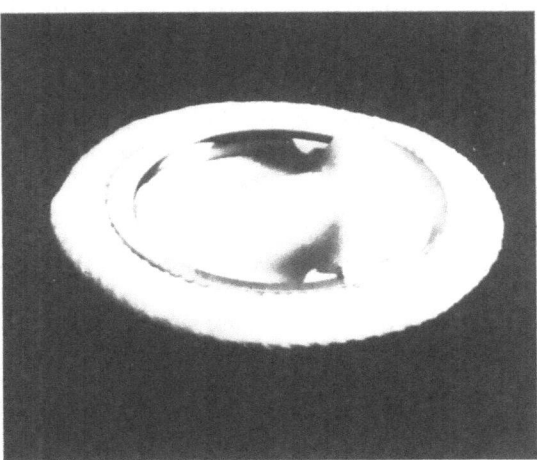

Figure 6.1 Wada–Cutter hingeless disc heart valve. (Picture used with permission of Miles Laboratories, Inc.)

Table 6.1 Evolution of Bjork–Shiley valve prosthesis

Year	Cage	Sewing ring	Type	Disc Opening angle	Clearance
1969	Stellite	Teflon	Delrin	60° AV, 50° MV	0.003 (in)
1971	Ditto	Ditto	Pyrolite (flat)	60° MV too	0.001 (in)
1975	Inflow strut Part of ring	Ditto	Radiopaque marker, Convexo-concave	60	Ditto
1981	'Monostrut', no welds	Ditto	Ditto	70	Ditto

hinge for the disc. The titanium inner ring extends as a lip onto the outflow and inflow surfaces. The base ring has two notches. The radiolucent solid Teflon (polyethylene) disc is vaguely Z-shaped in profile and occludes the orifice by having part of the disc seating on both surfaces. The larger portion of the disc seats on the outflow side of the titanium ring. The smaller portion of the disc overlaps onto the inflow side of the ring. The disc tilts open to an angle of 75–80°. The valve was used in the mitral, tricuspid and aortic positions. Problems encountered included early disc wear[2], massive thrombosis[3], thromboembolism, paraprosthetic leaks and poppet embolization. These complications led to this prosthesis being abandoned.

BJORK–SHILEY VALVE

Dr V. O. Bjork of Sweden combined with Mr D. Shiley of Shiley Inc. to develop the Bjork–Shiley prosthetic valve. The valve was tested experimentally in 1968 and was first used clinically in 1969[4,5]. The initial valve had two curved, roughly U-shaped, bare Stellite struts, which were heat-fused to the ring. The struts are bent apart for insertion of the disc, which is held in place by fitting the outflow strut into a central depression on the disc. Delrin was initially used to construct the disc, but it absorbed moisture during steam autoclaving with resultant swelling of the poppet. In 1971 the disc material was changed to graphite coated with pyrolytic carbon, and the edge was made thicker. The disc tilts open to 60 degrees and does not overlap the valve ring on closure. This allows a degree of regurgitant flow through the closed valve (10%, versus 3% for the Starr–Edwards valve) so as to keep the valve free of thombi. This design gives an optimal orificial diameter and area for a given tissue diameter and is less traumatic to erythrocytes with minimal incompetence. Table 6.1 outlines the various models of the Bjork–Shiley valve prosthesis.

Initially, in the mitral prosthesis the disc was designed to open only to 50° to prevent it touching the ventricular endocardium. Later, the angle was changed to 60° (Figure 6.2) to improve postoperative haemodynamics and to better wash the venricular side of the disc during diastole. Turning of the disc *in vivo* was expected to prolong the life of the disc. From late 1975 a radiopaque tantalum foil loop marker was incorporated into the disc to assist in the diagnosis of thrombosis[6].

There is no fabric on the struts or on the primary orifice. The aortic

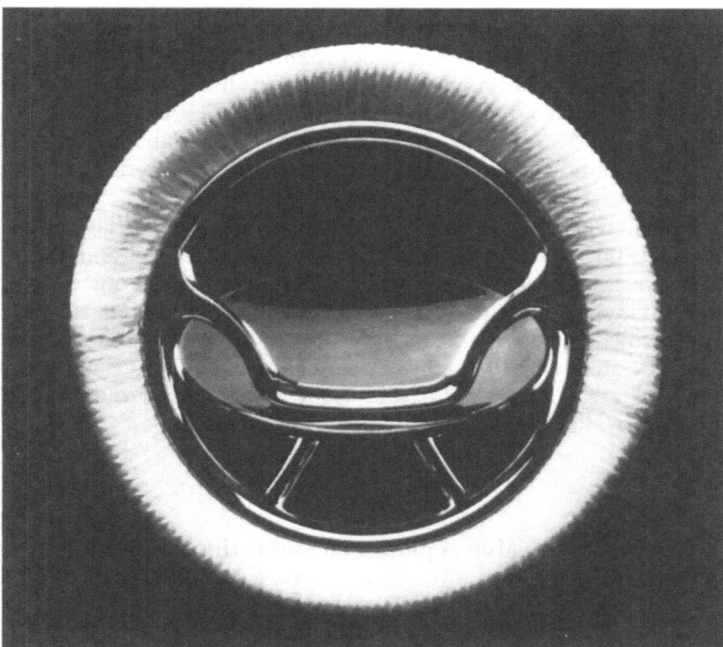

Figure 6.2 Bjork–Shiley 60 degree convexoconcave disc (mitral) valve with pyrolytic carbon poppet and Teflon sewing ring. (Picture courtesy Shiley Inc.)

prosthesis has a vertical, thin-walled base and a rectangular sewing ring, which serve to give a greater internal orifice in relation to the valve's external diameter. The mitral valve has a more horizontal, L-shaped sewing ring profile. Despite the theoretical advantage of the absence of a central occluder in the Bjork–Shiley valve, the flow pattern through the valve is primarily through the major orifice. Also the flow pattern is directly laterally and not centrally as in natural valves or with bioprostheses.

The Bjork–Shiley valve may be easily implanted in the aortic root and its low profile makes coronary arterial reimplantation into a Dacron graft easier. Durability has been very good and strut fracture is rare. The thin, unpadded sewing rings makes paraprosthetic leakage in a rigid aortic root more likely. The prime weakness of the tilting disc valve is the close association between the mobile poppet and the thrombogenic valve ring[7]. Thrombus on the ring can easily interfere with poppet motion and lead to sudden, catastrophic failure. In an attempt to reduce the flow stagnation zone on the outflow side of the disc, the design was later altered to a convexoconcave disc and the pivot point was moved 2.5 mm downstream to reduce obstruction by any thrombus that might form[8].

Since a modification in the manufacturing process in 1976 there has been a disturbing number of cases of early fracture at the welding point of the outlet strut in the Bjork–Shiley mitral valve prosthesis in sizes 29–33 mm[9].

The estimated incidence of strut fracture in models manufactured between February 1982 and March 1983 was approximately 0.3%, which is approximately three times the previous incidence. Shiley Incorporated have recalled all unimplanted valves manufactured before 28 February, 1982. Later a prosthesis with a 70° opening angle was introduced. Subsequent reports of outlet strut fracture[10,11] in patients with later manufactured valves did not still worries regarding the outlet strut welds.

In 1981 a new type of 'monostrut' Bjork–Shiley valve (Figures 6.3 and 6.4), which has no welding points, was introduced. The inlet and outlet struts are part of the same metal since the valve is machined from one piece of cobalt alloy (Haynes 25). The product name 'monostrut' refers to the valve's outlet strut which is now a single projecting finger of metal, rather than the U shape associated with the concavoconvex valves. This new strut has a cross-sectional area 3.5 times greater than the old wire outlet strut. The pyrolytic carbon disc occluder opens to 70 degrees.

Pathology of cardiac valve replacement with the Bjork–Shiley tilting-disc valve prosthesis

Between 1970 and 1985 a total of 292 patients had Bjork–Shiley valve prostheses implanted at Groote Schuur Hospital, Cape Town. At 5–6 years after implantation of a Bjork–Shiley prosthesis at this hospital 68.3% of patients were alive, and 80% of these patients were clinically free of significant embolism events.

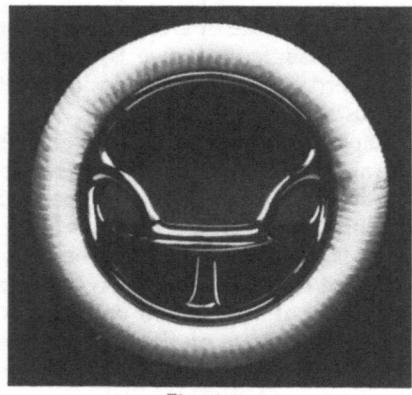
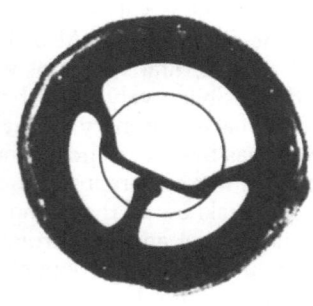

Fig. 6.3   Fig. 6.4

Figure 6.3   Bjork–Shiley monostrut (mitral) valve which has no welding points. The outlet strut consists of a single finger of metal. (Picture courtesy of Shiley Inc.)
Figure 6.4   Radiograph of Bjork–Shiley monostrut valve with radiopaque marker ring within the disc which opens to 70°

Aortic valve replacement

Seven of 12 autopsied patients with Bjork–Shiley aortic valve prostheses were males. The mean age of the 12 patients was 35.2 (SD = 15.2) years with a range of 2–60 years. The mean postoperative survival period was 110 (SD = 203) days with a range of 0–720 days. All patients received an anticoagulant (Warfarin) postoperatively. Only one of the 12 patients had scanty platelet and fibrin thrombus on the edge of the sewing ring (outflow aspect) of the Bjork–Shiley prosthesis. Table 6.2 gives the principal causes of death in the patients with Bjork–Shiley aortic valve prostheses.

Group 1

The six patients in this group (three males and three females) had a mean age of 34 years (SD = 19.3) with a range of 2–60 years. The principal causes of death are given in Table 6.2. The mean postoperative survival period was 2.6 days (SD = 3.8) with a range of 0–9 days.

Group 2

Four of these six late surviving patients were males. The mean age was 36.5 years (SD = 11.4) with a range of 25–50 years. The mean postoperative survival was 218 days (SD = 251) and the range was from 90 to 720 days. The principal causes of death are given in Table 6.2.

Mitral valve replacement

1. Only one patient with a Bjork–Shiley mitral valve prosthesis was autopsied. The patient was a 13-year-old female with rheumatic fever, whose mitral valve was replaced with a Carpentier–Edwards bioprosthesis. Within 2 years the bioprosthesis had undergone cuspal calcification which

Table 6.2 Principal causes of death in 12 patients with Bjork–Shiley aortic valve prostheses

Group 1	
Pulmonary hypertension	1
Stone heart	1
Unrecognized subaortic stenosis	1
Bleeding	1
Shock lung syndrome	1
Pneumonia	1
Group 2	
Stone heart	1
Dehiscence of prosthesis	1
Ruptured mycotic aneurysm	1
Infected prosthesis	1
Post-perfusion ostial stenosis	1
Motor vehicle accident	1

rendered it stenotic. The valve was replaced with a Bjork–Shiley valve. Free-floating thrombus was noted in the left atrium at operation; the patient did not survive the operation. Autopsy revealed recent occlusion of the left main coronary artery by a thromboembolus.

2. Surgically excised Bjork–Shiley mitral valve prostheses may show a variety of changes. One patient's prosthetic disc was dislodged during cardiac catheterization when the catheter passed through the lesser orifice. Emergency mitral valve replacement was performed and the disc was recovered from the aortic bifurcation. Host pannus may grow over the base ring and narrow the effective orifice of the Bjork–Shiley prosthesis. Maximal encroachment often involves the lesser orifice (Figure 6.5) and may lead to thrombotic obstruction (see Colour Plate J). Histology of the host tissue overgrowth shows compacted fibrin and fibrous tissue. The prosthesis may be totally immobilized by an overgrowth of host pannus tissue (see Figure 6.5).

Double valve replacement

A single patient was autopsied with Bjork–Shiley prostheses replacing both the mitral and tricuspid valves. The patient, a 44-year-old female with chronic rheumatic heart disease, died 4 hours postoperatively due to a massive haemorrhage from acute gastric erosions. Scanty fibrin thrombus was noted on the atrial aspect of the sewing ring of the tricuspid prosthesis.

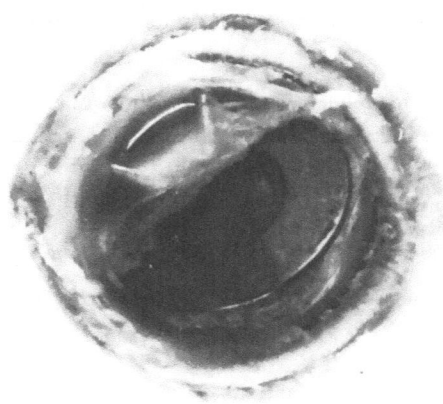

Figure 6.5 Pannus overgrowth occludes lesser orifice of Bjork–Shiley valve and limits disc mobility

Principal causes of death in 14 autopsied patients with Bjork–Shiley valve prostheses

The principal causes of death were as follows: (a) due to error in preoperative diagnosis, 2; (b) due to error in operative technique, 5; (c) due to problems inherent in the Bjork–Shiley valve, 1; (d) due to postoperative complications, 2; (e) unrelated to the cardiac operation, 2; (f) unknown causes, 1. The death of the 14th patient, who did not survive reoperation, was attributable to calcific stenosis of the previous xenograft valve.

Comment

The number of patients with Bjork–Shiley valve prostheses autopsied at our institution is too small for any definite conclusions to be made regarding the frequency of fatal complications. None of the prostheses examined showed evidence of significant wear or variance. Errors in operative technique accounted for 39% of the deaths, and valve-related problems were responsible for only 8% of the deaths.

Thromboembolism is the commonest and most dreaded complication of cardiac valves[12] including the Bjork–Shiley[13-15]. Thrombosis (Colour Plate J) of the Bjork–Shiley prosthetic cardiac valve may occur in any valve position and regardless of anticoagulant status[16]. The cumulative incidence of thrombosis of Bjork–Shiley prostheses is about 2% in the aortic position and about 4% in the mitral position. Prevention of this complication is dependent upon continuous anticoagulation; even temporary interruption or alteration of anticoagulation regimen may be detrimental. Although changes in anticoagulant therapy may rarely precipitate sudden thrombosis, in most cases a period averaging 10 months is required for pannus of organized thrombus to build up enough to cause acute catastrophic thrombosis and valve malfunction[16].

Operation to remove the thrombus or to replace the prosthesis is usually needed for left-sided cardiac prostheses, but thrombosed valves in the tricuspid position may be successfully treated with fibrinolytic medical therapy. Peterffy et al.[17] suggest that red thrombus on Bjork–Shiley valves may be amenable to such therapy, which should not be prolonged for more than 24 hours and, if unsuccessful, the patient should undergo valve replacement. Others[18] stress that, as soon as obstruction of the prosthesis is recognized, the patient should undergo immediate surgery. With regard to thrombosed, left-sided disc valves, Ledain et al.[19] recommend that fibrinolytic treatment (with its risk of embolism) should be reserved for critically ill patients who are too sick to undergo immediate surgery. Copans et al.[18] recommend that the Bjork–Shiley valve should only be used in the mitral area if excellent control of anticoagulation can be guaranteed.

Bjork and Henze[20], in reviewing 300 Bjork–Shiley aortic valvular implants, state that they encountered no cases of encapsulation or massive thrombosis in patients who were adequately anticoagulated. Two of their patients who developed massive thrombosis on their Bjork–Shiley aortic valves had received no anticoagulants. One patient underwent valve replacement and the other had operative removal of the thrombus only. This was facilitated by temporary removal of the disc. These authors stress that this method cannot be recommended for general use as an inexperienced surgeon may bend the struts so that the disc will not function properly after reinsertion. A decade later, thrombectomy[21,22] has been proposed as the treatment of choice for a thrombosed Bjork–Shiley prosthesis, but others[23] question whether thrombectomy is desirable.

Thrombosis has been a particular problem with Bjork–Shiley valves in the tricuspid position and in patients with multiple Bjork–Shiley prostheses. The cumulative incidence of thrombosis in patients with multiple prostheses is 26.8% at 6 years[24]. Several papers discuss the early diagnosis of thrombosis of the Bjork–Shiley valve prosthesis[25–27].

Yoganathan et al.[28] attributed thrombus formation and tissue overgrowth to the stagnation zone and the low shear in the minor outflow region. A ring-shaped radiopaque marker was incorporated into the disc in 1977 to assist in diagnosing massive thrombosis of this type of prosthesis[29]. Dale[30] found that the Bjork–Shiley and Lillehei–Kaster disc valves were equally thrombogenic, and that the rate was not lower than that in patients with Starr–Edwards aortic ball-valves.

The clinical and haemodynamic features of Bjork–Shiley prostheses have been described[31-33]. Other specific problems include immediate postoperative regurgitation of a Bjork–Shiley aortic valve due to interfering Teflon of a ventricular septal defect repair, prosthetic dehiscence, haemolysis due to paraprosthetic leak or death due to complete prosthetic detachment.

Obstruction of the Bjork–Shiley valve[34] by chordal tissue, sutures, early postoperative pannus ingrowth, tissue detached from the aortic intima, and septal interference of mitral Bjork–Shiley prosthesis have also occurred. Acute malfunction of a Bjork–Shiley aortic valve prosthesis due to a large thromboembolus, which originated in the left atrium, has also been reported[35]. Silver[36] observed wear in Bjork–Shiley prostheses recovered at autopsy or at operation.

Fracture of a Bjork–Shiley disc has been rarely reported[37]. Strut fractures in the Bjork–Shiley prosthesis[38,39] have been more common. The basic problem was a lack of durability of strut welding points[39]. The problem has persisted with a later model[10,11]. Strut fracture may have disastrous clinical consequences, but some patients have been saved by emergency valve replacement[40]. The latest model (monostrut) Bjork–Shiley valve has no weld points. Echocardiography has been used to detect dehiscence[41] and thrombosis[42] of Bjork–Shiley prostheses. Cineradiography may be used to assess the opening angle of Bjork–Shiley valves[43].

Henze et al.[44] describe the cause of death and the main pathological findings in 20 patients following 161 Bjork–Shiley aortic valve implant operations. Myocardial failure (nine patients) was the predominant cause of death. The remainder died of cerebral haemorrhage (three patients), malignancy (three patients), infection (two patients), dissecting aortic aneurysm (one patient), hepatorenal syndrome (one patient) and thromboembolism (one patient).

Roberts and Hammer[45] describe the clinical and autopsy findings in 46 patients who had one or more cardiac valves replaced with Bjork–Shiley prostheses and compared the latter with the findings in patients with caged-ball, caged-disc, and trileaflet prostheses. The Bjork–Shiley valves gave less problems with regard to disproportion, haemolysis (as judged by renal haemosiderosis), and prosthetic thrombi. No instance of prosthetic wear or variance was noted over the relatively short 3 to 30 months (mean = 11) follow-up period. Forty per cent of their early deaths (less than 2 months postoperation) were due to unknown causes, 18% were due to bleeding, coronary heart disease accounted for 15%, uncorrected associated valvular disease 12%, infection 9%, and prosthetic dysfunction was encountered in 6%. The latter figure is similar to the 8% incidence of valve-related deaths in my autopsy patients. Principal causes of the 13 late deaths reported by these authors[42] were as follows (my percentages): prosthetic valve endocarditis, 31%; unknown, 23%; prosthetic valve thrombosis, 23%; aortic regurgitation, 15%; and coronary heart disease, 8%. Roberts and Hammer[45] and others[46,47] caution that even mild aortic incompetence may cause cocking of the mitral disc of a caged-disc prosthesis. Roberts and Hammer[45] suggest that aortic incompetence may prevent proper opening of a mitral tilting-disc prosthesis and lead to mitral prosthetic dysfunction.

An up to 3-year follow-up of 268 patients with monostrut Bjork–Shiley valves revealed no thrombosis or mechanical failure[48]. A recent cumulative follow-up study of 4125 patient-years experience with the Bjork–Shiley valve confirmed the excellent long-term performance of this prosthesis[49].

LILLEHEI–KASTER VALVE

Lillehei and colleagues performed one of the first human heart valve replacements ever attempted using a bicuspid silicone rubber flap-valve aortic prosthesis[50]. An engineer called Robert Kaster, working in Lillehei's laboratory, tried to design an improved heart valve prosthesis. He and Dr A. Cruz produced the *Cruz–Kaster* pivoting-disc valve which had a concavoconvex shaped disc that tilted open to 85°. However, blood flowed mainly on one side of the disc, predisposing to thrombosis on the other side. It was tested experimentally from 1963, but was never used clinically. In 1965 the pivotal axis was moved towards the centre, so allowing blood flow on both aspects of the disc. The struts were altered and then abolished, yielding a cageless design with lateral guides to hold the disc in place[51]. The poppet was still a pivoting disc, but it was inclined at 18° when closed to aid rapid opening and closing.

The *Lillehei–Kaster* valve, which evolved from the above valve, was introduced in 1969. Medical Incorporated manufactured the 500S (mitral) and 300S (aortic) Lillehei–Kaster pivoting-disc valves. Delrin (acetal homopolymer) and various plastic discs were found to wear[52]. The valve was used clinically for the first time in 1970[53] and was made commercially available the following year. The Lillehei–Kaster valve prosthesis[7,54,55] has a pivoting disc (Figures 6.6 and 6.7) composed of a graphite centre covered by a thin layer (250 μm) of a carbon–silicone alloy (Pyrolite). The pyrolytic carbon disc is retained by a titanium housing that allows the disc to open to a maximum angle of 80°

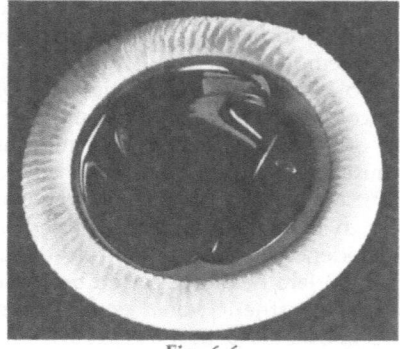 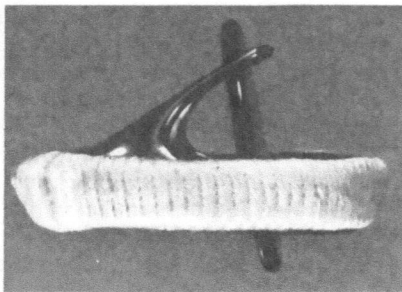

Fig. 6.6   Fig. 6.7

Figure 6.6   Lillehei–Kaster pivoting disc valve prosthesis. (Picture courtesy of Medical Inc.)
Figure 6.7   Lillehei–Kaster prosthesis with cloth sewing ring attached, viewed from the side to show disc tilted to its maximum angle of 80°. (Picture courtesy of Medical Inc.)

from its closed position of 18° to the horizontal (62° of movement). The disc seats in the prosthesis lumen at its equator. The metal housing can be rotated within the Teflon cloth sewing ring to permit optimal alignment of the disc after sewing ring fixation[54]. The effective diameter of the valve orifice is smaller than the diameter of the disc. The inner ring consists of bare metal.

Two tear-shaped, bare titanium struts project from the sewing ring at an angle of less than 90° to form an open cage. Three tiny metal feet project into the valve orifice from the inner ring on the surface opposite the cage; two act as hinges and the third functions as a disc stopper. The disc is free to distribute wear by moving around, and it is held in place within the housing by its own diameter during ventricular systole. The two long struts prevent the disc escaping through the outflow orifice. When closed the disc just barely overlaps the seat[7].

The valve gave good early results[7], but cardiac catheterization has revealed no superior function of this prosthesis compared to several other types

Table 6.3   Principal causes of death in nine patients with Lillehei–Kaster aortic valve prostheses

Group 1	
Anaesthetic mishap	1
Operative technique error	1
Myocardial failure	1
Unknown cause	1
Group 2	
Error in preoperative diagnosis	1
Operative error	1
Thrombosed prosthesis	1
Infected prosthesis	1
Coronary thrombosis	1

Table 6.4 Principal causes of death in seven patients with Lillehei–Kaster mitral valve prostheses

Unknown	2
Anticoagulant excess bleeding	2
Thrombosed prosthesis	2
Infected prosthesis	1

of valve prostheses. Catastrophic thrombosis was a common complication[55-58].

Pathology of cardiac valve replacement with the Lillehei–Kaster prosthesis

At 5–6 years after implantation of a Lillehei–Kaster valve prosthesis at Groote Schuur Hospital, Cape Town the survival rate was 63.5%, and 72.4% of these patients were clinically free of significant embolic events.

Aortic valve replacement

Nine patients with Lillehei–Kaster aortic valve prostheses were autopsied; five of the nine patients were females and the nine patients had a mean age of 43.4 years (SD = 16.4). The mean postoperative survival period of the whole group was 366.8 (SD = 596.7) days with a range of from 1 to 1800 days. The principal causes of death are indicated in Table 6.3.

In two of the patients in group 1 thrombus involved the sewing ring and extended into the lesser orifice of the prosthesis. Two patients in group 2 also had thrombi on their Lillehei prostheses. This filled the lesser orifice of one valve and totally immobilized the other prosthesis. The latter patient had received no anticoagulation postoperatively.

Principal causes of death

Four of the nine patients died due to either an error in preoperative diagnosis or to errors in operative technique. Thrombosis, when present, favoured the lesser orifice of the prosthesis.

Mitral valve replacement

Seven autopsy patients with Lillehei–Kaster mitral valve prostheses had a mean age of 27.4 years (SD = 15.2) with a range of 18–59 years. All seven patients underwent heart valve replacement for post-rheumatic mixed mitral valve disease. The mean postoperative survival was 453 days (SD = 552) with a range of 4–1350 days. Two patients survived 7 days or less and the other five survived 38 days or longer postoperatively.

Principal causes of death are given in Table 6.4. Thrombus was noted on two of the Lillehei–Kaster mitral valve prostheses. In two patients abundant thrombus filled the lesser orifice (Colour Plate K, and Figures 6.8 and 6.9) and led to almost total immobilization of the prosthesis. Scantier thrombus was present on both aspects of the sewing ring and within the greater orifice.

Double valve replacement with the Lillehei–Kaster prosthesis

Two patients came to autopsy with Lillehei–Kaster prostheses in both the aortic and mitral positions. The first patient, who was operated upon for infective endocarditis, died 210 days postoperatively of myocardial failure. Both Lillehei prostheses bore abundant bland antemortem thrombi on the sewing ring and 'horns' of the prosthesis. Thrombus was more plentiful on the mitral prosthesis.

The second patient died of cardiac failure 6.5 months after cardiac surgery. Both aspects of the Lillehei mitral prosthesis were covered by large amounts of antemortem thrombus, which was also continuous with left atrial thrombi. Thrombus produced severe orificial obstruction in the mitral prosthesis. Scanty antemortem thrombus was detected on the inferior aspect of the Lillehei aortic valve prosthesis.

Principal causes of death in patients with mitral and double valve replacement

Five out of the seven patients' deaths were due to problems directly related to the Lillehei–Kaster mitral valve prosthesis itself.

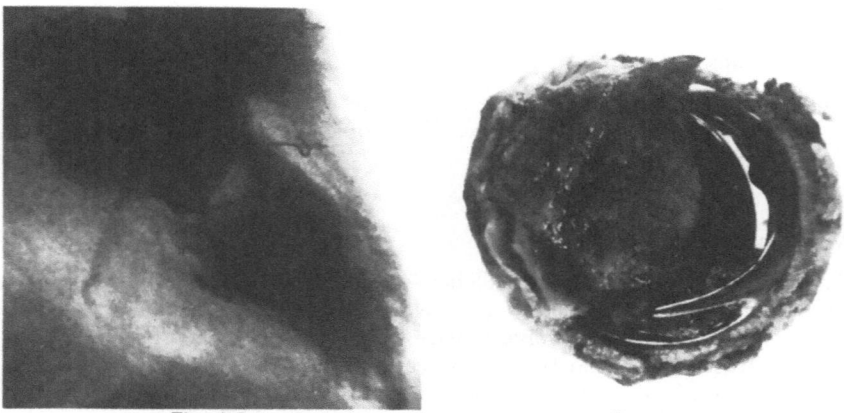

Fig. 6.8   Fig. 6.9

Figure 6.8 Angiogram (right anterior oblique view) of patient with thrombosed Lillehei–Kaster mitral valve prosthesis. Thrombus creates a radiolucent zone in the contrast medium inferior to the prosthesis
Figure 6.9 Appearance of explanted thrombosed Lillehei–Kaster valve shown in Figure 6.8. Bulky thrombus occludes the lesser orifice and partially obstructs the greater orifice

Comment

Lillehei and Kaster[59,60] introduced the concept of a pivoting-disc prosthetic valve in an attempt to improve on the haemodynamic performance of caged-ball prostheses. In our autopsy patients with Lillehei–Kaster valves, prosthesis-related principal causes of death were more commonly encountered in patients with mitral valve prostheses and in longer-surviving patients with aortic valve prostheses. Myocardial failure may have favoured the development of thrombi on some of the valvular prostheses. Conversely, thrombosis upon the prosthesis may have produced sufficient obstruction in some cases to account for the cardiac failure. Non-infected thrombus on the Lillehei–Kaster prosthesis was primarily situated within and around the lesser orifice of the valve.

The phonocardiographic and the echocardiographic characteristics[61], as well as the clinical and haemodynamic features, of the Lillehei–Kaster valve have been published[62,63]. Rao et al.[64] compared the incidence of chronic haemolysis following mitral valve replacement with the Lillehei–Kaster valve and with some other cardiac valvular prostheses. In isolated mitral valve replacement 66% showed compensated haemolysis, compared to 42% in Bjork–Shiley valves, 85% in composite seat Starr–Edwards valves and none in frame-mounted homograft valves. Poppet jamming of a Lillehei–Kaster prosthesis due to impaction of a left atrial monitoring line during mitral valve replacement has been described[7]. Behle and Brown[65] described a case with late snaring of a Lillehei–Kaster prosthesis by a fragment of left atrial monitoring catheter.

Nitter-Hauge[66] reported favourable results after a short follow-up period of 1 year in patients with a Lillehei–Kaster aortic valve prosthesis. Lillehei–Kaster valves implanted in the mitral position[67] gave similarly good results with up to 24 months follow-up. Intraoperative haemodynamic evaluation of the Lillehei–Kaster valve showed it to have better haemodynamics than caged-ball valves[68]. In vivo evaluation showed that the maximum opening angle of 80° was not reached; opening angles ranged from 57 to 74° without evidence of disc malfunction[69]. Forman et al.[70] catheterized 26 patients with Lillehei–Kaster valves and showed no advantage over other types of prosthetic valves.

In the discussion of a paper by Starek et al.[71], Lillehei warned against inserting too large a Lillehei–Kaster prosthesis in the mitral area, since a small left ventricle may lead to one of the struts becoming embedded in the myocardium. This may provoke scar tissue ingrowth, which may slowly impede disc motion. Mitha et al.[72] reported a disturbing incidence of thrombosis in their patients with Lillehei–Kaster valves involving at least 10% of the mitral implants and 5% of the aortic; in 1974 they stopped using the prosthesis. Thrombosis was attributed to late prosthetic disproportion following shrinkage in size of the heart postoperatively. Minimal impingement and cocking of the disc on the ventricular endocardium results in thrombosis of the prosthesis and of the left atrium. Mitha et al[72] postulate that insertion of smaller mitral prostheses may have obviated thrombosis.

Roberts et al.[73] noted that the regurgitant jet of blood from unsuspected severe aortic incompetence may interfere with the opening of disc valves. Dale[74] reported that arterial thromboembolic complications are a significant problem with both the Lillehei–Kaster and Bjork–Shiley disc valves, including those in the aortic position. Zwart[75] found an incidence of thromboembolism of 5.0 per 100 patient-years and the actuarial survival was 81% at 5 years with the Lillehei–Kaster prosthesis. Silver et al.[76] observed metal wear on the luminal aspect of the struts of Lillehei–Kaster valve prostheses. Despite the abundant clinical reports on the Lillehei–Kaster prosthesis, the pathology has not been well described.

LILLEHEI MEDICAL VALVE

This valve was introduced by Lillehei et al.[77] in order to overcome the problems with the Lillehei–Kaster prosthesis. The titanium components which characterized the latter were replaced by pyrolytic carbon layered over a graphite substrate. The base of the valve was made thinner to incorporate the advantage of the Bjork–Shiley valve regarding the inner-to-outer diameter ratio. The disc was also thinner than before. The design abolished struts and the cage was much shorter.

HAMMERSMITH VALVE

The Hammersmith low-profile prosthetic valve[78–80] was introduced in 1964 by Melrose and his colleagues. The valve had evolved from an earlier design of a self-retaining ball-valve[79]. The Hammersmith mitral valve was designed to open so that most of the blood flow was directed to the area next to the left ventricular septum below the aortic outflow tract. This meant creating a mechanism similar in action to a hinged flap, but without the disadvantages of a hinge joint. The initial tilting-disc valve had steel retaining pins loosely secured within a plastic ring as the hinge mechanism. Another arrangement repositioned the retaining elements; there were no steel pins and the ring was modified. This design was similar to the original ball-valve except that there were only two, not three legs attached to the disc, and two stops protruded from the inner aspect of the ring. Three types of Hammersmith mitral valve prosthesis have been manufactured.

The Mark I valve (used in animal experiments), had three legs of equal length supporting a large trap door. The Mark II valve used clinically had only two legs and a lighter trap door, which opened to one side only. Thus the valve had to be very accurately placed in the heart so that it opened into the left ventricular outflow tract, because one side was completely occluded when the trap door was open. The Mark III valve has three legs, two long and one short, so that the trap door opens all around its circumference. Positioning of the valve is less critical with this version. An extension of the ring prevents rotation of the disc.

Shaw et al.[81] reported sudden mechanical malfunction of Hammersmith mitral valve prostheses due to wear of the polypropylene material at the site of contact between the short leg of the disc and the valve ring. Such malfunction resulted from detachment of the disc from the ring, or the disc sticking in the open position. Polypropylene has a low resistance to abrasion and it is not suitable for prostheses in which the design predisposes to localized wear.

HALL–KASTER (MEDTRONIC–HALL) VALVE

Medtronic Blood Systems Inc. have manufactured the Medtronic–Hall A7700 (aortic) and M7700 (mitral) pivoting-disc valve prostheses from 1977 to the present time. The Hall–Kaster prosthetic design (Figure 6.10) aimed to have the least possible obstruction to flow when open and to increase the size of the small orifice[82]. All projections into the orifice, including the central disc guide strut, are open-ended to prevent thrombogenesis at these sites. The new pivotal-disc mechanism was so designed that when open the disc split the total valve orifice into two nearly equal parts. The disc has a composite, two-part movement. There is a large range of movement and in the aortic position the disc opens to 75°. The disc is less than 2 mm in thickness, with an aperture at the centre, and it is made of a graphite substrate containing tantalum which makes the disc radiopaque. It is Pyrolite-coated for maximum wear, polishability, and has electronegativity. The titanium valve housing includes an annular valve base, a pair of inflow pivots, a single outflow pivot, and an S-shaped disc guide strut with a disc stop (Figure 6.10). The disc is fitted to the guide strut, which controls the movement of the disc throughout its travel.

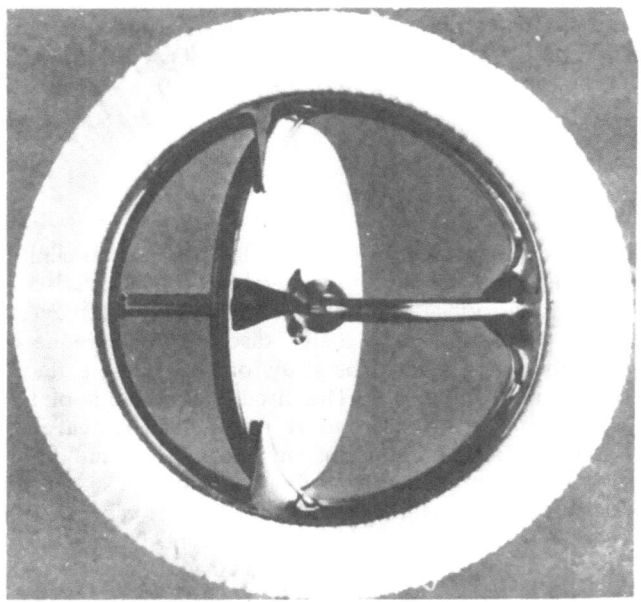

Figure 6.10 Medtronic–Hall (Medtronic–Kaster, Hall–Kaster) valve prosthesis has a disc having a central hole through which passes a U-shaped disc guide strut

The Hall–Kaster valve has no welds or bends[83]. The sewing ring is made of knitted Teflon. In the closed position the disc is parallel to the plane of the valve base and rests within the orifice on the two inflow pivots and the disc stop. To open, the disc lifts slightly, then pivots about the curved end of the outflow pivot through a arc of 75° in the aortic model. Soon after its clinical introduction in 1977, the clearance between the edge of the disc and the ring was reduced in order to lower the degree of regurgitation and theoretically to reduce the amount of haemolysis. The diameter of the sewing ring was reduced by 1 mm to allow insertion of a valve with a larger internal orifice in a given annulus.

Semb et al.[84] reported the first in vivo haemodynamic observations with this prosthesis in both acute and chronic experiments following implantation of the valve in the mitral position in dogs. These studies showed a low transvalvular pressure gradient, an effective opening angle of about 70° and good diastolic flow through both the large and small orifices of the prosthesis. Aasen et al.[85] used anticoagulants and antibiotics to develop a long-term canine model for studying the Hall–Kaster valve in the mitral position.

One study[86] reported the occurrence of intermittent aortic regurgitation in four of 160 patients with Hall–Kaster aortic prostheses. In all four patients mechanical obstruction to free movement of the disc was excluded. Wide opening of the occluder beyond the axis of blood flow appeared to be responsible for non-closure of the valve during diastole. The aortic incompetence was corrected by reorientation of the major orifice of the prosthesis. Such incompetence may be impossible to detect prior to closure of the aorta and discontinuation of cardiopulmonary bypass. Ideally the major orifice should face the anterior commissure, i.e. between the left and right aortic cusps. Hall et al.[87] reported encouraging results with more than 1000 Medtronic–Hall valves implanted since 1977.

OMNISCIENCE VALVE

The Omniscience valve prosthesis (Figure 6.11) has been in clinical use since August 1978. The valve has four tiny metal struts with angled ends which project into the valve orifice[88]. Closure of the orifice is achieved by a thin, curvilinear black pyrolytic carbon-coated disc with radiopaque core, which pivots between the metal struts. The struts on the inflow surface also angle upwards from the metal inner ring. The disc lies at an angle of 12° when the prosthesis is closed. The seamless suture ring, which is available in supra-, intra-, and sub-annular configurations, incorporates suture guide markers. Despite a short follow-up period, Rabago et al.[89] noted a significant incidence of valvular dysfunction, which led them to discontinue using the Omniscience prosthetic valve. Cortina et al.[90] found no significant difference regarding the incidence of prosthetic infection, paravalvular leak of anticoagulant-related haemorrhage when they compared Omniscience, Medtronic–Hall and Bjork–Shiley (70°) prostheses in mitral valve replacement. DeWall et al.[91] reported a low incidence of thromboembolic complications in patients studied

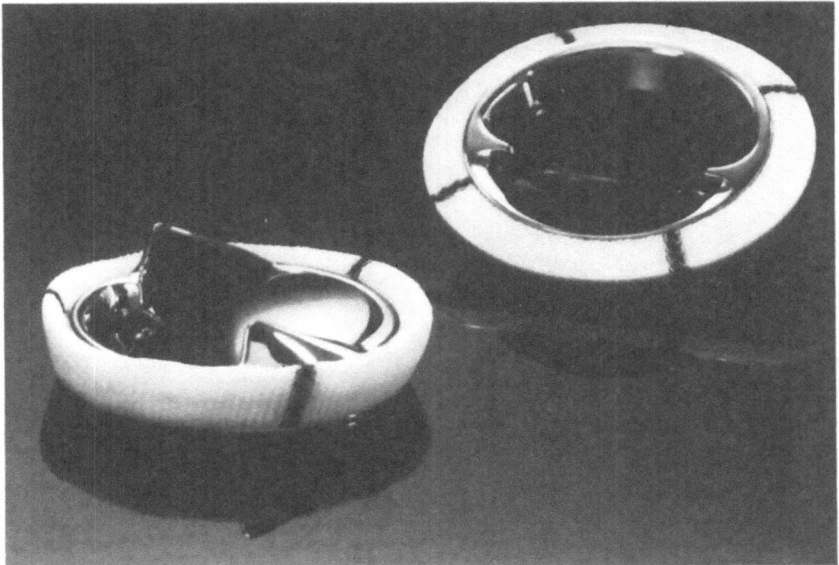

Figure 6.11 Omniscience 'advanced cardiac valve prosthesis,' aortic (left) and mitral (right). (Picture courtesy of Medical Inc.)

for 5 years (650 patient-years).

The pre-market approval application data base summary based on a 65-month eight-centre evaluation of 448 patients showed that 94.2% of patients with aortic prostheses and 95.1% with mitral prostheses are free of thrombotic complications at 5 years[92].

OMNICARBON VALVE

This prosthesis is similar to the Omniscience valve described above. Both prostheses are manufactured by Medical Incorporated, which was founded in 1971 to manufacture the Lillehei–Kaster valve prosthesis. The Omnicarbon valve is the first all-Pyrolite, hingeless prosthetic cardiac valve. An initial design had all portions of the valve, including the sewing ring, covered with black pyrolytic carbon. The dark-coloured sewing ring had two or three white marks on it for assisting with the orientation of the valve at the time of implantation[88]. The manufacturers have deferred clinical testing of the Omnicarbon prosthesis with coated sewing ring fabric due to concern that low-temperature vapour deposition of carbon-type surface layers on synthetic material may not produce films which are continuous, resilient and strongly adherent to the yarn surface. The abrasive and flexural stresses of implant suturing may cause 'dusting' of the deposited layer with resulting risk of embolism.

The Omnicarbon valve with an uncoated sewing ring (Figure 6.12) is

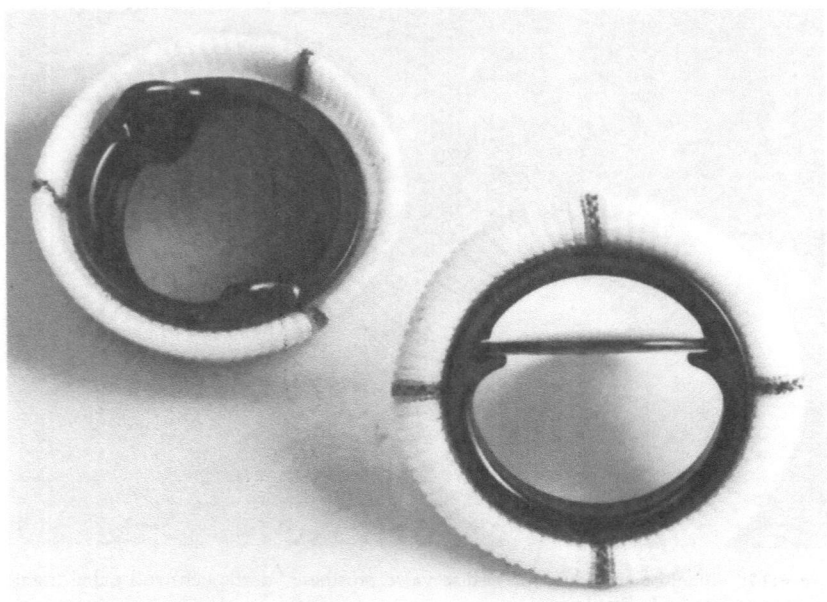

Figure 6.12 Omnicarbon 'advanced cardiac valve prosthesis', aortic (left) and mitral (right). (Picture courtesy of Medical Inc.)

presently being offered in selected international markets for clinical evaluation. The Teflon fabric sewing ring is available in five different configurations. The suture ring design allows for postimplantation rotation of the valve within the annulus and guide markers present on the ring (three for aortic and four for mitral) facilitate rapid, uniform suture placement.

SORIN VALVE

The Sorin valve has been used in Italy and prosthetic thrombosis has been reported[87].

BILEAFLET HEART VALVE PROSTHESES

Kalke–Lillehei double leaflet valve

The first rigid, bileaflet prostheses were described by Kalke and Lillehei in the mid-1960s[94,95]. This new design was tested in the pulse duplicator, in experimental animals and by cineradiography. The valve had excellent flow characteristics, and haemodynamics were better than existing designs. The leaflets and housing were made of titanium and the sewing ring of Teflon.

The leaflets opened to an angle of 60°, permitting flow through both the central and lateral areas of the orifice. Each leaflet had two ball-like knobs laterally that pivoted within ovoid recesses in the titanium housing. Thus, while opening, the leaflets slid laterally to increase the central orifice as they rotated. During closure the leaflets again moved to meet in the midline, leaving only a narrow linear gap. This prosthetic design was further refined and the valve was made totally of pyrolytic carbon. The prosthesis, now called the St Jude Medical valve, was ready for *in vitro* and animal testing in 1976[96].

St Jude Medical valve

This is a low-profile, lightweight, bileaflet, central-flow device made entirely of pyrolytic carbon (Figure 6.13, and Colour Plates L and M). It has two semicircular (D-shaped) discs[97] that open to an angle of 85 ° from a closed position in which the leaflets lie at 30–35 ° to the valve housing. A pivot mechanism eliminates the need for supporting struts. The two housings containing the pivoting ends of the discs protrude as smooth elevations on the inflow aspect of the valve[88]. All portions of the valve (except the sewing ring) are covered with black pyrolytic carbon. Each leaflet contains tungsten (5–10% by weight) to ensure a degree of radiopacity. Controlled leakage aims to minimize thrombosis. A pressure of only 0.8 mmHg is needed to open or close the valve. There is a seamless, double velour Dacron sewing cuff. The valve design allows for a high ratio of flow orifice to tissue annulus diameter.

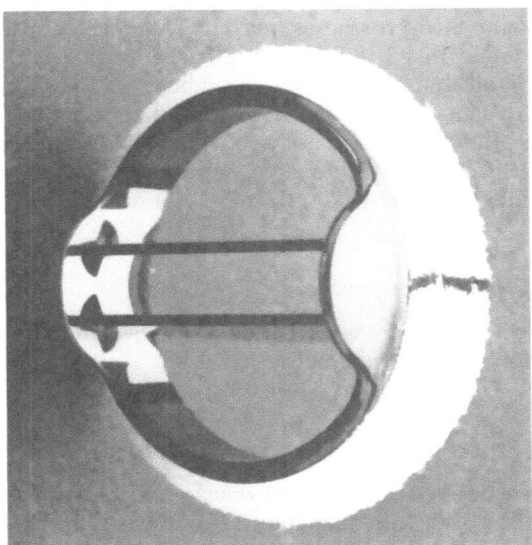

Figure 6.13 St Jude Medical heart valve prosthesis with aortic cuff. (Picture courtesy of St Jude Medical, Inc.)

In vitro tests[98] showed that the St Jude Medical valve was safe and had a superior haemodynamic function compared to other valvular prostheses. *In vivo* testing of the valve in calves[99] showed equally promising results. The St Jude Medical valve has undergone extensive worldwide clinical trials. Early postoperative catheterization studies at several centres showed excellent hydraulic function[100].

Groote Schuur Hospital experience of cardiac valve replacement with the St Jude Medical valve prosthesis

Stevens[101] from our institution reported that in a 40-month period (February 1979 to August 1981) 333 patients received 399 St Jude Medical (SJM) valves (118 aortic, 149 mitral, 59 aortic and mitral, three tricuspid plus mitral, two tricuspid, mitral and aortic, and two isolated tricuspid). The age range was 1.5–75 years (mean 34). There were 177 males and 156 females. The operative mortality was 4.8% and 306 patients were followed from 1 to 39 months (mean 15.4). Seventeen valve failures occurred: 13 had acute thrombotic obstruction (Figure 6.14), three had haemolysis immediately postoperatively and one had a late paravalvular leak needing reoperation. Of the 13 obstructed valves, seven had emergency reoperation, with one death. Five died suddenly in pulmonary oedema, and one had echocardiographic and auscultatory evidence of an obstructed tricuspid valve. None of these patients was on anticoagulants.

Fifty embolic events occurred in 42 patients within the first 30 days, and 26 when anticoagulation was unsatisfactory. Seventeen patients had severe anticoagulation-induced bleeding. Restudy of 33 patients showed small mean gradients across the SJM prostheses (mitral 0–6 mmHg, aortic 0–26 mmHg). Stevens[101] concluded that the SJM valve has good haemodynamics, a low incidence of emboli, but the sudden thrombosis of the valve in the non-anticoagulated patients stresses the need for anticoagulant therapy.

At 5–6 years after implantation of a SJM valve at Groote Schuur Hospital, Cape Town, 79.4% of patients are alive, and 81.3% of these patients are free of significant embolism events[34].

St Jude Medical aortic valve prosthesis

Ten patients (six of whom were males) with St Jude Medical prostheses replacing the aortic valve were autopsied.

Group 1

Seven patients who died less than 30 days postoperatively had a mean age of 47.4 years (SD = 18) with a range of 19–66 years. The mean postoperative survival period was 9.5 days (SD = 9.9) with a range of 17 hours to 25 days. Only one of the seven prostheses showed scanty antemortem thrombi on the sewing ring. The principal causes of death are given in Table 6.5.

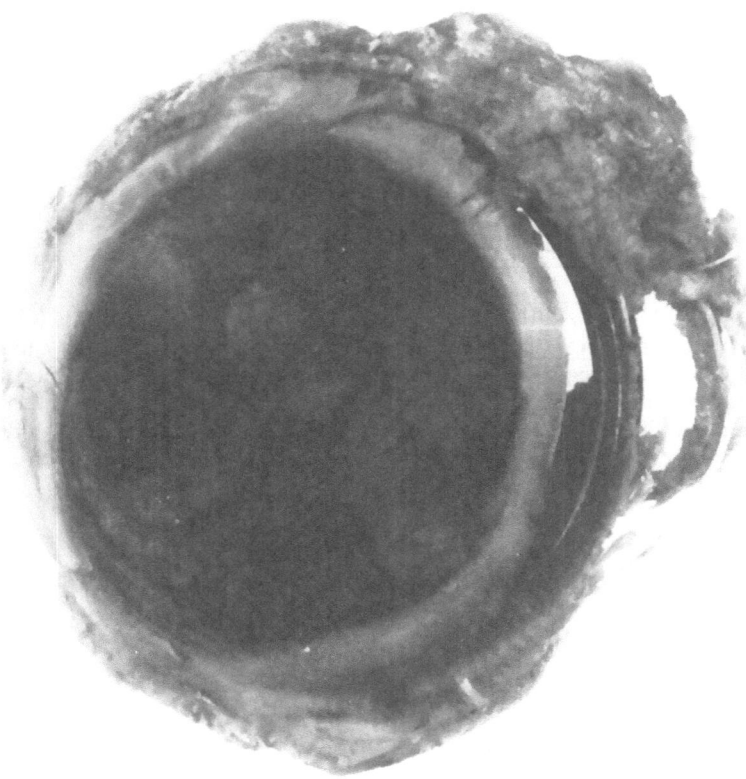

Figure 6.14 View of outflow aspect of explanted, thrombosed St Jude Medical valve prosthesis

Table 6.5 Principal causes of death (one per patient) in 10 patients with St Jude Medical aortic valve prostheses

Group 1	
Unknown	3
Bleeding (haematological abnormality)	1
Myocardial failure	1
Ruptured mycotic aneurysm (present preoperatively)	1
Infected pulmonary infarcts (present preoperatively)	1
Group 2	
Infective endocarditis	3

Group 2

The three patients who survived longer than 1 month postoperatively (Table 6.5) were three women aged 33, 67 and 71 years. Postoperative survival was

Table 6.6 Principal cause of death (one per patient) in nine patients with St Jude Medical mitral valve prostheses

Group 1	
Unknown	4
Anticoagulant excess, bleeding	1
Paraprosthetic leak	1
Group 2	
Anticoagulant excess, bleeding	1
Myocardial failure	1
Pneumonia	1

32, 42 and 120 days. All three patients died of infective endocarditis (Colour Plate M). Predisposing factors for infection were the presence (one each) of the following diseases in these three patients: diverticulitis, septic abortion with infective endocarditis preoperatively, and postoperative wound infection. Culture grew *Staphylococcus aureus*, *Pseudomonas* and coliforms. Two patients had ring abscesses and the patient with the staphylococcal infection had two mycotic aneurysms in the aortic root.

Mitral valve replacement
Nine patients with St Jude prostheses in the mitral position were autopsied.

Group 1

The six patients who died less than 30 days postoperatively had a mean age of 23.5 years (SD = 18.2) and a range of 6–59 years. Four of the six subjects were females. The mean postoperative survival period was 7.7 days (SD = 10.2) with a range of 36 hours to 28 days. Scanty thrombi were present on the left atrial (inflow) aspect of the sewing ring in two out of the six prostheses. Table 6.6 gives the principal cause of death in these six patients.

Group 2

Three patients died more than 30 days postoperatively. Postoperative survival was 38, 59 and 180 days respectively. Principal causes of death are indicated in Table 6.6. The patient who died of myocardial failure showed very extensive thrombus lining most of the left atrium, as well as on both aspects of the St Jude mitral valve prosthesis and the septal and inferior walls of the left ventricle. The primary abnormality was myocardial failure with the formation of stasis thrombi at these sites, rather than primary thrombotic occlusion of the St Jude prosthesis.

Aortic and mitral valve replacement with St Jude Medical prostheses

Autopsies were performed upon eight patients with St Jude Medical prostheses in both the aortic and the mitral positions. Five of the eight patients were females.

Table 6.7 Principal causes of death (one per patient) in eight patients with St Jude Medical prostheses in the aortic and mitral positions

Group 1	
Bleeding	1
Air embolism	1
Hepatitis	1
Septicaemia	1
Infective endocarditis	1
Group 2	
Thrombosed mitral prosthesis	2
Anticoagulant excess, bleeding	1

Group 1

The five patients who died early postoperatively had a mean age of 29.3 years (SD = 14.3) with a range of 15–46 years. Mean postoperative survival was 15 days (SD = 13) with a range of 20 hours to 30 days. All five St Jude mitral valve protheses were free of thrombi, but one out of the five St Jude aortic prostheses bore infected vegetations. Table 6.7 lists the principal cause of death in these patients.

Group 2

The three patients who died more than 30 days postoperatively were aged 30, 34 and 28 years. Two of the three were females. Two of the three mitral valve prostheses in this group of patients were immobilized by thrombosis (Figure 6.14 and Colour Plate L) on both aspects of the prosthesis. The third patient had a low prothrombin index (13%) and bled spontaneously into her brain and vulva. The principal causes of death in these three patients are listed in Table 6.7. Both patients who died of thrombosed prostheses had inadequate anticoagulant control. All of the deaths in this group were attributable to problems adherent in the design and structure of the St Jude prosthesis.

St Jude Medical prosthetic valve replacement of the mitral and tricuspid valves

One patient, a 16-year-old female with Marfan's syndrome, had both her mitral and tricuspid valves replaced by St Jude Medical valves. Two weeks postoperatively the patient underwent reoperation for thrombotic obstruction of the St Jude tricuspid valve. The patient did not survive reoperation. The left anterior descending coronary artery contained calcified, embolic material and the ventricles showed myocytolysis.

Tricuspid valve replacement with a St Jude Medical prosthesis

One patient, an 18-month-old female, underwent isolated tricuspid valve replacement with a St Jude prosthesis due to severe tricuspid valve incompetence following an episode of infective endocarditis. Death on the second postoperative day was due to severe thromboembolic pulmonary hypertension. The St Jude prosthesis appeared normal.

Summary of principal causes of death in 29 patients with St Jude Medical valves

There were no deaths due to an error in preoperative diagnosis. Three patients died due to an error in operative technique and the deaths of nine were due to problems directly related to the St Jude Medical valve. Six patients died of postoperative complications, four died of complications unrelated to the cardiac operation and the cause of death was unknown in seven patients.

Comment

The St Jude Medical (SJM) prosthetic valve has gained wide acceptance since its clinical introduction in 1977[102–104]. Lillehei[105,106] has summarized the worldwide experience with the SJM prosthetic valve. *In vitro* haemodynamic studies[107–110] show that, in general, the SJM valve represents a clear improvement in valve design with a low level of stenosis and a low regurgitant fraction. Catheterization data after SJM implantation in patients were also favourable[101]; the SJM haemodynamics are claimed to be superior to those of any other valve. Colman *et al.*[111] state that the SJM valve is the prosthesis of choice over a bioprosthesis for mitral valve replacement under the following conditions: (a) a small valve ring, i.e. all that would accept only a prosthesis below 27 mm diameter; (b) elevated left ventricular end-diastolic pressure, including all forms of cardiomyopathies; or (c) giant left atrium. Kinsley[104] inserted a SJM aortic valve obliquely in six patients as a simple method for aortic root enhancement.

In vitro the SJM valve is less vulnerable to leaflet entrapment[112] than other disc valves, which can be totally immobilized by a single interference anywhere around their circumference. The SJM valve is vulnerable only at the areas immediately adjacent to the two pivot guards. Small thrombi at these critical points may cause failure of the valve (Colour Plate L). Salvatore *et al.*[113] reported a case wherein a chordal remnant had immobilized one leaflet of a SJM mitral valve prosthesis in a partially closed position and the patient was in no distress. When fully open to 85 ° the large effective orifice area of the SJM valve, free of any struts, is separated into approximate thirds, with complete washing over each leaflet during the cardiac cycle. A slow cardiac rate or rhythm disturbance may produce occasional slight leaflet asynchrony, which is detectable by high-speed cinefilm or echocardiography[114,15]. Since tissue valves are contraindicated in children and young persons, especially due to their propensity to undergo calcification (see Chapter 8), the SJM valve may have an important role to play in this group of patients[116].

Thrombotic occlusion of SJM prostheses in the mitral[117], tricuspid[118] and aortic[119] positions have been reported[120]. Hunt *et al.*[121] reported that thromboembolic complications occurred less frequently in patients with St Jude valves than in reports of similar patients with other prostheses, provided that anitcoagulation was maintained. Joyce *et al.*[122] successfully dissolved thrombus on a thrombosed SJM tricuspid valve in a 16-month-old child and restored normal valve function.

Thromboembolic complications were significantly more frequent with the Bjork–Shiley valve replacements than with the St Jude valve[123]. Wada and Kasagi[124] reported 3.7 thromboembolic episodes per 100 patient-years in their experience with 132 implanted SJM prostheses. Three of the five thromboembolic episodes were considered to be due to poor anticoagulation control and the cause was unknown in two instances. Duncan et al.[125] reported that the risk of thromboembolism for aortic and mitral SJM valves is 2.1% per patient-year in each group.

Ziemer et al.[126] reported an intrinsic manufacturing fault in a SJM valve. Minimal disproportion between the leaflets and the valve ring caused intermittent inhibition of leaflet motion leading to reoperation. A paraprosthetic leak may mimic entrapment of a leaflet in a SJM mitral valve prosthesis[127]. Other reported complications include partial detachment of a SJM aortic valve, escape of a leaflet from a SJM mitral prosthesis due to a pivot area fracture and a remnant of papillary muscle impinging on the prosthesis.

Principal disadvantages of the SJM valve are the poor design of the valve holder and the need for long-term anticoagulation[128]. Nicoloff et al.[129] noted a low incidence of bacterial endocarditis and thromboemboli and an absence of mechanical failure. D'Alessandro et al.[130] established that the SJM valve is durable for at least 4 years. Sauvage[131] found that there are no significant differences regarding hospital mortality for the old-style Bjork–Shiley, the St Jude, or the Hancock valves. However, valve-related deaths within 2 years were higher in the patients with Hancock valves compared to those with Bjork–Shiley or SJM valves. Jones et al.[132] reported that the complication rate with the St Jude valve is as low or lower than that for any other mechanical prosthetic cardiac valve available in the world today. Further clinical reports on this valve have recently appeared[133,134].

Duromedics bileaflet valve

Hemex Scientific Inc. started manufacturing this low-profile pivoting concave bileaflet valve prosthesis in 1982. The leaflets consist of pyrolitic carbon layered over a tungsten-enriched graphite substrate. Pyrolitic carbon with a Stellite stiffener ring comprises the housing structure. The sewing ring is composed of Dacron which is available with or without a Biolite coating. Radiography easily demonstrates the curved leaflets, the radiopaque base ring and the serrated suture ring retainer. The valve is undergoing FDA clinical investigation in America.

REFERENCES

1. Pierce, W. S., Behrendt, D. M. and Morrow, A. G. (1968). A hinged prosthetic cardiac valve fabricated of rigid components: experimental evaluations in vitro and in vivo. *J. Thorac. Cardiovasc. Surg.*, **56**, 229
2. Bjork, V. O. (1970). Experiences with the Wada–Cutter valve prosthesis in the aortic area. One-year follow-up. *J. Thorac. Cardiovasc. Surg.*, **60**, 26
3. Cokkinos, D. V., Voridis, E., Bakoulas, G. and Skalkeas, G. D. (1971). Thrombosis of two high-flow prosthetic valves. *J. Thorac. Cardiovasc. Surg.*, **62**, 947

4. Bjork, V. O. (1969). A new tilting disc valve prosthesis. *Scand. J. Thorac. Cardiovasc. Surg.*, **3**, 1

5. Bjork, V. O. (1970). The central-flow tilting disc valve prosthesis (Bjork–Shiley) for mitral valve replacement. *Scand. J. Thorac. Cardiovasc. Surg.*, **4**, 15

6. Bjork, V. O., Henze, A. and Heindmarsh, T. (1977). Radiopaque marker in the tilting disc of the Bjork–Shiley heart valve. *J. Thorac. Cardiovasc. Surg.* **73**, 563

7. Lefrak, E. A. and Starr, A. (1979). *Cardiac Valve Prostheses.* (New York: Appleton-Century-Crofts)

8. Bjork, V. O. (1978). The improved Bjork–Shiley tilting disc valve prosthesis. *Scand. J. Thorac. Cardiovasc. Surg.*, **12**, 81

9. Goldstein, J. A., Zucker, R. P. and Lee, B. Y. (1986). Echocardiographic demonstration of outlet strut fracture of a Bjork–Shiley mitral prosthesis. *J. Am. Coll. Cardiol.*, **7**, 949

10. Wolfe, S. M. and Greenberg, A. (1985). Strut fractures with the Bjork–Shiley valve (letter). *N. Engl. J. Med.*, **312**, 314

11. Sacks, S. H., Northeast, A. D. R. and Watkins, J. (1984). Late strut fracture in a Bjork–Shiley valve prosthesis (current series). *Br. Heart J.*, **51**, 578

12. Bozer, A. Y. and Karamehmetoglu, A. (1972). Thrombosis encountered with Bjork–Shiley prosthesis. *J. Cardiovasc. Surg.*, **13**, 141

13. Moreno-Cabral, R. J., McNamara, J. J., Mamiya, R. T., Brainard, S. C. and Chung, G. K. T. (1978). Acute thrombotic obstruction with Bjork–Shiley valves. Diagnostic and surgical considerations. *J. Thorac. Cardiovasc. Surg.*, **75**, 321

14. Olinger, G. N., Thompson, M. A. and Keelan, M. H. Jr. (1982). Optimal management of suspected thrombosis of standard Bjork–Shiley unmarked tilting disc mitral valve prosthesis. *Am. Heart J.*, **103**, 440

15. Ben-Zvi, J., Hildner, F. J., Chandraratna, P. A. and Samet, P. (1974). Thrombosis on Bjork–Shiley aortic valve prosthesis. Clinical, arteriographic, echocardiographic and therapeutic observations in seven cases. *Am. J. Cardiol*, **34**, 538

16. Wright, J. O., Hiratzka, L. F., Brandt, B. III and Doty, D. B. (1982). Thrombosis of the Bjork–Shiley prosthesis: illustrative cases and review of the literature. *J. Thorac. Cardiovasc. Surg.*, **84**, 138

17. Peterffy, A., Henze, A., Savidge, G. F. *et al.* (1980). Late thrombotic malfunction of the Bjork–Shiley tilting disc valve in the tricuspid position. Principles for recognition and management. *Scand. J. Thorac. Cardiovasc. Surg.*, **14**, 33

18. Copans, H., Lakier, J. B., Kinsley, R. H. *et al.* (1980). Thrombosed Bjork–Shiley mitral prostheses. *Circulation*, **61**, 169

19. Ledain, L. D., Ohayon, J. P., Colle, J. P., Lonent-Roudaut, F. M. and Besse, P. M. (1986). Acute thrombotic obstruction with disc valve prostheses: diagnostic considerations and fibrinolytic treatment. *J. Am. Coll. Cardiol.*, **7**, 743

20. Bjork, V. O. and Henze, A. (1973). Encapsulation of the Bjork–Shiley aortic valve prosthesis caused by the lack of anticoagulant treatment. *Scand. J. Thorac. Cardiovasc. Surg.*, **7**, 17

21. Ayusu, L. A., Juffe, A., Rufilanchas, J. J., Babin, F., Burgos, R. and Figuera, D. (1982). Thrombectomy: surgical treatment of the thrombosed Bjork–Shiley prosthesis. Report of seven cases and review of the literature. *J. Thorac. Cardiovasc. Surg.*, **84**, 906

22. Venugopal, P., Kaul, U., Iyer, K. S., Rao, I. M., Balram, A., Das, B., Sampathkumar, A. *et al.* (1986). Fate of thrombectomized Bjork–Shiley valves. A long-term cinefluoroscopic, echocardiographic and hemodynamic evaluation. *J. Thorac. Cardiovasc. Surg.*, **91**, 168

23. Moulton, A. L. (1984). Thrombectomy for clotted Bjork–Shiley prostheses: is it really a proven procedure? (Letter) *J. Thorac. Cardiovasc. Surg.*, **87**, 147

24. Mattingly, W. T. Jr., O'Connor, W., Zeok, J. V. and Todd, E. P. (1983). Thrombotic catastrophe in the patient with multiple Bjork–Shiley prostheses. *Ann. Thorac. Surg.*, **35**, 253

25. Sabbagh, A. H. (1983). Clotted Bjork–Shiley mitral valve prostheses: early detection and surgical management. *Cardiovasc. Res. Cent. Bull.*, **21**, 101

26. Boskovic, D., Pechacek, L. W. and Krajcer, Z. (1983). Thrombosis of a Bjork–Shiley aortic valve prosthesis diagnosed by two-dimensional echocardiography. *J. Clin. Ultrasound*, **11**, 165

27. Beeuwswaert, R., Denef, B. and De Geest, H. (1983). Diagnosis and treatment of obstruction of a tricuspid Bjork–Shiley prosthesis. *Acta Cardiol.*, **38**, 13
28. Yoganathan, A. P., Corcoran, W. H., Harrison, E. C. and Carl, J. R. (1978). The Bjork–Shiley aortic prosthesis: flow characteristics, thrombus formation and tissue overgrowth. *Circulation*, **58**, 70
29. Bjork, V. O., Henze, A. and Heindmarsh, T. (1977). Radiopaque marker in the tilting disc of the Bjork–Shiley heart valve. *J. Thorac. Cardiovasc. Surg.*, **73**, 563
30. Dale, J. (1977). Arterial thromboembolic complications in patients with Bjork–Shiley and Lillehei–Kaster aorticd disc valve prostheses. *Am. Heart J.*, **93**, 715
31. Bharadwaj, B., Wall, R. and Nutting, S. (1980). Long-term follow-up of patients who underwent single valve replacement with Bjork–Shiley prosthesis. *Can. J. Surg.*, **23**, 183
32. Daenen, W., Nevelsteen, A., van Cauwelaert, P., de Maesschalk, E., Willems, J. and Stalpaert, G. (1983). Nine years' experience with the Bjork–Shiley prosthetic valve: early and late results of 932 valve replacements. *Ann. Thorac. Surg.*, **35**, 651
33. Marshall, W. G. Jr, Kouchoukos, N. T., Karp, R. B. and Williams, J. B. (1983). Late results after mitral valve replacement with the Bjork–Shiley and porcine prostheses. *J. Thorac. Cardiovasc. Surg.*, **85**, 902
34. Rose, A. G. (1984). Pathology of heart valve replacement by valvular prostheses. *MD thesis*, University of Cape Town.
35. Koops, E. and Puschel, K. (1979). Thromboembolic malfunction of a Bjork–Shiley aortic valve prosthesis. *Thorac. Cardiovasc. Surg.*, **27**, 319
36. Silver, M. D. (1980). Wear in Bjork–Shiley heart valve prostheses recovered at necropsy or operation. *J. Thorac. Cardiovasc. Surg.*, **79**, 693
37. Norenberg, D. D., Evans, R. W., Gundersen, A. E. and Abellera, R. M. (1977). Fracture and embolization of a Bjork–Shiley disc. Fatal failure of a prosthetic mitral valve. *J. Thorac. Cardiovasc. Surg.*, **74**, 925
38. Brubakk, O., Simonsen, S., Kallman, L. *et al.* (1981). Strut fracture in the new Bjork–Shiley mitral valve prosthesis. *Thorac. Cardiovasc. Surg.*, **29**, 108
39. Larrieu, A. J., Puglia, E. and Allen, P. (1982). Strut fracture and disc embolization of a Bjork–Shiley mitral valve prosthesis: localization of embolized disc by computerized axial tomography. *Ann. Thorac. Surg.*, **34**, 192
40. Sethia, B., Quin, R. O. and Bain, W. H. (1983) Disc embolisation after minor strut fracture in a Bjork–Shiley mitral valve prosthesis. *Thorax*, **38**, 390
41. Wang, R., Lee, W. T. and Mok, C. K. (1982). Two-dimensional echocardiographic features of Bjork–Shiley aortic prosthetic valve dehiscence. *Thorax*, **37**, 540
42. Lewis, B. S., Aganthangelou, N. E., Dos Santos, L. A. and Antunes, M. J. (1983). Real-time 2-dimensional echocardiographic visualization of thrombus on a Bjork–Shiley mitral valve prosthesis. Emergency cesarean section and mitral valve replacement in late pregnancy. *Am. J. Cardiol*, **51**, 908
43. Verdel, G., Heethaar, R. M., Jambroes, G. *et al.* (1983). Assessment of the opening angle of implanted Bjork–Shiley prosthetic valves. *Circulation*, **68**, 355
44. Henze, A., Carlsson, S. and Bjork, V. O. (1973). Mortality and pathology following aortic valve replacement with the Bjork–Shiley tilting disc valve. *Scand. J. Thorac. Cardiovasc. Surg.*, **7**, 7
45. Roberts, W. C. and Hammer, W. J. (1976). Cardiac pathology after valve replacement with a tilting disc prosthesis (Bjork–Shiley type). A study of 46 necropsy patients and 49 Bjork–Shiley prostheses. *Am. J. Cardiol*, **37**, 1024
46. Roberts, W. C., Bulkley, B. H. and Morrow, A. G. (1973). Pathologic anatomy of cardiac valve replacement: a study of 224 necropsy patients. *Prog. Cardiovasc. Dis.*, **15**, 539
47. Hammermeister, K. E., Dillard, D. H. and Kennedy, J. W. (1969). Severe, intermittent, mitral regurgitation in a Cross–Jones valve. Report of a case with angiographic and hemodynamic observations. *J. Thorac. Cardiovasc. Surg.*, **58**, 575
48. Vogel, J. H. K. (1985). The monostrut Bjork–Shiley heart valve. *J. Am. Coll. Cardiol.*, **6**, 1142
49. Sethia, B., Turner, M. A., Lewis, S., Rodger, R. A. and Bain, W. H. (1986). Fourteen years' experience with the Bjork–Shiley tilting disc prosthesis. *J. Thorac. Cardiovasc. Surg.*, **91**, 350

50. Long, D. M. Jr, Sterns, L. P., De Riemer, R. H. *et al.* (1960). Subtotal and total replacement of the aortic valve with plastic valve prostheses: experimental investigation and successful clinical application utilizing selective cardiac hypothermia. *Surg. Forum,* **10,** 660

51. Kaster, R. L. and Lillehei, C. W. (1967). A new cageless free-floating pivoting disc prosthetic heart valve: design, development and evaluation. *Digest. 7th Int. Conf. Biol. Eng.,* Stockholm, p. 387

52. Kaster, R. L., Lillehei, C. W. and Starek, P. J. K. (1970). The Lillehei–Kaster pivoting disc aortic prosthesis and a comparative study of its pulsatile flow characteristics with four other prostheses. *Trans. Am. Soc. Artif. Intern. Organs,* **16,** 233

53. Lillehei, C. W., Kaster, R. L., Coleman, M. *et al.* (1974). Heart-valve replacement with Lillehei–Kaster pivoting disc prosthesis. *N.Y. State Med. J.,* **74,** 1426

54. Byrne, J. P., Behrendt, D. M., Kirsh, M. M. and Orringer, M. B. (1977). Replacement of heart valves by prosthetic devices. In Joachim, H. L. (ed.) *Pathobiology Annual.* Vol. 7. p. 83. (New York: Appleton-Century-Crofts)

55. Chun, P. K. C. and Nelson, W. P. (1977). Common cardiac prosthetic valves. *J. Am. Med. Assoc.,* **238,** 401

56. Christo, M. C., Figueroa, C. C. S. and Souza, J. M. (1975). Nossa experiencia com a substituicao de valvas cardiacas por proteses pivotantes de disco de Lillehei–Kaster. *Argu. Bras. Cardiol.,* **28,** 149

57. Costa, I. A., Faraco, D. L. and Sallum, F. S. (1976). Disfuncao de protes de Lillehei–Kaster em posicao mitral. *Rev. Bras. Med.,* **33,** 33

58. Buffolo, E., Forte, V. and Silva de Andrade, J. C. (1975). Results of valvular replacements by Lillehei–Kaster prostheses. Presented at 3 Congresso Nacional de Chirurgia Cardiaca, Rio de Janeiro, Brazil

59. Kaster, R. L. and Lillehei, C. W. (1967). A new cageless free-floating pivoting disc prosthetic heart valve: design, development and evaluation. *Digest of the 7th International Conference of Medical and Biological Engineering,* Stockholm, Sweden, p. 387

60. Lillehei, C. W., Kaster, R. L., Starek, P. J., Bloch, J. H. and Rees, J. R. (1970). A new central flow pivoting disc aortic and mitral prosthesis: initial clinical experience. (Abstract). *Am. J. Cardiol.,* **26,** 668

61. Gibson, T. C., Starek, P. J. K., Moos, S. *et al.* (1974). Echocardiographic and phonocardiographic characteristics of the Lillehei–Kaster mitral valve prosthesis. *Circulation,* **49,** 434

62. Nitter-Hauge, S., Hall, K. V. and Froysaker, K. V. (1977). Mitral valve replacement. A comparative clinical and haemodynamic study of the new Lillehei–Kaster and Bjork–Shiley prostheses. *Scand. J. Thorac. Cardiovasc. Surg.,* **11,** 111

63. Uhrenholdt, A., Jensen, G. and Lauridsen, P. (1980). Hemodynamic findings after insertion of the Lillehei–Kaster valve in the mitral ostium. *Scand. J. Thorac. Cardiovasc. Surg.,* **14,** 185

64. Rao, K. M., Learoyd, P. A., Rao, R. S. *et al.* (1980). Chronic haemolysis after Lillehei–Kaster valve replacement. Comparison with the findings after Bjork–Shiley and Starr–Edwards mitral valve replacement. *Thorax,* **35,** 290

65. Behle, P. R. and Brown, A. H. (1983). Late snaring of Lillehei–Kaster prosthesis by a fragment of left atrial monitoring catheter. *Thorax,* **38,** 879

66. Nitter-Hauge, S., Hall, K. V., Froysaker, T. and Efskind, L. (1974). Aortic valve replacement: one-year results with Lillehei–Kaster and Bjork–Shiley disc prosthesis. *Am. Heart J.,* **88,** 23

67. Nitter-Hauge, S., Froysaker, T. and Hall, K. V. (1977). Clinical and haemodynamic results following mitral valve replacement with the new Lillehei–Kaster pivoting disc valve prosthesis. *Scand. J. Thorac. Cardiovasc. Surg.,* **11,** 15

68. Starek, P. J. K., Wilcox, B. R. and Murray, G. F. (1976). Hemodynamic evaluation of the Lillehei–Kaster pivoting disc valve in patients. *J. Thorac. Cardiovasc. Surg.,* **71,** 123

69. Sigwart, U., Schmidt, H., Gleichman, U. *et al.* (1976). *In vivo* evaluation of the Lillehei–Kaster heart valve prosthesis. *Ann. Thorac. Surg.,* **22,** 213

70. Forman, R., Gersh, B. J., Fraser, R. and Beck, W. (1978). Hemodynamic assessment of Lillehei–Kaster tilting disc aortic and mitral prostheses. *J. Thorac. Cardiovasc. Surg.,* **75,** 595

71. Starek, P. J. K., McLaurin, L. P., Wilcox, B. R. and Murray, G. F. (1976). Clinical evaluation of the Lillehei–Kaster pivoting-disc valve. *Ann. Thorac. Surg.,* **22,** 362

72. Mitha, A. S., Matisonn, R. E., Le Roux, B. T. and Chesler, E. (1976). Clinical experience with the Lillehei–Kaster cardiac valve prosthesis. J. Thorac. Cardiovasc. Surg., **72**, 401
73. Roberts, W. C., Fishbein, M. C. and Golden, A. (1975). Cardiac pathology after valve replacement by disc prosthesis. A study of 61 necropsy patients. Am. J. Cardiol, **35**, 740
74. Dale, J. (1977). Arterial thromboembolic complications in patients with Bjork–Shiley and Lillehei–Kaster aortic disc valve prostheses. Am. Heart J., **93**, 715
75. Zwart, H. H. J., Hicks, G., Schuster, B., Nathan, M., Tabrah, F., Wenzke, F., Ahmed, T. and DeWall, R. A. (1979). Clinical experience with the Lillehei–Kaster valve prosthesis. Ann. Thorac. Surg., **28**, 158
76. Silver, M. D., Koppenhof, H., Heggtveit, H. A. and Reif, T. H. (1985). Metal wear in Lillehei–Kaster heart valve prostheses. Artif. Organs, **9**, 270
77. Lillehei, C. W. (1977). Heart valve replacement with the pivoting disc: appraisal of results and description of a new all-carbon model. J. Assoc. Advance. Med. Instr., **11**, 85
78. Melrose, D. G., Bentall, H. H., McMillan, I. K. R., Flege, J. B., Diaz, F. R. A., Nahas, R. A., Fautley, R. and Carson, J. (1964). The evolution of a mitral valve prosthesis. Lancet, **2**, 623
79. Bentall, H. H., McMillan, K. R. and Melrose, D. G. (1963). A new mitral valve prosthesis. J. Physiol., **167**, 7P
80. Raftery, E. B., Dayem, M. K. A. and Melrose, D. G. (1968). Mechanical performance of Hammersmith mitral valve prosthesis. Br. Heart J., **30**, 666
81. Shaw, T. D. R., Gunstensen, J. and Turner, R. W. D. (1974). Sudden mechanical malfunction of Hammersmith mitral valve prostheses due to wear of polypropylene. J. Thorac. Cardiovasc. Surg., **67**, 579
82. Hall, K. V., Kaster, R. L. and Woien, A. (1979). An improved pivotal disc-type prosthetic heart valve. J. Oslo City Hosp., **29**, 3
83. Nitter-Hauge, S., Enge, I., Sembe, B. K. H. and Hall, K. V. (1978). Primary clinical experience with the Hall–Kaster valve in the aortic position. Results at 3 months including hemodynamic studies. Circulation, **60**, (Suppl. I), I-55
84. Semb, B. K. H., Aasen, A., Woxholt, G. et al. (1979). In vivo haemodynamic evaluation of the Hall–Kaster central flow prosthetic heart valve. Scand. J. Clin. Lab. Invest., **39**, 731
85. Aasen, A. O., Resch, F., Semb, B. J. et al. (1980). Development of a canine model for long-term studies after mitral valve replacement with the Hall–Kaster prosthesis. Europ. Surg. Res., **12**, 199
86. Antunes, M. J., Colsen, P. R. and Kinsley, R. H. (1982). Intermittent aortic regurgitation following aortic valve replacement with the Hall–Kaster prosthesis. J. Thorac. Cardiovasc. Surg., **84**, 751
87. Hall, K. V., Nitter-Hauge, S. and Abdelnoor, M. (1985). Seven and one-half years' experience with the Medtronic-Hall valve. J. Am. Coll. Cardiol., **6**, 1417
88. Silver, M. D. and Wilson, G. W. (1983). Pathology of cardiovascular prostheses including coronary artery bypass and other vascular grafts. In Silver, M. D. (ed.) Cardiovascular Pathology, Vol. 2, p. 1225. (New York: Churchill Livingstone)
89. Rabago, G., Martinell, J., Fraile, J., Andrade, I. G. and Montenegro, R. (1984). Results and complications with the Omniscience prosthesis. J. Thorac. Cardiovasc. Surg., **87**, 136
90. Cortina, J. M., Martinell, J., Artiz, V., Fraile, J. and Rabago, G. (1986). Comparative clinical results with Omniscience (STM1), Medtronic–Hall, and Bjork–Shiley convexo-concave (70 degrees) prostheses in mitral valve replacement. J. Thorac. Cardiovasc. Surg., **91**, 174
91. DeWall, R., Pelletier, L. C., Panebianco, A., Hicks, G., Schuster, B., Bonan, R., Martinau, J. P. and Yip, L. (1984). Factors influencing thromboembolic complications in Omniscience cardiac valve patients. Europ. Heart J., **5**, (Suppl. D), 53
92. Agozzini, L., Bellitti, R., Schettini, S. et al. (1984). Acute thrombosis of Sorin tilting disc mitral prostheses. Int. J. Cardiol., **5**, 351
93. Mikhail, A. A. (1984). Omniscience cardiac valve prosthesis comprehensive clinical review. 65-month 8-center evaluation. (PMAA Data Base Summary). A publication by Medical Incorporated, pp. 1-8
94. Kalke, B. R., Carlson, R. G. and Lillehei, C. W. (1968). Hingeless double-leaflet prosthetic heart valve for aortic, mitral or tricuspid positions: experimental study on replacement in the mitral position. Biomed. Sci. Instr., **4**, 190

95. Kalke, B. R., Lillehei, C. W. and Kaster, R. L. (1969). Evaluation of a double leaflet prosthetic heart valve of new design for clinical use. In Brewer, L. A. III (ed.) *Prosthetic Heart Valves*, p. 285. (Springfield, Illinois: Charles C. Thomas)

96. Palmquist, W. E., Nicoloff, D. M., Emery, R. W. et al. (1978). St Jude Medical, Inc., all pyrolytic carbon heart valve. Presented at the Association for Advancement of Medical Instrumentation 13th Annual Meeting. Washington, DC, 28 March – 1 April.

97. Bonchek, L. I. (1981). Current status of cardiac valve replacement: selection of a prosthesis and indications for operation. *Am. Heart J.*, **101**, 96

98. Emery, R. W., Palmquist, W. E., Mettler, E. et al. (1978). A new cardiac valve prosthesis: in vitro results. *Trans. Am. Soc. Artif. Intern. Organs*, **24**, 550

99. Emery, R. W., Mettler, E. and Nicoloff, D. M. (1979). A new cardiac prosthesis: the St Jude Medical cardiac valve. *In vivo* results. *Circulation*, **60** (Suppl. I), I-48

100. Status Report No. 10, St Jude Medical, Inc., St Paul, Minn., 17 July 1980

101. Stevens, J. E. (1982). The Cape Town experience with the Saint Jude prosthetic valve. Paper read at the XIII Southern African Cardiac Society Congress, Cape Town, 6–8 September

102. Nicoloff, D. M. and Anderson, R. W. (1979). Current status of the St Jude cardiac valve prosthesis. *Contemp. Surg.*, **15**, 11

103. Emery, R. W., Anderson, R. W. and Lindsay, W. G. (1979). Clinical and hemodynamic results with the St Jude Medical aortic valve prosthesis. *Surg. Forum*, **30**, 235

104. Emery, R. W., Mettler, E. and Nicoloff, D. M. (1979). A new cardiac prosthesis: the St Jude Medical cardiac valve. *In vivo* results. *Circulation*, **60**, 48

105. Lillehei, C. W. (1982). Worldwide experience with the St Jude Medical aortic valve prosthesis: clinical and hemodynamic results. *Contemp. Surg.*, **20**, 17

106. Lillehei, C. W. (1982). Worldwide experience with the St Jude Medical valve prosthesis: clinical and hemodynamic results. *Nippon Kyobu Geka Gakkai Zasshi*, **30**, 466

107. Gabbay, S., Yellin, L., Frishman, W. H. et al. (1980). *In vitro* hydrodynamic comparison of St Jude, Bjork–Shiley and Hall–Kaster valves. *Am. Soc. Artif. Intern. Organs*, **16**, 231

108. Gottwik, M. G., Tessari, R., Neumeier, K. et al. (1981). *In vitro* comparison of Bjork–Shiley and St Jude Medical valvular prosthesis in aortic position in a new pulse duplicator. In Bircks, W., Ostermeyer, J. and Schutte, H. D. (eds.) *Cardiovascular Surgery 1980. Proceedings of the 29th International Congress of the European Society of Cardiovascular Surgery.* (Berlin: Springer-Verlag)

109. Kasagi, Y. and Wada, J. (1981). Hemodynamic characteristics of the St Jude Medical valve in mock circulation – one year follow-up of our initial 230 St Jude Medical valve implantations. *Proceedings of the Second International Symposium on the St Jude Valve.* San Diego, California, 11–14 March, p. 254

110. Kinsley, R. H. (1981). Aortic root enhancement and the St Jude prosthesis. *Proceedings of the Second International Symposium on the St Jude Valve.* San Diego, California, 11–14 March, p. 135

111. In Bircks, W., Ostermeyer, J. and Schutte, H-D. (eds). *Cardiovascular Surgery 1980.* the selection of the St Jude Medical prosthesis as a mitral valve substitute. *Proceedings of the Second International Symposium on the St Jude Valve.* San Diego, California, 11–14 March, p. 295

112. Starek, P. J. K. (1981). Immobilization of disc heart valves by unravelled sutures. *Ann. Thorac. Surg.*, **31**, 66

113. Salvatore, L., Paolini, G. and Benedetti, M. (1981). Cardiac valvular replacement with the St Jude Medical prosthesis in 160 patients. Clinical and hemodynamic results. *Proceedings of the Second International Symposium on the St Jude Valve.* San Diego, California, 11–14 March, p.187

114. Castaneda-Zuniga, W., Nicoloff, D. M., Jorgensen, C., Nath, P. H., Zollikofer, C. and Amplatz, K. (1980). *In vivo* radiographic appearance of the St Jude valve prosthesis. *Radiology*, **134**, 775

115. Tri, T. (1980). Echocardiographic evaluation of the St Jude Medical prosthetic valve. *Radiology*, **134**, 229

116. Baudet, E. M. (1980). Cardiac valve replacement in children with St Jude Medical prostheses. *Radiology*, **134**, 149

117. Commerford, P. J., Lloyd, E. A. and De Nobrega, J. A. (1981). Thrombosis of St Jude Medical cardiac valve in the mitral position. *Chest.* **80**, 326

118. Bowen, T. E., Tri, T. B. and Wortham, D. C. (1981). Thrombosis of a St Jude Medical tricuspid prosthesis. (Case report). *J. Thorac. Cardiovasc. Surg.*, **82**, 257

119. Moulton, A. L., Singleton, R. T., Oster, W. F., Bosley, J. and Mergner, W. (1982). Fatal thrombosis of an aortic St Jude Medical valve despite 'adequate' anticoagulation: Anatomic and technical considerations. *J. Thorac. Cardiovasc. Surg.*, **83**, 472

120. Ledain, L. D., Ohayon, J. P., Colle, J. P., Lorient-Roudat, F. M., Roudat, R. P. and Besse, P. M. (1986). Acute thrombotic obstruction with disc valve prostheses: diagnostic considerations and fibrinolytic treatment. *J. Am. Coll. Cardiol.*, **7**, 743

121. Hunt, D., Sloman, G. and Sutton, L. (1981). The St Jude Medical valve – the Australian experience. *Med. J. Aust.*, **2**, 276

122. Joyce, L. D., Boucek, M. and McGough, E. C. (1983). Urokinase therapy for thrombosis of tricuspid prosthetic valve. *J. Thorac. Cardiovasc. Surg.*, **85**, 935

123. Horstkotte, D., Korfer, R., Seipel, L., Bircks, W. and Loogen, F. (1983). Late complications in patients with Bjork–Shiley and St Jude Medical heart valve replacement. *Circulation*, **68**, II–75

124. Wada, J. and Kasagi, Y. (1983). A new mechanical valve: SJM. *Int. Surg.*, **68**, 935

125. Duncan, J. M., Cooley, D. A., Livesay, J. J., Ott, D. A., Reul, G. J., Walker, W. E. and Frazier, O. H. (1983). The St Jude Medical valve: early clinical results in 253 patients. *Texas Heart Inst. J.*, **10**, 11

126. Ziemer, G., Luhmer, I., Oelert, H. and Borst, H. G. (1982). Malfunction of a St Jude Medical heart valve in mitral position. *Ann. Thorac. Surg.*, **33**, 391

127. Guttierez, F. R., Tiefenbrunn, A. J., McKnight, R. C. and Clark, R. E. (1982). Periprosthetic leak mimicking entrapment of a leaflet in a St Jude Medical mitral valve prosthesis: case report. (Letter). *J. Thorac. Cardiovasc. Surg.*, **83**, 471

128. DeBakey, M. E., Lawrie, G. M. and Morris, G. C. (1982). Experience with 366 St Jude valve prostheses in 346 patients. *Proceedings of the Third International Symposium on the St Jude Medical Heart Valve*, November 1982, Scottsdale, Arizona, (USA: Yorke Medical Books), p. 14

129. Nicoloff, D. M., Lindsay, W. G. and Arom, K. V. (1982). Four and a half years with the St Jude prosthesis. *Proceedings of the Third International Symposium on the St Jude Medical Heart Valve*, November 1982, Scottsdale, Arizona, (USA: Yorke Medical Books), p. 25

130. D'Alessandro, L. C., Baruffi, and Giordani, F. (1982). Italian experiences with the St Jude Medical valve. *Int. Surg.*, **68**, 41

131. Sauvage, L. R. (1982). A comparison of the first 24 months of 65 St Jude, 65 Bjork–Shiley, and 49 Hancock aortic and mitral valve prostheses. *Int. Surg.*, **68**, 108

132. Jones, T. W., Thomas, G. I., Stavney, L. S. and Manhas, D. R. (1984). The St Jude experience. *Am J. Surg.*, **147**, 593

133. D'Angelo, G. J., Kish, G. F., Sardesai, P. G. and Tan, W. S. (1986). Clinical assessment of the St. Jude Medical cardiac prosthesis. A 5-year experience. *Am. Surg.*, **52**, 101

134. Ribeiro, P. A., Al Zaibag, M., Idris, M., Al Kasab, S., Davies, G., Mashat, E., Wareham, E. and Al Fagih, M. (1986). Antiplatelet drugs and the incidence of thromboembolic complications of the St Jude Medical aortic prosthesis in patients with rheumatic heart disease. *J. Thorac. Cardiovasc. Surg.*, **91**, 92

TISSUE VALVES

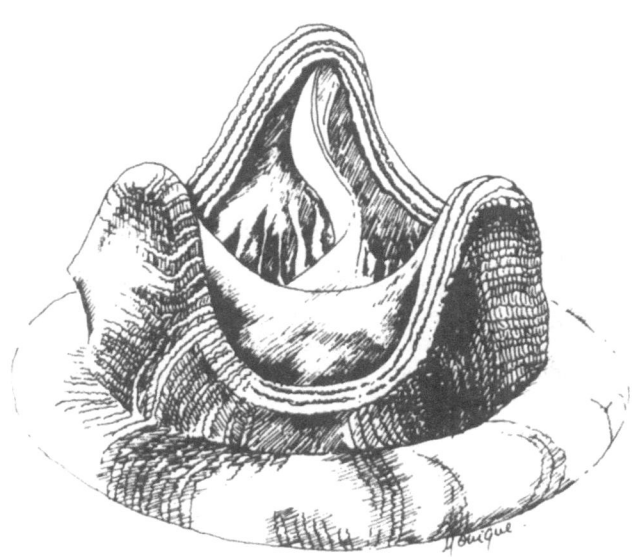

7
Homograft and Xenograft Aortic Valves, Fascia Lata and Dura Mater Valves

There is some confusion over exact definitions of non-chemically treated tissue valves. Homograft valves[1,2] vary according to the method and timing of collection, sterilization, methods of valve storage, technique of implantation, and use of a free graft or one on a supporting stent. Ross[3], and Barrat-Boyes[4] independently were the first to successfully implant a homograft aortic valve orthotopically. Heimbecker et al.[5] also showed that aortic valve homografts were a feasible long-term therapy.

HOMOGRAFT AORTIC VALVES

Fresh homograft aortic valve

Fresh valves are usually obtained between 4 and 48 hours after death, commonly from males aged between 18 and 40 years who did not die with infection. Cuspal fibroblasts are kept alive *in vitro* and theoretically should be capable of mitosis and collagen synthesis following implantation of the valve in a recipient. Fresh homograft aortic valves implanted in the sub-coronary position proved virtually free of thromboembolic complications without anticoagulant therapy[6]. Homograft valves mounted on a stent can be implanted in other intracardiac positions[7] and the stent aids insertion of the graft in the aortic position[8,9].

Sterilized homograft aortic valve

At first the valves were removed from cadavers using either sterile precautions or clean conditions. To ensure the sterility of the excised valve severe methods[10] were initially used, e.g. exposure to ethylene oxide or beta-propiolactone sterilization, irradiation, freezing and freeze-drying. Such treatment abolished valve viability. Surface sterilization using formaldehyde vapour, or the use of *in vitro* antibiotics in high concentrations, led to successful sterility, but also yielded a non-viable valve. Euthermic incubation of valves in antibiotic solutions achieved satisfactory sterilization with only a 15% reduction in cuspal viability[11]. Fungi were not affected by such treatment. Some reports have shown continued donor cell survival in fresh allograft leaflets implanted into dogs[12], whereas others have reported rapid cell loss after implantation[13,14].

The problem of ensuring viability is compounded by the need for having a means of storing valve homografts of different sizes until they are required. A variety of storage processes have been tried, including hypothermic storage in tissue culture medium, glycerol or dimethylsulphoxide. Freeze-drying and storage at room temperature was unsuccessfully used from 1962 to 1968.

Fortunately, such homograft valves were not widely used, since those subjected to the rigorous sterilization and storage techniques in use up to 1968 had a high failure rate[2]. Antibiotic sterilization has been applied more recently and about 50% of such patients have normal valve function 5 years after implantation[2]. The freedom from embolism, anticoagulation, noise and haemolysis justify the use of aortic valve homografts.

The use of a rigid stent leads to greater stresses on the homograft valve with resultant accelerated leaflet degeneration[9]. A pliable stent may reduce the magnitude of this problem[15]. Pulmonary valve homografts implanted in the mitral position have been most unsuccessful[16]. The pathology of the human aortic valve homograft[17-20] includes thickening of the bases of the cusps of aortic valve homografts, calcification, 'degenerative' changes in the cuspal collagen and rupture or performation of the cusps. Aparicio et al.[19] studied the microscopic changes in valvular homografts and pig aortic xenografts sterilized by various methods. The freeze-dried valves showed structural changes due to physicochemical degradation of the collagen due to improper preservation of the graft prior to insertion. Calcification was observed in this group, but not in homografts treated with gamma-radiation. The latter valves showed fewer and less severe morphological alterations.

XENOGRAFT AORTIC VALVES

Unfixed xenograft valves

In 1965 Duran and Gunning[21] reported on the behaviour of freeze-dried pig aortic valves transplanted into the descending thoracic aorta of 17 dogs. Although no animal survived for more than 18 months, the xenograft cusps were all in good condition. Duran and Gunning transplanted a xenograft aortic valve into a patient in 1964. This patient, cited by Binet et al.[22], died 24 hours later from causes unrelated to the xenograft. At necropsy the valve was competent and in good condition. Encouraged by this, Binet et al.[22] treated xenograft aortic valves with 3 days immersion in a mercurial solution prior to implanting them into five patients. Four patients received pig aortic valves and one was given a calf aortic valve. All five patients were doing well when documented about 3 months later.

Fresh sheep aortic valves, stored in a lactate-Ringer antibiotic solution and then implanted into the descending aorta of dogs, showed thrombosis, cuspal atrophy and fibrosis[23]. Freeze-dried valves showed a marked tendency for the grafts to rupture through the heterologous aortic wall cuff. Sweatt *et al.*[24] transplanted aortic valves of sheep and pigs into the descending thoracic aorta of dogs. The valves were fresh, freeze-dried, or treated with propiolactone. Half of the recipient dogs received azathioprine. The following conditions gave the best results: (a) transplantation of a minimum of aortic wall with the valve; (b) good initial alignment and movement of the cusps; (c) administration of azathioprine for 8 weeks; and (d) support of the graft by a Dacron tube, preventing rupture and separating the graft from ingrowing host tissue. Drury *et al.*[25] showed that 50–80% sucrose solution is acceptable for the long-term preservation of biological valves.

Formaldehyde-preserved xenograft

Obtaining aortic valve grafts from animals overcomes the logistical problems encountered with procuring cadaveric human aortic valves. Fresh valves have the potential problem of rejection. Various means of pretreating the xenograft valve in order to render it less antigenic have been used, e.g. mercurial salts[26] or 4% buffered formaldehyde solution. In 1968 Warren Hancock, of Hancock Laboratories, California, and William Angell of Cutter Laboratories, California, produced the first commercially prepared tissue valve. This was a formalin-tanned, stent-mounted porcine xenograft. Long-term follow-up was disappointing. The University of Cape Town formaldehyde-treated porcine xenografts yielded similarly disappointing results (see below). Formalin fixation by cross-linking of valvular collagen was found to be reversed *in vivo*, resulting in stretching, thinning and tearing of the leaflets when the cusp degenerated[11,27].

Pathology of the University of Cape Town formaldehyde-treated porcine xenograft bioprosthesis

The mitral valve was replaced by a formaldehyde-preserved, stent-mounted porcine aortic valve in 33 patients at Groote Schuur Hospital. Usually there was a gradual onset of dysfunction of the prosthesis, which allowed for timeous replacement of the failed xenografts by another valve substitute[28]. Eleven of the failed xenograft prosthetic valves were studied, and two patients came to autopsy.

The 11 patients ranged in age from 18 to 59 years. The valves had been *in situ* for a mean period of 9.9 months (SD = 8.6) and the range was from 2 to 32 months. Table 7.1 summarizes the clinicopathological details of the 11 patients. The cusps of the xenograft prostheses showed varying degrees of stretching and deformation with resultant valvular incompetence (Colour Plate N). No cusp had perforated and no thrombi were seen with the naked eye. A single prosthesis, which had been implanted for 32 months, showed a torn commissure. Microscopically eight out of the 11 valves had a thin layer of platelet-fibrin thrombus on the arterialis (concave) surface of the cusps. No viable donor cells were present within the cusps. Some cusps had isolated mononuclear cells on their surface.

Table 7.1 Clinicopathological details of 11 patients whose failed xenografts were examined

Patients			Pig aortic valve grafts				
						Microscopic appearance	
No.	Age	Sex	Duration (months)	Macroscopic appearance	Cells	Collagen reduction	Thrombus
1	20	F	2	*	Surface	+ +	Nil
2	56	F	3	*	+ + + Plasma Cells	+	Nil
3	23	F	4	*	Surface	+ +	+
4	59	F	4	*	Nil	+	+
5	49	M	4	*	Nil	+ +	+
6	25	M	9	*	Surface	+ Two cusps + + One cusp	+
7	43	F	12	*	Surface	+ +	+
8	42	M	12	*	Nil	+ +	+
9	18	F	13	*	Surface	+	+
10	40	F	14	*	Surface	+	Nil
11	58	M	32	*T	+ Plasma Cells	+	+

+ = Scanty, + + = moderate, + + + = numerous
* All cusps showed varying degrees of stretching with resultant valvular incompetence;
T = torn commissure.

A variable loss of the cuspal collagen was noted in each of the 11 valves. The collagen acquired an amorphous, hyaline or fibrinoid appearance and stained less intensely with the van Gieson stain. The fibrosa was often no longer distinguishable as a distinct layer within the cusp. An immune-mediated cellular response to the graft was noted in two valves only (cases 2 and 11). The pathology of valves which failed early (4 months or less after insertion) was the same as those failing later (after 9 months).

The cusps of unused control valves (Figures 7.1 and 7.2) meet together in a triradiate fashion with a wide area of apposition, and have clearly discernible valve pockets. The contact areas of the cusps lie in a vertical plane at a level superior to that of the sewing ring. The failed xenograft valves (Colour Plate N and Figure 7.3) had stretched cusps, which hung down below the level of the sewing ring and rendered the valve incompetent. In a few of the xenografts one cusp (often the one with muscle in its base) showed a greater degree of prolapse than did the other two.

The host cellular response in nine of the 11 cases consisted of scanty mononuclear cells at the base of the cusp, where it contacted the host tissue. There was no sign of a host immune response to the acellular, denatured collagen of the cusp in these nine valves. In the remaining two xenografts the cellular response was more florid (Figures 7.4a and 7.4b) and there were indications of a possible host immune response as evidenced by the presence of plasma cells and pyroninophilic lymphocytes migrating out from the base towards its free margin. The cellular infiltrate had eroded the cusp in areas.

None of the valves was infected or calcified. The cuspal elastic tissue and acid mucopolysaccharide appeared normal. Electron microscopy of unused, stent-mounted control pig valves revealed that the collagen fibres were poorly preserved, but their structural integrity appeared to be intact and most still

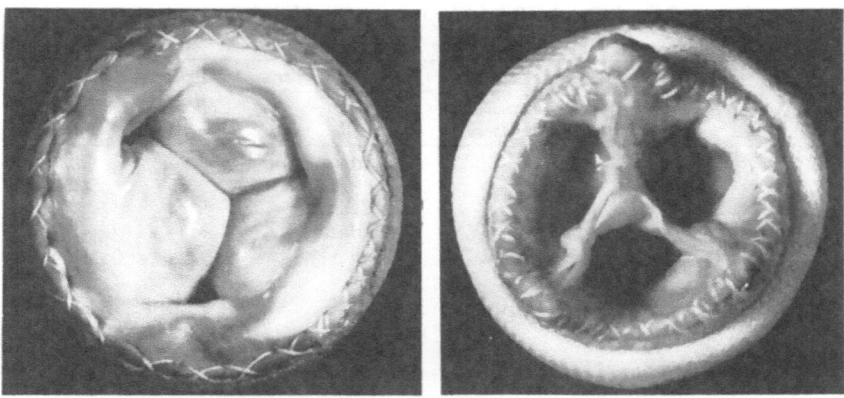

Fig. 7.1   Fig. 7.2

Figure 7.1 Inflow aspect of unused, stent-mounted, formaldehyde-treated porcine aortic valve xenograft prosthesis
Figure 7.2 Outflow aspect of the same formaldehyde-preserved porcine xenograft valve prosthesis seen in Figure 7.1, showing good cuspal apposition

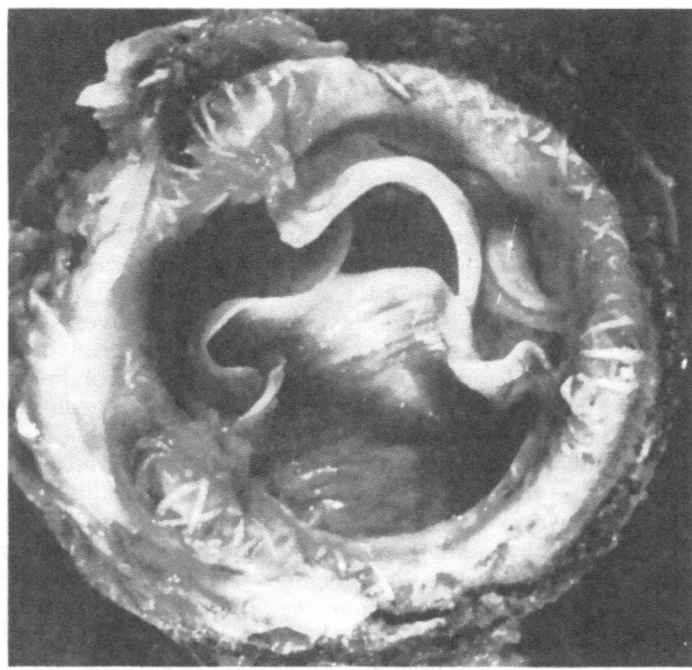

Figure 7.3 Explanted failed (incompetent) formaldehyde-preserved porcine xenograft valve showing downward prolapsing, stretched cusps

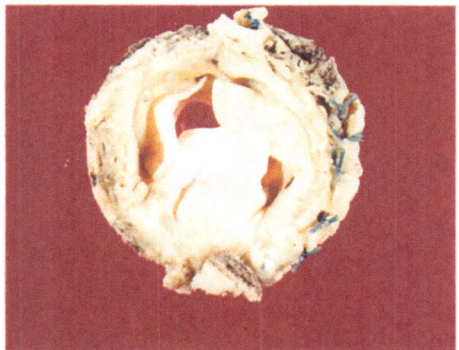

Plate N Stretching of the cusps has led to severe incompetence of this formaldehyde-preserved porcine aortic valve prosthesis, which is seen from the inflow aspect

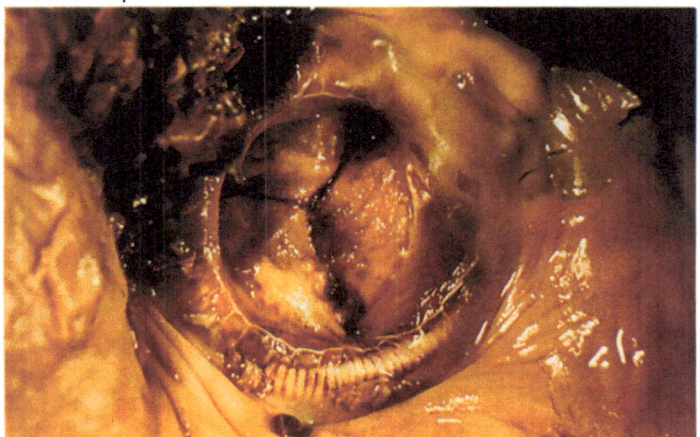

Plate O Left atrial aspect of severely calcified, stenotic Hancock mitral bioprosthesis. Left atrial thrombus is present too

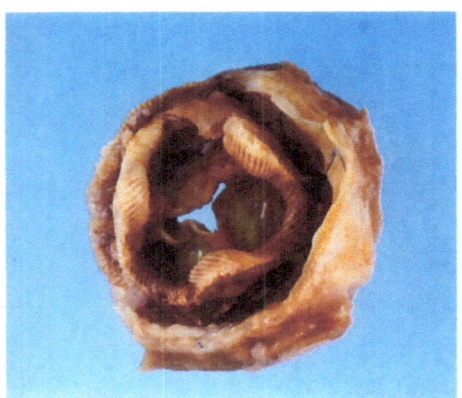

Plate P Inward stent bending due to 'polymer creep' in Hancock bioprosthesis

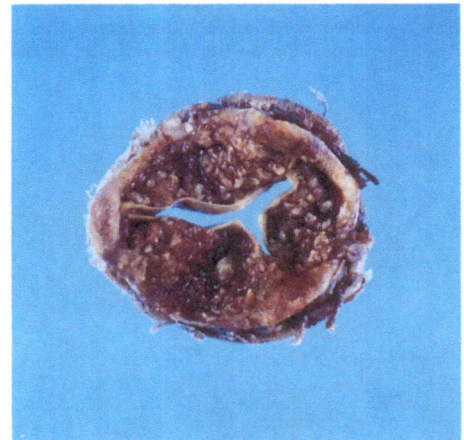

Plate Q Massive thrombotic deposits fill the cuspal pockets of a Carpentier–Edwards aortic valve prosthesis. The patient had received no anticoagulants in the early post-operative period

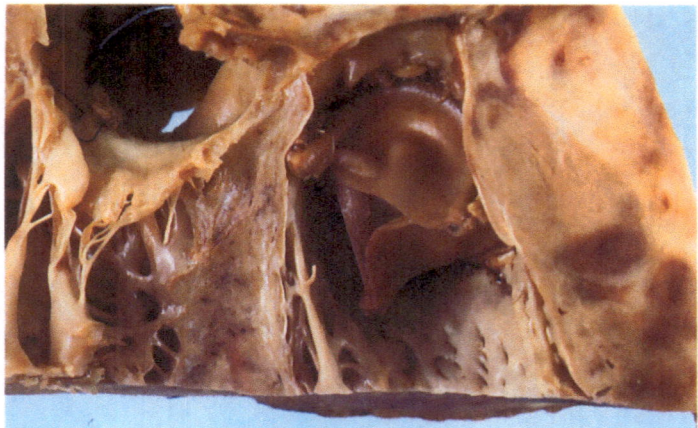

Plate R A sewing ring suture looped around a supporting post of an Ionescu–Shiley mitral bioprosthesis is producing some stenosis of the prosthesis. The supporting post is indenting the septal endocardium

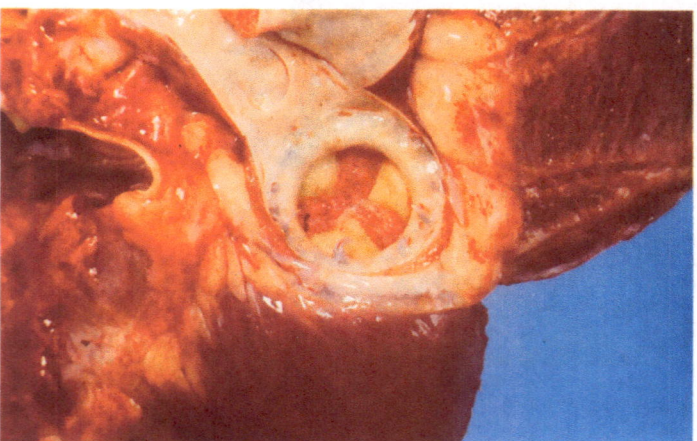

Plate S Mitroflow Medical mitral bioprosthesis implanted in a baboon heart shows a triradiate pattern of thrombus deposition on the inflow aspect of the valve

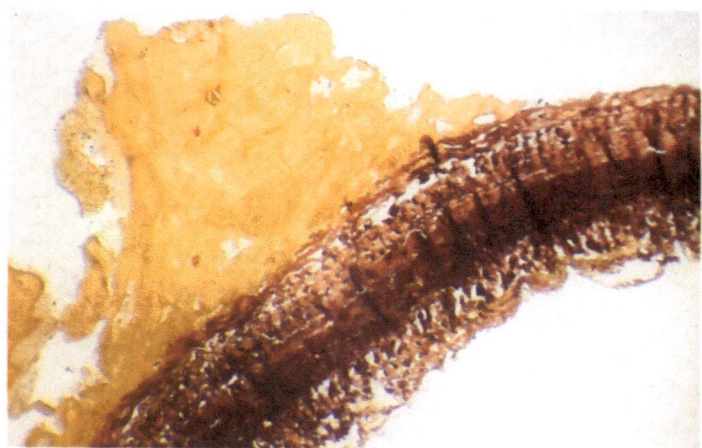

Plate T Histological appearance of bland thrombus on Mitroflow Medical valve. Elastic van Gieson, × 150

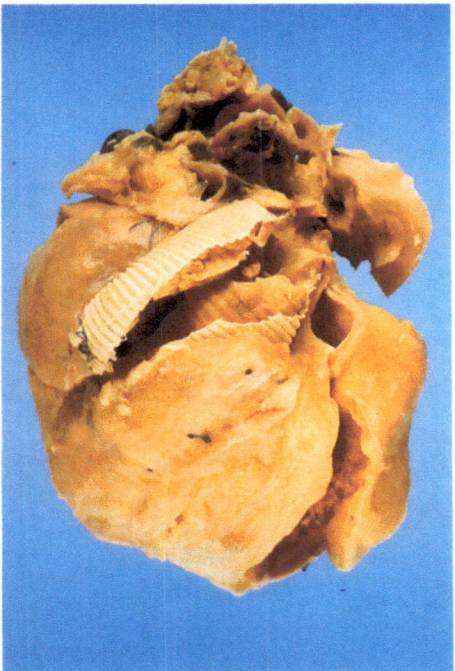

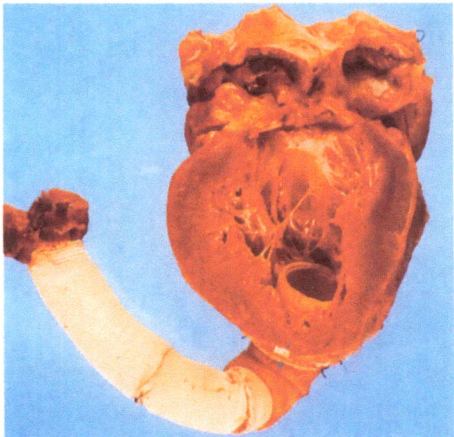

Plate V Tube graft links left ventricular apex to thoracic aorta. Death was due to rupture at the aortic anastomosis

Plate U Thrombus partially obstructs tubed conduit linking right ventricle to main pulmonary artery

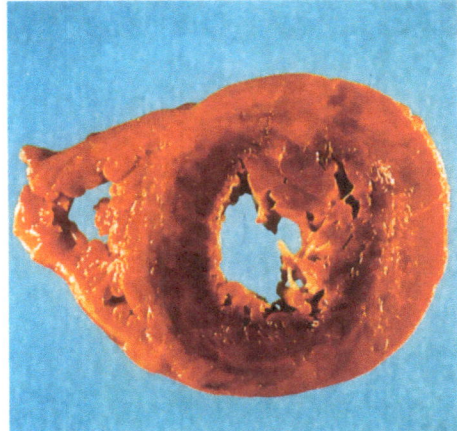

Plate X Concentric haemorrhagic necrosis of the left ventricle in a patient with a Starr–Edwards aortic valve prosthesis

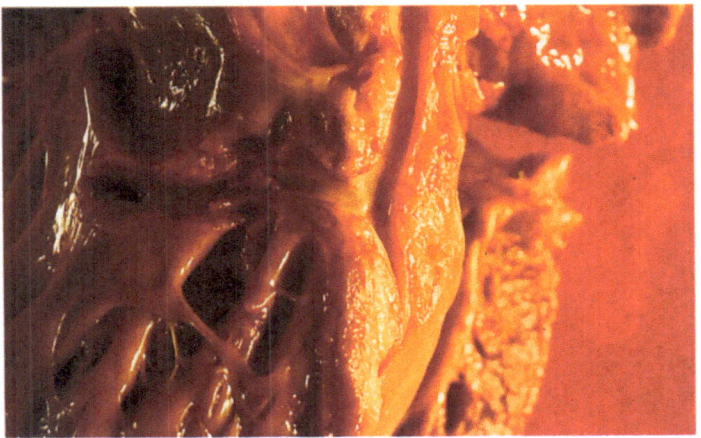

Plate W Thromboembolus lies within a septal perforator branch of the left anterior descending coronary artery. Such arteries are seldom examined at autopsy and may only be adequately assessed by postmortem coronary angiography.

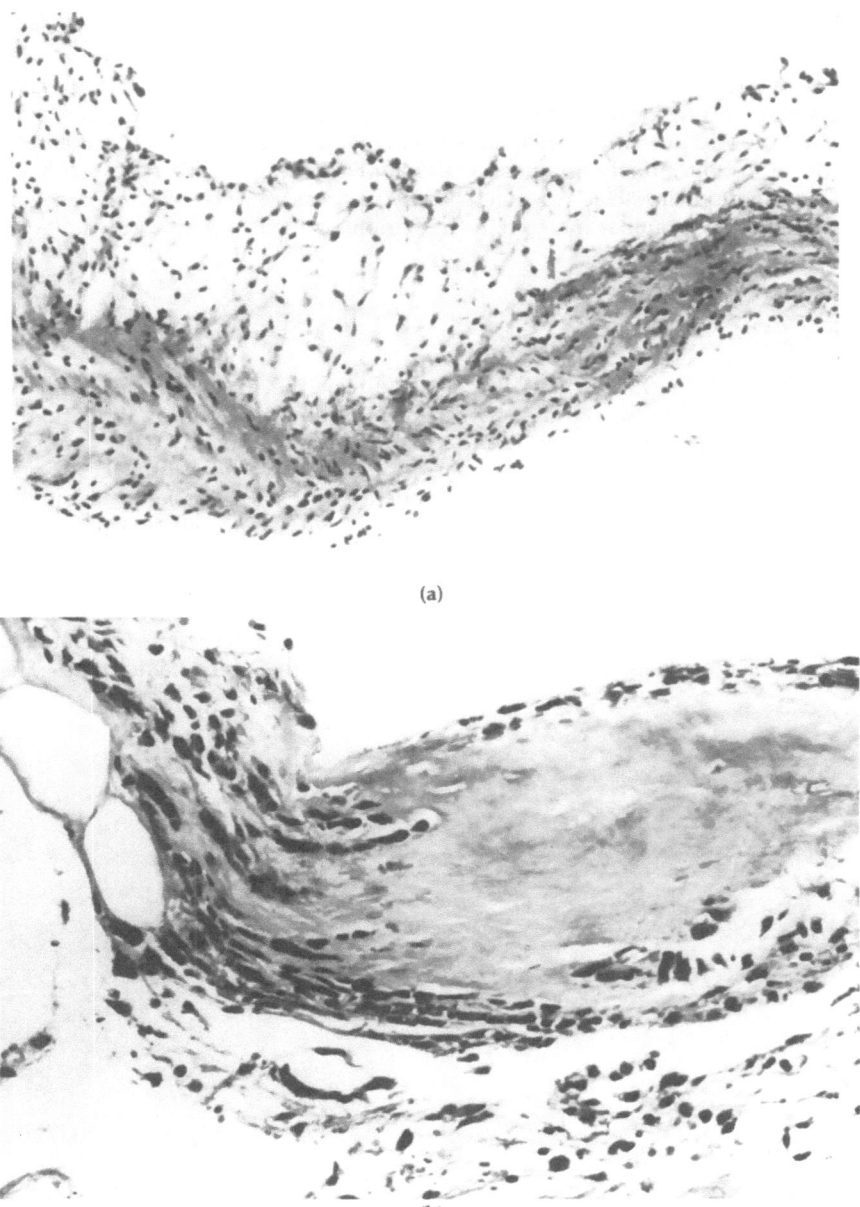

(a)

(b)

Figure 7.4 **(a)** Histology of cusp of an unused, formaldehyde-preserved porcine aortic valve xenograft prosthesis. The collagenous fibrosa constitutes the darker-stained layer. (Haematoxylin–eosin, × 150)
(b) Host cellular assault against fibrosa of formaldehyde-treated porcine aortic valve cusp. (Haematoxylin–eosin, × 150)

119

showed a regular periodicity (Figure 7.5). The collagen fibres of the xenograft valve of patient. 10 had an ultrastructural appearance similar to that of the controls. However, electron microscopy of the collagen present in the valve of patient 2 (one of the two valves eliciting an immune response) revealed that the poorly preserved collagen fibres in many areas seemed to disintegrate into amorphous, finely granular material (Figure 7.6). Few fibres showed residual periodicity. Electron microscopy of areas of total loss of collagen revealed finely granular material in the region normally occupied by collagen fibres.

Comment

Stretching of the valve cusps was the cause of the incompetence in all 11 failed aortic valve xenografts, with a torn commissure contributing to the regurgitation in one patient. Tearing of the substance of the cusps was not noted. A similar problem of stretching of aortic valve homograft cusps was encountered by Davies et al.[18]. My experience in these 11 patients[29] is similar to that of Wright et al.[30] and Stimmel et al.[31], who reported that implanted formalin-preserved porcine xenograft valves showed valvular insufficiency in 35% of cases within 1 year of operation because of tissue disruption.

While there are many instances, both physiological and pathological, in which collagen is rapidly destroyed[32-34], it appears unnecessary to postulate active collagenolysis of the cuspal collagen of the failed xenografts. The

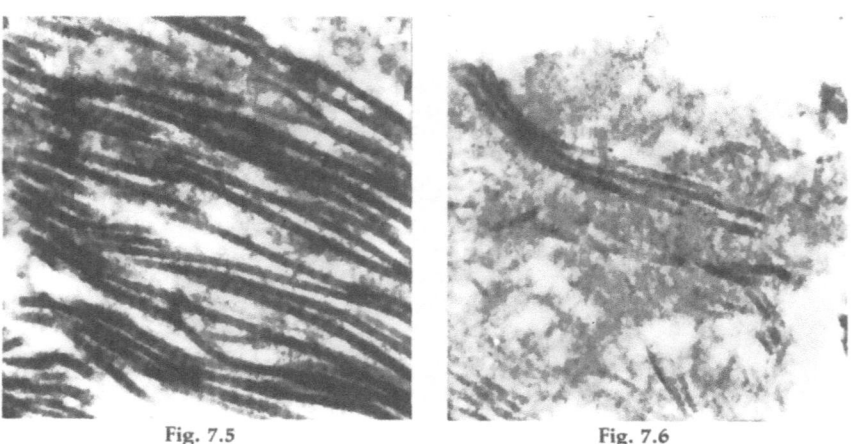

Fig. 7.5   Fig. 7.6

Figure 7.5   Transmission electron microscopy of an unused formaldehyde-preserved porcine aortic valve prosthesis shows mainly intact collagen fibres with regular periodicity. (Lead citrate and uranyl acetate, × 89 000)

Figure 7.6   Poorly preserved collagen fibres in cusp of a formaldehyde-preserved porcine aortic valve xenograft prosthesis, which had been implanted in a patient for 2 months. Periodicity is lacking and the fibres are disintegrating to yield amorphous, finely granular material. (Lead citrate and uranyl acetate, × 129 000)

inert and denatured collagen in the transplanted pig valve has a limited durability. No living cells are present within the valve substance, thus no new collagen can be produced. The breakdown of the valvular collagen, which is not prevented by the formaldehyde treatment, is a function of time, augmented perhaps by the increased mechanical stress that the valve is subjected to in the mitral position.

Ionescu et al.[35] postulated that calcification would be less prone to occur due to the low pH inside the formaldehyde-treated transplant. The absence of calcification in our xenografts appears to confirm this, but this finding may simply be due to their short duration. It is doubtful that the pH within the formalin-treated xenograft aortic valve cusps would remain low for many months, since the valve is in intimate contact with the circulating blood. Calcification has been frequently observed in aortic homografts transplanted in the fresh state[17].

Another possible explanation for the absence of calcification may be that formaldehyde acts as a tanning substance by combining readily with the epsilon-amino group of the lysine residues in collagen with the formation of a methylol compound[36]. These groups, which are important in tissue mineralization such as calcification, may thus be blocked by the action of the formaldehyde. As we shall see later (Chapter 8), cuspal calcification is a serious complication limiting the use of glutaraldehyde-treated xenografts in young persons.

The low incidence of an immune response in formaldehyde-treated xenograft valves is probably because the cuspal tissue is low in cell membrane elements, contains denatured protein and is a non-living graft. Collagen possesses a low antigenicity even if untreated. This premise has been borne out by cardiac transplantation in which the donor myocardium readily evokes a host rejection response, whilst the donor heart valves seldom stimulate rejection. Autograft, homograft and xenograft valves usually fail to evoke a destructive immunological or inflammatory response in the host.

Glutaraldehyde-treated porcine xenograft aortic valves

Carpentier prosthesis

Carpentier[37] showed that the durability of a preserved tissue valve depends upon its own structural integrity. The underlying concept of the porcine aortic valve was changed from that of a graft to that of a bioprosthesis, i.e. the tissues used to construct the valves are pretreated in such a way that they become non-antigenic and stable like a synthetic material. Unlike a graft, the durability of the bioprosthesis depends upon the stability of the biological material rather than host cell regeneration. Sodium metaperiodate oxidation of mucopolysaccharides and glycoproteins reduces antigenicity, and glutaraldehyde prevents collagen denaturation. The new glutaraldehyde-treated porcine aortic valve was first implanted by Carpentier in 1968 using an asymmetrical stent to support the muscular component of the right coronary cusp[38]. Unfortunately, Carpentier's first glutaraldehyde-treated xenografts were hampered by poor leaflet mobility and tissue fatigue due to the oxidation step in the tanning process[39].

Hancock glutaraldehyde-preserved porcine xenograft valve

Although formaldehyde is unsuitable for treatment of biological valves because it weakens the chemical cross-linkage bonds in collagen, glutaraldehyde enhances formation of collagen covalent cross-linkage bonds and increases tissue strength[40]. Following the promising results obtained by Carpentier's glutaraldehyde-treated xenograft valve, three glutaraldehyde-treated xenograft valves were made commercially available by Hancock Laboratories, American Edwards Laboratories and Shiley Incorporated.

These three companies manufacture the porcine bioprosthesis in a similar manner. Differences in techniques of tissue handling and valve mounting probably account for the main differences between these valve types[26,41]. In the case of the Hancock glutaraldehyde-treated xenograft valve (Figure 7.7), the Stellite and polypropylene stent has a symmetrical and uniform design. The stent is covered with Dacron. A 0.2% glutaraldehyde solution is used for pressure fixation of the valve in the closed position prior to suturing of

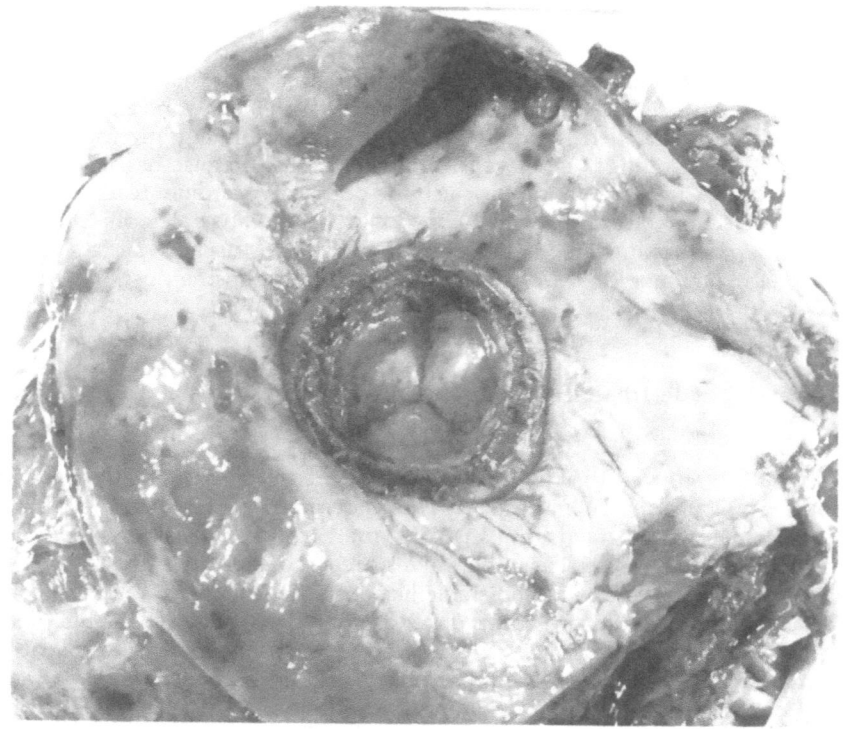

Figure 7.7 Opened left atrium showing Hancock porcine bioprosthesis in the mitral position. The patient's death was unrelated to the prosthesis

the valve (by continuous and interrupted sutures) to the cloth-covered, semi-flexible stent and for subsequent storage of the manufactured bioprosthesis. A silicone rubber (Silastic) insert within the Dacron cloth ring acts as a cushion to facilitate coaption of the bioprosthesis to the patient's valvular annulus. The prosthesis is radiolucent apart from the metallic ring in the base. The aortic prosthesis (model 242) and the atrioventricular valve (model 342) differ only in the shape of their sewing margins. Due to the obstructive effect within the stent of the muscular component to the porcine right coronary cusp, Hancock Laboratories produced a valve (model 250) in which this cusp was replaced by a non-muscular cusp. This yielded a composite prosthesis with a larger flow orifice.

Pathology of valve replacement with the Hancock porcine xenograft bioprosthesis
Seventy-one per cent of patients with Hancock valves implanted at Groote Schuur Hospital, Cape Town, between 1977 and 1982 inclusive were alive at 5–6 years after the operation, and 72% were free of significant embolism events.

Mitral valve replacement
Only eight patients with Hancock mitral valve bioprostheses were autopsied. Their mean age was 38.9 years (SD = 19.4 years) with a range of 16–63 years. Four patients were males. Mean postoperative survival was 95.4 days (SD = 171.1 days) with a range of 0-318 days. The principal causes of death in these patients are indicated in Table 7.2. One patient developed calcification of the xenograft prosthesis (Colour Plate O).

Only one of the eight Hancock prosthetic valves bore thrombi, which were situated on the atrial side of the sewing ring and between one stent of the prosthesis and the left ventricular wall.

Aortic valve replacement
A solitary autopsy patient had a Hancock aortic valve prosthesis. The patient, a 68-year-old male with aortic medionecrosis, had developed aortic incompetence due to ring dilatation and underwent successful aortic valve replacement with a Hancock prosthesis. Death 7.5 months after surgery was due to a ruptured dissecting aneurysm of the aorta. The Hancock prosthesis appeared normal.

Double valve replacement
Three patients had Hancock prostheses inserted in both the aortic and the mitral positions for rheumatic valvular disease. The first patient, a 22-year-old male, did not survive the operation, during which surgically induced

Table 7.2 Principal causes of death in eight patients with Hancock mitral valve prostheses

No cause found	3
Calcified Hancock xenograft	1
Poor preoperative condition	1
Unoperated severe aortic stenosis	1
Myocardial necrosis	1
Surgical disruption of valve ring	1

complete heart block followed insertion of the mitral prosthesis. At autopsy the Hancock valves were normal.

The second patient, a 37-year-old male, survived 13 days after surgery. The Hancock aortic valve was normal, but the mitral prosthesis was covered with abundant infected *(Staphylococcus aureus)* vegetations, which narrowed the effective orifice of the prosthesis by as much as 60%. Partial dehiscence had occurred where sewing ring sutures had torn free from the infected host tissue.

The third patient, a 21-year-old male, suffered severe acute myocardial ischaemia during cardiopulmonary bypass with coronary perfusion (? operative air embolism) and survived only 3 hours postoperatively. Autopsy revealed extensive biventricular myocyte necrosis. No significant coronary arterial disease was present. The Hancock prostheses appeared normal.

Principal causes of death in 12 patients with Hancock prostheses

The principal causes of death in the 12 patients with Hancock valve prostheses were as follows: due to error in preoperative diagnosis, 1; due to error in operative technique, 2; due to problems related to the prosthetic valve, 2; due to postoperative complications, nil; unrelated to the cardiac operation, 3; and cause unknown, 4. Prosthesis-related complications were the cause of only 17% of the 12 deaths, but the mean postoperative duration of the patients with implanted prostheses was only 83.5 days (SD = 149.2).

Comment

Many of the comments made here are equally applicable to other tissue valves. Cohn et al.[42] compared the Hancock porcine valve prosthesis with a prosthetic Harken discoid valve for isolated mitral valve replacement. They concluded that there is a significant reduction in morbidity and mortality, primarily from reduced thromboembolism, if a porcine valve is used for mitral replacement. They recommend that anticoagulants should be used in patients with atrial fibrillation and enlarged left atria regardless of the type of valve used. Stahmann et al.[43] reported a patient with transient cerebral ischaemic attacks due to release of thromboemboli from the worn stent cloth.

Unexplained primary thrombosis of a Hancock prosthesis has occasionally been encountered[44]. Pipkin et al.[45] reported that only one of six late deaths of patients with Hancock prostheses was due to a valve-related problem. Their actuarial analysis predicted 84% survival at 3 years. The Hancock valve appears capable of good function for at least 5–6 years[46–48]. Valve failure is more likely to be encountered in the mitral position. Zusman et al.[49] found that the Hancock modified orifice valve (model 250) has a good hydraulic performance and a low embolic rate without the need for anticoagulation. It may be used for the elderly patient with a small aortic root.

Several reports document structural changes in Hancock valve prostheses[50–53]. Spray and Roberts[51] observed the following histological changes in 44 bioprostheses: (a) fibrin deposits on the inflow and outflow surfaces of the cusps; (b) inflammatory cellular infiltrates; (c) histiocyte deposition; (d) giant cell formation and (e) focal disruption of the fibrocollagenous structure of the cusps. Their observations indicate that porcine bioprostheses are not biologically inert in the human circulation. Valve failure was rare up to the period of 72 months studied. Dysfunction of Hancock prosthetic valves due to degeneration, disruption and/or thrombosis has been documented by others[54,55]. Bortoloti et al.[56] reported two cases of late Hancock prosthetic stenosis due to fibrous tissue overgrowth on the atrial aspect of the cusps. Schoen et al.[57] described a patient with the carcinoid syndrome who had his mitral and tricuspid valves replaced by Hancock valve prostheses. He died 8 months later of tumour-related complications, and carcinoid plaques had extended onto both prostheses from the atria.

Regarding infective endocarditis of Hancock prostheses, Magilligan et al.[58] concluded that the Hancock porcine xenograft is (a) as resistant to infection as are rigid prostheses in active infective endocarditis; (b) resistant to early postoperative bacteraemias; and (c) easier to sterilize than rigid prostheses and more durable than other tissue valves (e.g. fascia lata, homograft or pericardial valves) in the face of prosthetic valve endocarditis.

Mycobacterium chelonei contamination of the Hancock porcine valve prosthesis occurred in a few lots manufactured between October 1975 and August 1976. Some patients developed endocarditis due to this latent infection[59]. Bortolotti et al.[60] studied 10 infected Hancock valves removed from nine patients. Causative organisms included Gram negative bacteria in three patients (*Klebsiella, Enterobacter* and *Serratia*), Gram-positive organisms in two patients (*Staphylococcus aureus* and *Streptococcus viridans*) and fungi in four (*Candida* in three and an *Aspergillus* species in one). Prosthetic incompetence was the commonest type of dysfunction resulting from the infection. The mortality of prosthetic valve endocarditis is very high, and a high incidence of infection-related deaths occurs when endocarditis involves porcine xenografts.

Salomon et al.[61] reported an unusual complication of the Hancock valve, namely strut compression by a too small aortic root resulting in the struts being angled centrally into the aortic lumen. Impedance of central flow had led to subsequent valve thrombosis. In a similar case reported by Magilligan et al.[62] the inward bending of the stents was associated with severe haemolysis. Inward stent-post bending (Colour Plate P) of a Hancock bioprosthesis may be due to 'polymer creep'[63], which is an ageing characteristic of polypropylene.

Arbustini et al.[52] described a case in which lipid infiltration of the cusps of a Hancock mitral valve prosthesis 8 years after implantation was so diffuse and severe that it, by itself, led to commissural detachment and significant valve incompetence. Histology revealed cholesterol clefts in the spongiosa and fibrosa, interspersed with amorphous material. Scanning electron microscopy showed erythrocytes, platelets and macrophages on the cuspal surface, which was partially devoid of endothelial cells. Transmission electron microscopy revealed large lipid droplets between bundles of collagen fibres.

Pre- and post-implantation ultrastructural changes in Hancock porcine valvular xenografts were described by Ferrans et al.[53]. Unimplanted, commercially available valves showed loss of endothelium and acid mucopolysaccharides. Short-term post-implantation changes included insudation of plasma proteins, penetration of erythrocytes into surface crevices, formation of a thin surface fibrin layer and deposition of macrophages, giant cells and a few platelets. Longer-term changes consisted of progressive disruption of collagen, erosion of the valvular surfaces, platelet deposition and accumulation of lipid. They concluded that progressive breakdown of collagen is a critical factor in the long-term durability of glutaraldehyde-treated porcine valvular xenografts.

Carpentier–Edwards glutaraldehyde-treated porcine xenograft valve

The first series of xenograft aortic valves produced by American Edwards Laboratories incorporated an oxidation step with sodium metaperiodate before glutaraldehyde fixation. This step was abandoned in the mid-1970s. The second series of valves was treated with glutaraldehyde alone. The first such valve was implanted by Dr Carpentier in March 1975 and the prosthesis was marketed from 1976.

The Carpentier–Edwards valve (Figure 7.8) is treated in a stronger glutaraldehyde solution (0.625% glutaraldehyde in phosphate buffered saline, pH 7.4) than is the Hancock valve[2,39]. The compliant metal stent consists of Elgiloy (an alloy of cobalt and nickel). A flat sheet of mylar is laser cut and sewn onto the wireform as a support for the cloth covering and the sewing ring. The entire stent (i.e. the supporting posts and base frame) is flexible. The inflow orifice is contoured to support the partly muscular, porcine right coronary cusp. The commissural supports are not equidistant and slant inwards at an angle to conform with the anatomical configuration of the porcine aortic valve. The asymmetry allows the use of a larger pig valve for a given stent diameter. The strength and flexibility of Elgiloy allows the use of a thinner metal frame, resulting in an improved orifice-to-annulus ratio[2] of 0.91 (compared to 0.76 for the Hancock valve).

The metal frame is covered with porous, knitted Teflon cloth to facilitate tissue invasion and encapsulation. The sewing ring consists of reemay and sponge rings, which are covered by Teflon cloth. As in the Hancock valve,

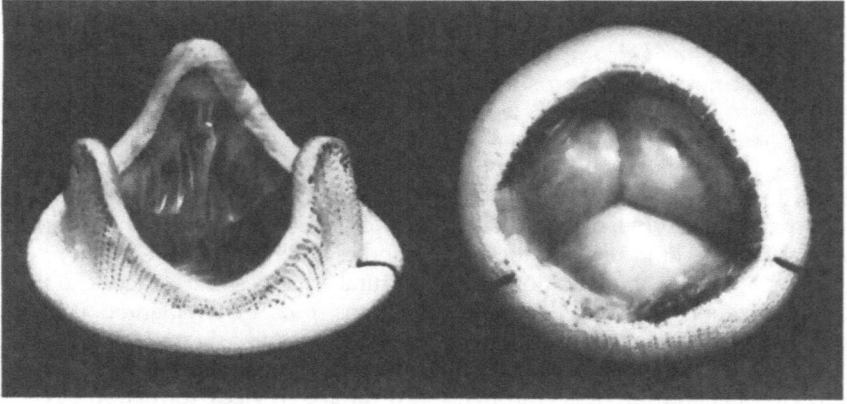

Figure 7.8 Carpentier–Edwards glutaraldehyde-treated porcine aortic valve xenograft prosthesis. (Picture courtesy of American Edwards Laboratories)

the compliant sewing ring allows coaption between the valve and an often irregular or calcified tissue bed. The pig valve is atttached to the stent by both interrupted and continuous sutures.

The models 2625 aortic and 6625 mitral Carpentier–Edwards bioprostheses have been used worldwide since March 1975. American Edwards Laboratories in November 1968[64] reported that 0.625% glutaraldehyde is an effective sterilizing agent against a wide variety of organisms including *Escherichia coli, Staphylococcus aureus, Streptococcus pyogenes, Candida albicans* and five species of mycobacteria. Only the mature spore of *Chaetomium globosum* was found to be resistant to 0.625% glutaraldehyde. Glutaraldehyde in concentrations of up to 10% proved to be ineffective against this organism's mature spore, but 4% formaldehyde killed the spores. Since glutaraldehyde-induced tissue cross-linkage is not reversed after short-term exposure to 4% formaldehyde, this step was added to the valve preparation as an additional sterilization precaution. The recent Carpentier–Edwards valves are thus treated with both glutaraldehyde and formaldehyde. Experiments with ^{14}C-labelled formaldehyde showed that formaldehyde is not incorporated into the protein structure of the valve.

The asymmetric design of the Carpentier–Edwards valve, plus the thinner sewing ring, provide better hydraulic function than the standard Hancock valve. However, the transvalvular gradients, especially in the small sizes, are still higher than those of mechanical valves.

Recently American Edwards Laboratories have introduced the Carpentier–Edwards SAV bioprosthesis that pairs low pressure fixation (< 4 mmHg) with a specially modified stent post composed of Mylar, which is flared between the commissures to accommodate the wider opening low-pressure fixed leaflets. This aims to reduce the risk of abrasion of the aortic valve leaflets against the stent. The Carpentier–Edwards SAV prosthesis has a 30% lower profile compared to the models 6625 and 2625 Carpentier–Edwards bioprostheses. Lower commissural supports aim to improve coronary artery flow in the aortic position and reduce the risk of ventricular perforation when implanted in the mitral position. An increase in the effective orifice area is aimed at in this valve, and the aortic sewing ring is specially designed for supra-annular placement. Clinical trials with this valve have been encouraging[65].

Pathology of cardiac valve replacement with the Carpentier–Edwards porcine xenograft bioprosthesis
At 5–6 years after implantation of a Carpentier–Edwards valve at Groote Schuur Hospital (years 1977 to 1982 inclusive) 74.5% of patients were alive, and 75% of these patients were clinically free of significant embolism.

Aortic valve replacement
Fifteen patients with isolated replacement of the aortic valve with a Carpentier–Edwards bioprosthesis were autopsied. Eleven patients died 30 days or less after operation (group 1) and only four died later (group 2).
Group 1. These 11 patients had a mean age of 57.8 years (SD = 11.9) and their ages ranged from 39 to 82 years. Postoperative survival ranged from

0.8 to 15 days, with a mean of 4.3 days (SD = 5.5). None of the 11 Carpentier–Edwards prostheses bore naked-eye thrombus.

Group 2. These four patients had a mean age of 43.7 years (SD = 14.2) and the range was 31–59 years. The mean postoperative survival period was 106.8 days (SD = 119.2) with a range of 35–285 days. The prostheses were all free of thrombus. Table 7.3 lists the principal causes of death in the 14 patients with Carpentier–Edwards aortic prostheses.

Histologically, the valve cusps of the prostheses in the group 1 patients showed well-preserved cuspal collagen with ghost outlines of pre-existing fibroblasts and scanty fibrin deposits on both aspects of the cusps. A few host monocytes and lymphocytes were attached to the cuspal surfaces. The four prostheses implanted in the group 2 patients also showed well-preserved collagen, but the cuspal collagen in the prosthesis of the longest survivor (who was murdered 285 days postoperatively) stained less intensely with the van Gieson stain. A few valve cusps contained scanty interstitial fibrin deposits, but there was no sign of calcification or of infection. All valves were devoid of endothelial cells and only an isolated host cell was attached to the cuspal surfaces. No intracuspal haematomas were seen.

Mitral valve replacement
Sixteen patients with Carpentier–Edwards mitral valve prostheses were autopsied. Twelve patients died 30 days or earlier postoperatively (group 1) and four survived longer (group 2).

Group 1. The 12 patients comprising this group had a mean age of 36.2 years (SD = 13.7) and an age range of 16–62 years. Their mean postoperative survival was 7.7 days (SD = 8.4) with a range of 0–30 days. Four of the 12 Carpentier–Edwards mitral prostheses bore scanty, non-obstructive thrombi (two on the sewing ring and two on the concave aspects of the cusps).

Histologically, all of the prosthetic cusps showed acellular, well-preserved collagen. Scanty focal, surface fibrin deposits were present on nearly all of the valves examined. No calcification was detected and none of the valves had elicited a foreign-body giant cell response. Electron microscopy of three randomly selected prostheses, which had been implanted for periods of 1 day, 8 days and 30 days, revealed normal-looking collagen fibres.

Table 7.3 Principal causes of death in five patients with Carpentier–Edwards aortic valve prostheses

Unknown	3
Prosthesis blocks coronary ostium	1
Operatively induced myocardial damage	2
Iatrogenic coronary dissection	1
Ruptured aortotomy wound	3
Cerebral haemorrhage	1
Mediastinal abscess	1
Myocardial failure	1
Myocardial infarction (atherosclerosis)	1
Traumatic death	1

Group 2. The four group 2 patients had a mean age of 33 years (SD = 32) with a range of 13–70 years. The mean postoperative survival was 1725 days (SD = 430) with a range of from 1170 to 2220 days. Two of the four prostheses showed surface thrombotic deposits; scanty fibrin-platelet deposits on the sewing ring in one patient and abundant similar thrombus filled the concavities of the three cusps in another. All four porcine valves had poorly preserved cuspal collagen. Focal fibrin deposits permeated the interstitium of the cusps and there appeared to be a total loss of acid mucopolysaccharide. No intracuspal haematomas were seen. Electron microscopy performed upon a porcine valve which had been implanted for 1740 days revealed evidence of focal dissolution of collagen fibres. Table 7.4 lists the principal causes of death in the 16 patients with Carpentier–Edwards mitral prostheses.

More than one Carpentier-Edwards valve prosthesis in the same heart

Seven patients with more than one Carpentier–Edwards prosthetic heart valve in the same heart were autopsied.

Group 1. Four of six patients who died less than 1 month postoperatively were males. The mean age of the six patients was 29 years (SD = 14.3) with a range of 14–51 years. Mean postoperative survival was 2.2 days (SD = 2.4) with a range of 0–6 days. One patient had both the aortic and the mitral valves replaced; three patients had their aortic, mitral and tricuspid valves replaced, and the remaining two patients had both their mitral and tricuspid valves replaced. None of the 15 prostheses showed macroscopical thrombus.

Histology showed similar features to those observed in the group 1 patients with Carpentier–Edwards aortic and mitral prostheses, described above. The cause of death was unknown in five patients, and one patient died of infected pulmonary infarcts.

Group 2. The single patient was a 14-year-old female who died suddenly while at school 391 days after replacement of her aortic and mitral valves because of chronic rheumatic heart disease. Autopsy revealed extensive calcification and stenosis of the mitral prosthesis. Scanty fibrin-platelet thrombi were noted on the concave (non-contact) aspects of both bioprostheses, but there was no evidence of calcification of the aortic prosthesis, which had been implanted at the same time as the mitral prosthesis.

Table 7.4 Principal causes of death (one per patient) in 16 patients with Carpentier–Edwards mitral valve prostheses

Unknown	6
Operative air embolism	1
Infection	1
Calcified xenograft	1
Cerebral thromboembolism	3
Cerebral haemorrhage	1
Mediastinitis, septicaemia	1
Myocardial failure	1
Suicide	1

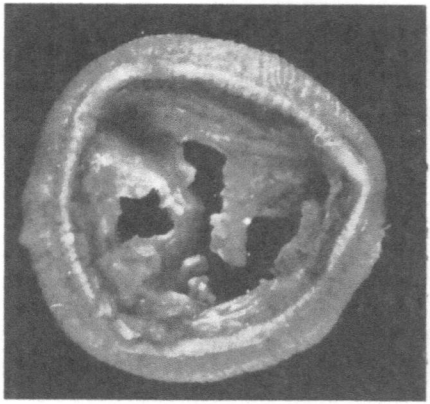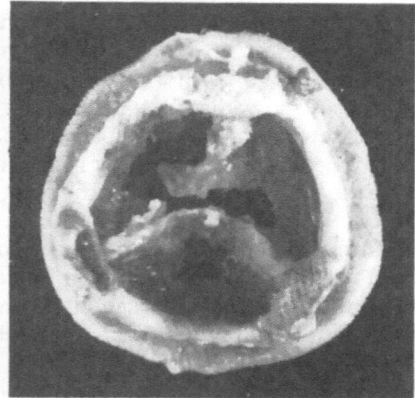

Figure 7.9 Inflow aspect *(left)* and outflow aspect *(right)* of Carpentier–Edwards bioprosthesis showing tears and holes in the substance of the cusps

Pathology of surgically resected Carpentier–Edwards valvular prostheses
Ten surgically removed Carpentier–Edwards valves were examined. Eight valves had been implanted in the mitral position, and two in the aortic position. The patients' ages ranged from 13 to 56 years at the time of initial operation, with a mean of 36 years (SD = 16). The prostheses had been implanted for periods ranging from 2 to 60 months (mean = 41 months). Five of the prosthetic valves were removed because of pure incompetence (Figures 7.9–7.11), one showed stenosis only, and two showed both stenosis and incompetence. Three of the five incompetent valves had tears near the commissures (type I lesion of Ishihara *et al.*[66]), and the other two had tears and/or holes (Figure 7.9) in the cuspal substance (types III and IV lesions of Ishihara *et al.*[66]). Three valves which showed cuspal calcification (Figure 7.10) had been implanted in three patients who were aged 13, 14 and 16 years at the time of their initial operation. Three other valves showed scanty surface fibrin deposits and one aortic prosthesis was removed 3 years after implantation, because of massive thrombosis (Colour Plate Q). The latter patient had received no anticoagulants postoperatively. One valve showed resolving infection of the cusps. In valves implanted for up to 36 months the collagen appeared histologically normal, but by 60 months there was a uniformly severe depletion of cuspal collagen.

Principal causes of death in all patients with Carpentier–Edwards porcine xenograft bioprostheses
The principal causes of death in the 38 patients with Carpentier–Edwards porcine aortic valve xenograft prostheses studied fell into the following categories: (a) error in preoperative diagnosis, nil; (b) error in operative technique, 5; (c) prosthesis-related problems, 9; (d) general postoperative complications, 6; (e) unrelated to cardiac operation, 4; and (f) unknown causes, 14.

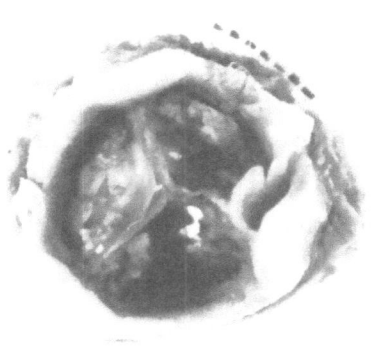 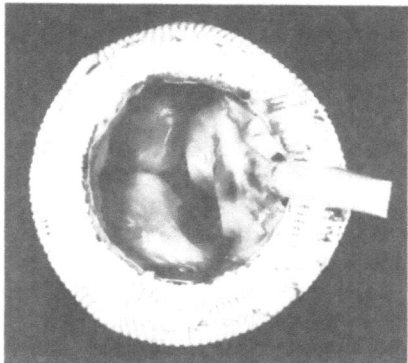

Fig. 7.10   Fig. 7.11

Figure 7.10 Calcified Carpentier–Edwards bioprosthesis. A small perforation is present in the substance of one cusp (bottom)
Figure 7.11 Probe indicates perforation at base of one cusp of non-calcified Carpentier–Edwards bioprosthesis

Comment

Between March 1975 and January 1978 an estimated 8000 Carpentier–Edwards bioprostheses were implanted worldwide and the following complications had been reported to the manufacturers, American Edwards Laboratories[67]: endocarditis 5, high gradient 5, thromboembolism 5, thrombosis 5, prosthetic calcification by the 17th postoperative day 1, periprosthetic leak 1, leaflet perforation 6 (related to handling with surgical instruments), haemolysis 1, regurgitation 2 (due to stent distortion produced by sutures, which spanned distances greater than 5 mm), miscellaneous 9 (e.g. sewing ring disruptions and loosening of tissue-to-stent suture line). In 1985 American Edwards Laboratories reported[68] on 355 patients with Carpentier–Edwards porcine bioprostheses followed up for an accumulative total of 1367 patient-years. Freedom from valve-related deaths was 97.3% (SD = 1.8) at 6 years, and freedom from all valve-related complications was 83.9% (SD = 4.9) at 6 years.

Haemodynamic studies[69] comparing Hancock and Carpentier–Edwards bioprostheses revealed that Carpentier–Edwards prostheses had significantly lower transvalvular gradients than the Hancock valves[70] and the differences in the design of bioprosthetic valves and that of natural valves are probably major factors in increasing the stress in the bioprostheses. Echocardiography has been useful in evaluating porcine aortic bioprostheses and detecting degeneration of such valves, vegetations, dehiscence and flail porcine valve leaflets.

Clinical experience with the Carpentier–Edwards porcine bioprosthesis indicated that it was a valid heart valve substitute[71,72]. Carpentier *et al.*[73] suggested that variations in histological structure and durability resulted in part from inadequate preservation of the valve during the shipping process and large variations in the intervals between harvesting and glutaraldehyde treatment, and in part too from high-pressure glutaraldehyde fixation. These authors expressed the hope that reduction of turbulence by the supra-annular concept and improved preservation of the valve would minimize the incidence of calcification.

Despite the low incidence of thromboembolic events in patients with tissue valves, there are a few reports of massive thrombosis in relation to Carpentier–Edwards prostheses[74,75]. In one of our patients[74], thrombosis (Colour Plate Q) involved the aortic valve prosthesis, but spared an identical type of prosthesis in the mitral position.

Angell and Angell[76] state that porcine valves undergo sterile degeneration 5–7 years postimplantation. Many of the degenerative changes are related to host reactivity, e.g. calcium deposition, and host phagocytic activity. The highest incidence of tissue failure occurs in young patients 6 years after implantation. Schoen et al.[77] noted that causes of valve failure included calcification-related cuspal tears, tears without calcium deposits, cuspal stiffening and thrombosis. Late primary dysfunction was most often due to degenerative processes, especially calcification, often with secondary tears. However, cuspal tears (without associated calcification or thombosis) predominated at shorter intervals. Warnes et al.[78] noted that later degenerative changes were more severe in bioprostheses in the mitral compared to the aortic position.

Excellent medium- and long-term results were obtained in older adults[79] in whom severe dysfunction occurred mainly with recurrent infective endocarditis. Thromboembolism occurred only in patients with mitral valve replacement, especially in those with atrial fibrillation, and if no anticoagulation was given. Sarabu and Parker[80] recorded an unusual functional abnormality of a porcine xenograft valve that may be difficult for a pathologist to detect on morphological examination alone. Two of their patients required reoperation because in each patient it was discovered that one of the cusps of the mitral prosthesis was in the fixed-open position with no evidence of a perivalvular leak. These authors presumed that the failure of the leaflet to close properly had been present from the operation.

Structural alterations in porcine xenografts described by Ashraf and Bloor[81] included fibrin deposits, erythrocyte trapping, disruption of the valve matrix, and interstitial oedema. Scanning electron microscopy demonstrated an absence of endothelial cells. Camilleri et al.[82] observed no significant evidence of tissue rejection in 29 xenograft bioprostheses which had been implanted for periods of up to 115 months. They emphasized three factors: (a) disruption of the endothelial cell barrier and lack of significant host endothelialization; (b) increased cuspal permeability, which favours calcification and lipid accumulation; (c) biodegradation of the collagen framework. Similar findings have been noted by others[83]. Cuspal perforations may be due to the abrasive effects of the cut ends of sewing ring sutures[84,85].

Forman et al.[86] correlated echocardiographic and pathological findings in malfunctioning porcine valves. Prolapse was associated with thinning of the leaflets, longitudinal tears close to the margin and acid mucopolysaccharide accumulation. Valve fracture was seen with and without prolapse, and consisted of small perforations or tears of the leaflet. A flail leaflet was seen with a linear tear of the free margin and was associated with calcific deposits.

Experimental evidence indicates that glutaraldehyde-preserved porcine heart valves are vulnerable to compressive flexure, which produces fatigue-induced damage, and this may limit long-term durability. Degenerative changes are more severe in the mitral than in the aortic valve position. This is probably related to the greater closing pressure that the mitral valve is subjected to. Spontaneous xenograft failure usually occurs in a progressive and gradual fashion, but occasionally acute, catastrophic, spontaneous xenograft failure has been encountered. Biodegradation of collagen is the commonest cause of failure, but occasionally manufacturing faults may be responsible, e.g. the case of Grehl et al.[87] in which two leaflets of a Carpentier–Edwards porcine xenograft valve tore away from the aortic wall.

Intracuspal haematomas[88] have been described in bioprosthetic valves implanted in the mitral position. The haematomas result from entry of blood into the space between the sewing ring and the most basilar region of the bioprosthetic tissue. This space extends along the entire circumference of the bioprosthesis and is continuous with the spongiosa in which the haematoma develops. Intracuspal haematomas were not found in porcine valvular prostheses mounted on aortic-type stents, in which the sutures are more protected and more closely spaced, or in bioprostheses made of tissues (e.g. pericardium or dura mater), which lack a spongiosa.

Glutaraldehyde-preserved porcine xenograft valves may become infected. Ferrans et al.[89] reported four cases and reviewed another 43 cases in the literature, including several patients with Hancock xenograft bioprostheses. They concluded that infection in such valves: (a) develops in the fibrin layer that covers the cusps; (b) can involve the cuspal collagen and (c) is rarely associated with valve ring abscesses. Considerable destruction of prosthetic tissue can result from the infection. Downham and Rhoades[90] encountered six patients with infective endocarditis associated with porcine valve xenografts. The infection was fatal in four of the patients. A nosocomial ocurrence was suggested by the fact that Staphylococcus epidermidis was the causative organism in all six patients.

The role and timing of surgical intervention after diagnosis of prosthetic valve endocarditis is not settled. However, early aggressive replacement of infected artificial valves appears to be an integral part of the therapy[91]. It has been shown that porcine valves can be used successfully to replace previously infected ones. Magilligan et al.[92] were able to cure porcine valve infective endocarditis readily with antimicrobial therapy alone. The main features of the patients cured by antibiotics alone include infection by streptococci, normal echocardiograms and normal haemodynamic function of the affected valve prosthesis. Those who died, or who required surgery, had more aggressive bacterial or fungal infections, thickening of the bioprosthetic leaflets or masses present on echocardiography, and severe transprosthetic gradients at cardiac catheterization. Obstruction of an infected bioprosthesis is a sign that the endocarditis cannot be cured by medical treatment alone.

Angell—Shiley valve

Dr W. W. Angell and co-workers started making glutaraldehyde-treated porcine aortic valve xenografts in 1970. In 1975 Shiley Incorporated marketed the Angell—Shiley xenograft valve. These valves were treated with 0.5% glutaraldehyde and had a flexible stent made of Delrin, which was totally covered by Dacron cloth. The stent has an anatomic design derived from castings of the most frequent porcine aortic valve configurations[93]. Each pig valve is matched to one of 70 different anatomic stent configurations, which vary in shape and size. This provides a natural position and support for the valve. The resulting annular sewing rim is not circular in shape and thus the orificial area of the bare stent is a calculated quantity.

Low-profile bioprosthesis

This low-profile, glutaraldehyde-fixed porcine aortic valve is produced by Cientifica Argentina of Buenos Aires, Argentina. Navia *et al.*[94] studied the hydraulic and haemodynamic features of this valve in 316 patients. In a later report Navia *et al.*[95] stated that the probability of freedom from embolism of the new flexible stent series at 48 months was 91% for mitral valve replacement and 93% for aortic valve replacement.

Xenomedica bioprosthesis

Gallo *et al.*[96] have reported disappointing results with this glutaraldehyde-preserved porcine xenograft. The mitral prostheses frequently became incompetent and also had high transvalvular gradients.

Tascon bioprosthesis

Tascon Medical Technology manufactures the Tascon heart valve bioprosthesis, which is composed of two components; namely a porcine aortic valve mounted in a Dacron-covered Elgiloy stent, and a separate sewing ring. The two components are connected by a plastic-threaded locking mechanism.

The dry, sterile sewing ring can be immediately sewn into the valve annulus. The valve-stent component is stored in a glutaraldehyde solution and has to be rinsed prior to insertion. The valve has been tested in animals by the manufacturers, and clinical trials were started in February 1984.

AUTOLOGOUS FASCIA LATA VALVE

Professor A. Senning[97] of Switzerland, in 1962 first implanted an unstented aortic valve prosthesis fabricated from fascia lata. While the patient was on cardiopulmonary bypass a strip of fascia was taken from the patient's thigh, cleaned and tailored to size. The strip was sutured into the aortic root using continuous sutures and the commissures were attached to the aortic wall by separate, Teflon-felt anchored sutures. Senning's favourable experience with such a valve stimulated others[98,99] to produce a series of stent-mounted fascia lata prostheses for use in the aortic, mitral, tricuspid and pulmonary positions. The early results showed a low rate of thromboembolism.

This encouraged many surgeons worldwide to implant home-made autologous fascia lata valves (Figure 7.12). Accumulating data soon began to sound a cautionary note regarding the durability and lack of thrombogenicity of the fascia lata valve. Such valves gave disastrous results when used in the mitral and tricuspid position[100,101] due to severe regurgitation. Within 3 years after implantation 90% of mitral valves and 20% of aortic valves had failed[2]. Removed valves often showed leaflet shrinkage, retraction and loss of mobility due to overgrowth by host tissue[102]. This type of valve is no longer used.

DURA MATER HOMOGRAFT VALVE

The external aspect of the dura mater has a smooth, shiny surface and the internal aspect is covered by a layer of arachnoidal endothelial cells. Since the dural double collagen layer has the collagen bundles arranged at right

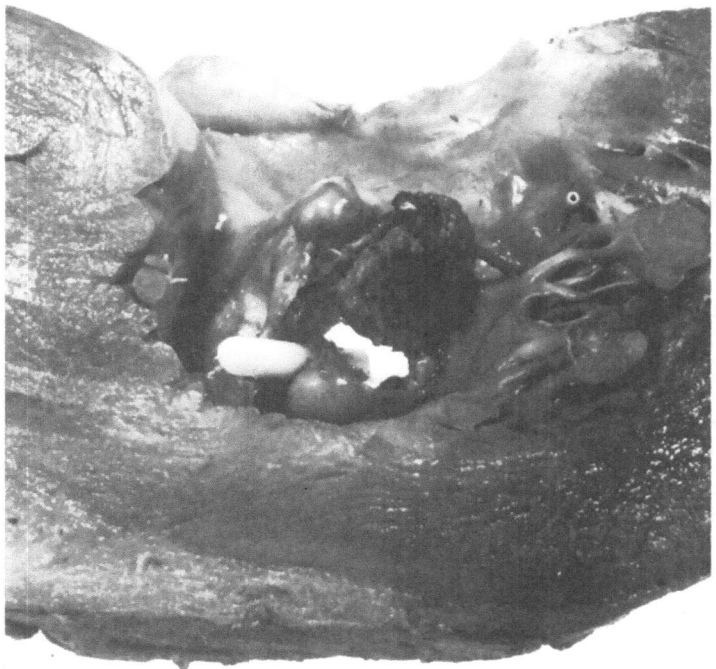

Figure 7.12 Infected autologous fascia lata valve prosthesis. A pin holds up a torn, infected cusp and a plastic probe passes through a perforation in another cusp

angles to each other it is stronger than fascia lata, in which there is only a single layer of collagen fibres arranged in parallel. The failure of the fascia lata valve led to attempts to fashion a valve from dura mater. This form of prosthesis was pioneered by Professor E. J. Zerbini and colleagues in Brazil[103,104].

Dura mater was obtained within 20 hours after traumatic death from human cadavers aged between 10 and 50 years. Cases of infective or degenerative diseases, as well as neoplasia, were excluded. The dura mater was removed at autopsy using sterile gloves and instruments. Thereafter it was washed for 1–2 hours in flowing water and then placed in a sterile container filled with 98% glycerol at room temperature for 10–20 days. At the end of this time a sample of the dura was cultured bacteriologically.

Before valve construction the tissue was rehydrated in sterile physiological saline and the valves were then fashioned under sterile conditions. The leaflets were separately cut from the dura selecting areas with a similar texture, thickness and vascularity. The separate cusps were mounted on a Dacron velour-covered, rigid, stainless steel stent and attached to each other by interrupted sutures augmented by Teflon strips. The dura mater was mounted on the outside of the struts with retention of the full central orifice. Completed prostheses were stored at 4°C in an antibiotic solution[2]. The radiopaque stent was readily recognizable on X-ray.

The dura mater valve has a low incidence of thromboembolism without anticoagulation[2]. Procurement of dura mater is a problem outside large metropolitan areas, where trauma victims are less plentiful. Sterility is another important problem, since glycerol is of dubious efficacy in this regard. The valve has shown a moderately high rate of early and late re-operation. Several reports[105–107] document the later history of the dura mater bioprosthesis, which is no longer used.

REFERENCES

1. Angell, W. W., Buch, W. S. and Shumway, N. E. (1972). The viable aortic homograft. In Ionescu, M. I., Ross, D. N. and Wooler, G. H. (eds) *Biological Tissue in Heart Valve Replacement.* p. 383 (London: Butterworths)
2. Lefrak, E. A. and Starr, A. (1979). *Cardiac Valve Prostheses.* (New York: Appleton-Century-Crofts)
3. Ross, D. N. (1962). Homograft replacement of the aortic valve. *Lancet,* **2,** 487
4. Baratt-Boyes, B. G. (1964). Homograft aortic valve replacement in aortic incompetence and stenosis. *Thorax,* **19,** 131
5. Heimbecker, R. A., Aldridge, H. E. and Lemire, G. (1968). The durability and fate of aortic valve grafts. An experimental study with long term follow-up of clinical patients. *J. Cardiovasc. Surg.,* **9,** 511
6. Baratt-Boyes, B. G. (1979). Cardiac surgery in the antipodes. *J. Thorac. Cardiovasc. Surg.,* **73,** 804
7. Angell, W. W., Angell, J. D. and Sywak, A. (1977). The tissue valve as a superior cardiac valve replacement. *Surgery,* **82,** 875
8. Bonchek, L. I. (1981). Current status of cardiac valve replacement: selection of a prosthesis and indications for operation. *Am. Heart J.,* **101,** 96
9. Angell, W. W., Wuerflein, R. D. and Shumway, N. E. (1967). Mitral valve replacement

with the fresh aortic valve homograft: experimental results and clinical application. *Surgery*, **62**, 807

10. Welch, W. (1969). A comparative study of different methods of processing aortic homografts. *Thorax*, **24**, 746

11. Angell, W. W., Angell, J. D. and Kosek, J. C. (1979). Clinical and experimental comparisons establishing the glutaraldehyde treated xenograft as the standard for tissue heart valve replacement. In Ionescu, M. I. (ed.) *Tissue Heart Valves*. p. 89. (London: Butterworths)

12. Buch, W. S., Kosek, J. C. and Angell, W. W. (1971). The role of rejection and mechanical trauma on valve graft viability. *J. Thorac. Cardiovasc. Surg.*, **62**, 696

13. Gavin, J. B., Herdson, P. B., Munro, J. L. and Baratt-Boyes, B. G. (1973). Pathology of antibiotic-treated human heart valve allografts. *Thorax*, **28**, 473

14. Wheatley, D. J. and McGregor, C. G. A. (1977). Post implantation viability in canine allograft heart valves. *Cardiovasc. Res.*, **11**, 78

15. Heng, M. K., Barratt-Boyes, B. G., Agnew, T. M., Brandt, P. W. T., Kerr, A. R. and Graham, K. J. (1977). Isolated mitral replacement with stent-mounted antibiotic-treated aortic allograft valves. *J. Thorac. Cardiovasc. Surg.*, **74**, 230

16. Somerville, J., Ross, D. N. and Ross, J. K. (1972). Mitral valve replacement with stored inverted pulmonary homograft valve. *Thorax*, **27**, 583

17. Smith, J. C. (1967). The pathology of the human aortic valve homograft. *Thorax*, **22**, 114

18. Davies, H., Missen, G. A. K., Blandford, G., Roberts, C. I., Lessof, M. H. and Ross, D. N. (1968). Homograft replacement of the aortic valve. *Am. J. Cardiol.*, **22**, 195

19. Aparicio, S. R., Donnelly, R. J., Dexter, F. and Dexter, D. A. (1975). Light and electron microscopy studies on homograft and heterograft heart valves. *J. Pathol.*, **115**, 147

20. Hudson, R. E. B. (1966). Pathology of the human aortic valve homograft. *Br. Heart J.*, **28**, 291

21. Duran, C. G. and Gunning, A. J. (1965). Heterologous aortic-valve transplantation in the dog. *Lancet*, **2**, 114

22. Binet, J. P., Duran, C. G., Carpentier, A. *et al.* (1965). Heterologous aortic valve transplantation. *Lancet*, **2**, 1275

23. Halseth, W. L., Nellis, N., Fraser, R. E., Thompson, R. G. and Paton, B. C. (1966). Heterotransplantation of the aortic valve into the descending aorta. (Abstract). *Circulation*, **33,34** (Suppl. 3), III-120

24. Sweatt, J. L., Allen, C. F., Kwong, K-H. and Paton, B. C. (1970). Influence of preparation and immunosuppression upon longevity of grafted aortic valves. *Arch. Surg.*, **101**, 658

25. Drury, P. J., Olsen, E. G. J. and Ross, D. N. (1982). Morphological assessment of sucrose preservation for porcine heart valves. *Thorax*, **37**, 466

26. Binet, J. P., Duran, C. G., Carpentier, A. and Langlois, J. (1965). Heterologous aortic valve transplantation. *Lancet*, **2**, 1275

27. Buch, W. S., Kosek, J. and Angell, W. W. (1970). Deterioration of formalin treated aortic valve heterografts. *J. Thorac. Cardiovasc. Surg.*, **60**, 673

28. Byrne, J. P., Behrendt, D. M., Kirsh, M. M. and Orringer, M. B. (1977). Replacement of heart valves by prosthetic devices. In Joachim, H. L. (ed.) *Pathobiology Annual*. Vol. 7. p. 83. (New York: Appleton-Century-Crofts)

29. Rose, A. G. (1972). Pathology of the formalin-treated heterograft porcine aortic valve in the mitral position. *Thorax*, **27**, 401

30. Wright, J. A., Stacey, R. and Horton, N. A. (1971). Heterograft mitral and tricuspid valve replacement in a review of seven grafts. *Med. J. Aust.*, **2**, 852

31. Stimmel, B., Stein, E., Katz, A., Litwak, R. S. and Donoso, E. (1972). Phonocardiographic manifestations of heterograft valve dysfunction in the mitral area. *Br. Heart J.*, **34**, 936

32. Perez-Tamayo, R. (1970). Collagen resorption in carrageenin granulomas. II: Ultrastructure of collagen resorption. *Lab. Invest.*, **22**, 142

33. Montfort, I. and Perez-Tamayo, R. (1961). Studies on uterine collagen during pregnancy and puerperium. *Lab. Invest.*, **10**, 1240

34. Lazarus, G. S., Daniels, J. R., Brown, R. S. *et al.* (1968). Degradation of collagen by a human granulocyte collagenolytic system. *J. Clin. Invest.*, **47**, 2622

35. Ionescu, M. I., Wooler, G. H., Whitaker, W., Smith, D. R., Taylor, S. H. and Hargreaves, M. D. (1968). Heart valve replacement with reinforced aortic heterografts. *J. Thorac. Cardiovasc. Surg.*, **56**, 333

36. Hall, D. A. (ed.) (1964). *International Review of Connective Tissue Research.* Vol. 2. p. 293. (New York: Academic Press)

37. Carpentier, A. (1971). Principles of tissue valve transplantation. In Ionescu, M. I., Ross, D. N. and Wooler, G. H. (eds) *Biological Tissue in Heart Valve Replacement.* p. 49. (London: Butterworths)

38. Carpentier, A., Lamaigre, C. G., Robert, L., Carpentier, S. and DuBost, C. (1969). Biological factors affecting long-term results of valvular heterografts. *J. Thorac. Cardiovasc. Surg.,* **58,** 467

39. Carpentier, A., Deloche, A., Relland, J., Fabiani, J. N., Forman, J., Camilleri, J. P., Soyer, R. and DuBost, C. (1974). Six-year follow-up of glutaraldehyde-preserved heterografts with particular reference to the treatment of congenital valve malformations. *J. Thorac. Cardiovasc. Surg.,* **68,** 771

40. Bonchek, L. I. (1981). Current status of cardiac valve replacement: selection of a prosthesis and indications for operation. *Am. Heart J.,* **101,** 96

41. *Carpentier–Edwards Bioprosthesis: Clinical Report.* American Edwards Laboratories. January 1985. Santa Ana, California

42. Cohn, L. H., Sanders, J. H. and Collins, J. J. (1981). Actuarial comparison of Hancock porcine and prosthetic disc valves for isolated mitral valve replacement. *Circulation,* **54,** (Suppl. 3), III-60

43. Stahmann, F., Knott, H. W. and Doty, D. B. (1979). Transient cerebral ischemic attacks associated with worn porcine heterograft prosthesis. Case report. *J. Thorac. Cardiovasc. Surg.,* **77,** 872

44. Croft, C. H., Buja, L. M., Floresca, M. Z., Nicod, P. and Estrera, A. (1986). Late thrombotic obstruction of aortic porcine bioprostheses. *Am. J. Cardiol.,* **57,** 355

45. Pipkin, R. D., Buch, W. S. and Fogarty, T. J. (1976). Evaluation of aortic valve replacement with a porcine xenograft without long-term anticoagulation. *J. Thorac. Cardiovasc. Surg.,* **71,** 179

46. Cohn, L. H., Koster, J. K., Mee, R. B. B. and Collins, J. J. (1979). Long-term follow-up of the Hancock bioprosthetic heart valve. A 6-year review. *Circulation,* **60** (Suppl. 1), I-87

47. Casarotto, D., Bortolotti, U., Thiene, G., Galluci, V. and Cevese, P. G. (1979). Long-term results (from 5 to 7 years) with the Hancock S-G-P bioprosthesis. *J. Cardiovasc. Surg.,* **20,** 399

48. Gallo, J. I., Ruiz, B., Carrion, M. F., Gutierrez, J. A., Vega, J. L. and Duran, C. M. G. (1981). Heart valve replacement with the Hancock bioprosthesis: a 6-year review. *Ann. Thorac. Surg.,* **31,** 444

49. Zusman, D. R., Levine, F. H., Carter, J. E. and Buckley, M. J. (1981). Hemodynamic and clinical evaluation of the Hancock modified-orifice aortic bioprosthesis. *Circulation,* **64** (Suppl. 2), II-189

50. Bolooki, H., Mallon, S., Kaiser, G. A., Thurer, R. J. and Kieval, J. (1983). Failure of Hancock xenograft valve: importance of valve position (4- to 9-year follow-up). *Ann. Thorac. Surg.,* **36,** 246

51. Spray, T. L. and Roberts, W. C. (1977). Structural changes in porcine xenografts used as substitute cardiac valves. Gross and histologic observations in 51 glutaraldehyde-preserved Hancock valves in 41 patients. *Am. J. Cardiol.,* **40,** 319

52. Arbustini, E., Bortolotti, U., Valente, M. *et al.* (1982). Cusp disruption by massive lipid infiltration. A rare cause of porcine valve dysfunction. *J. Thorac. Cardiovasc. Surg.,* **84,** 738

53. Ferrans, V. J., Spray, T. L., Billingham, M. E. and Roberts, W. C. (1977). Ultrastructure of Hancock porcine valvular heterografts. Pre- and post-implantation changes. *Circulation,* **58** (Suppl. 1), I-10

54. Hetzer, R., Hill, J. D., Kerth, W. J., Wilson, A. J., Adappa, M. G. and Gerbode, F. (1978). Thrombosis and degeneration of Hancock valves: clinical and pathological findings. *Ann. Thorac. Surg.,* **26,** 317

55. Brown, J. W., Dunn, J. M., Spooner, E. and Kirsh, M. M. (1978). Late spontaneous disruption of a porcine xenograft mitral valve. Clinical, hemodynamic, echocardiographic, and pathological findings. *J. Thorac. Cardiovasc. Surg.,* **75,** 606

56. Bortolotti, U., Galluci, V. and Casarotto, D. (1979). Fibrous tissue overgrowth on Hancock mitral xenografts: a cause of late prosthetic stenosis. *Thorac. Cardiovasc. Surg.*, **27**, 316
57. Schoen, F. J., Hausner, R. J., Howell, J. F., Beazley, H. L. and Titus, J. L. (1981). Porcine heterograft valve replacement in carcinoid heart disease. *J. Thorac. Cardiovasc. Surg.*, **81**, 100
58. Magilligan, D. J., Quinn, E. L. and Davila, J. C. (1977). Bacteremia, endocarditis and the Hancock valve. *Ann. Thorac. Surg.*, **24**, 508
59. Rumisek, J. D., Albus, R. A. and Clark, J. S. (1985). Late Mycobacterium chelonei bioprosthetic valve endocarditis: activation of implanted contaminant? *Ann. Thorac. Surg.*, **39**, 277
60. Bortolotti, U., Thiene, G., Milano, A., Panizzon, G., Valente, M. and Galluci, V. (1981). Pathological study of infective endocarditis on Hancock porcine bioprostheses. *J. Thorac Cardiovasc. Surg.*, **81**, 934
61. Salomon, N. W., Copeland, J. G., Goldman, S. and Larson, D. F. (1979). Unusual complication of the Hancock porcine heterograft: strut compression in the aortic root. *J. Thorac. Cardiovasc. Surg.*, **77**, 294
62. Magilligan, D. J., Fisher, E. and Alam, M. (1980). Hemolytic anemia with porcine xenograft aortic and mitral valves. *J. Thorac. Cardiovasc. Surg.*, **79**, 628
63. Schoen, F. J., Schulman, L. J. and Cohn, L. H. (1985). Quantitative analysis of 'stent creep' of explanted Hancock standard porcine bioprostheses used for cardiac valve replacement. *Am. J. Cardiol.*, **56**, 110
64. *Edwards Laboratories Data Sheet*, November 1978. Microbiology and biochemistry data associated with the Carpentier–Edwards bioprosthesis. Edwards Laboratories, Santa Ana, California.
65. Carpentier, A., Dubost, C., Lane, E. *et al.* (1982). Continuing improvements in valvular bioprostheses. *J. Thorac. Cardiovasc. Surg.*, **83**, 27
66. Ishihara, T., Ferrans, V. J., Boyce, S. W., Jones, M. and Roberts, W. C. (1981). Structure and classification of cuspal tears and perforations in porcine bioprosthetic cardiac valves implanted in patients. *Am. J. Cardiol*, **48**, 665
67. Clinical Report. *Summary of Clinical Results with the Model No. 6625 and Model 2625 Carpentier–Edwards Bioprostheses, July 1978.* American Edwards Laboratories, Santa Ana, California
68. Clinical Report. *Carpentier–Edwards Bioprosthesis, January 1985.* American Edwards Laboratories. Santa Ana, California.
69. Navia, J. A., Haller, J. D., Gimenez, C. *et al.* (1982). Low profile bioprosthesis for cardiac valve replacement: hydraulic and hemodynamic studies. *Med. Instr.* **16**, 57
70. Levine, F. H., Carter, J. E., Buckley, M. J. *et al.* (1981). Hemodynamic evaluation of Hancock and Carpentier–Edwards bioprostheses. *Circulation*, **64** (Suppl. 2), II-192
71. Carpentier, A., Deloche, A., Relland, J. *et al.* (1976). Valvular xenograft and valvular bioprosthesis: 1965–1975. In Kalmanson, D. (ed.) *The Mitral Valve.* p. 505. (Acton, Mass.: Publishing Sciences Group)
72. Gallo, I., Ruiz, B. and Duran, C. M. (1983). Clinical experience with the Carpentier–Edwards porcine bioprosthesis: short-term results (from 2 to 4.5 years). *Thorac. Cardiovasc. Surg.*, **31**, 277
73. Carpentier, A., Dubost, C., Lane, E., Carpentier, S., Relland, J., DeLoche, A., Fabiani, J-N., Chauvaud, S., Perier, P. and Maxwell, S. (1982). Continuing improvements in valvular bioprostheses. *J. Thorac. Cardiovasc. Surg.*, **83**, 27
74. Commerford, P. J., Curcio, C. A. and Rose, A. G. (1981). Thrombosis of a porcine xenograft in the aortic position. A case report. *Scand. J. Thorac. Cardiovasc. Surg.*, **15**, 239
75. Singh, S. V. and Wright, J. E. (1983). The Carpentier–Edwards bioprosthesis as replacement for human heart valves (seven years' experience). *Indian Heart J.*, **35**, 34
76. Angell, W. W. and Angell, J. D. (1980). Porcine valves. *Prog. Cardiovasc. Dis.*, **23**, 141
77. Schoen, F. J., Collins, J. J. Jr and Cohn, L. H. (1983). Long-term failure rate and morphologic correlations in porcine bioprosthetic heart valves. *Am. J. Cardiol*, **51**, 957
78. Warnes, C. A., Scott, M. L., Silver, G. M., Smith, C. W., Ferrans, V. J. and Roberts, W. C. (1983). Comparison of late degenerative changes in porcine bioprostheses in the mitral and aortic valve position in the same patient. *Am. J. Cardiol.*, **51**, 965

79. Magilligan, D. J. Jr, Lewis, J. W. Jr, Jara, F. M., Lee, M. W., Alam, M., Riddle, J. R. and Stein, P. D. (1980). Spontaneous degeneration of porcine bioprosthetic valves. *Ann. Thorac. Surg.*, **30**, 259
80. Sarabu, M. R. and Parker, F. B. Jr (1983). Unusual complication of porcine heterograft. *Ann. Thorac. Surg.*, **35**, 553
81. Ashraf, M. and Bloor, C. M. (1978). Structural alterations of the porcine heterograft after various durations of implantation. *Am. J. Cardiol*, **41**, 1185
82. Camilleri, J. P., Pornin, B. and Carpentier, A. (1982). Structural changes of glutaraldehyde-treated porcine bioprosthetic valves. *Arch. Pathol. Lab. Med.*, **106**, 490
83. Isomura, T., Yanai, T., Akagawa, H., Aoyagi, S., Kosuga, K., Ohishi, K. and Koga, M. (1986). Late pathological changes of Carpentier–Edwards porcine bioprostheses in the mitral position. *J. Cardiovasc. Surg.*, **27**, 307
84. Nunez, L., Iglesias, A., Aguado, M. G. *et al.* (1982). Early leaflet perforation as a cause of bioprosthetic dysfunction. *Scand. J. Thorac. Cardiovasc. Surg.*, **16**, 17
85. Jones, M., Rodrigues,, E. R., Eidblo, E. E. and Ferrans, V. J. (1985). Cuspal perforations caused by long suture ends in implanted bioprosthetic valves. *J. Thorac. Cardiovasc. Surg.*, **90**, 557
86. Forman, M. B., Phelan, B. K., Robertson, R. M. and Virmani, R. (1985). Correlation of two-dimensional echocardiography and pathologic findings in porcine valve dysfunction. *J. Am. Coll. Cardiol.*, **5**, 224
87. Grehl, T. M., O'Neill, M. B. Jr., Naifeh, J., Dajee, A., Hurley, E. J. and Riemenschneider, T. (1981). Spontaneous heterograft aortic valve failure. *Ann. Thorac. Surg.*, **31**, 274
88. Barnhart, G. R., Ishihara, T., Ferrans, V. J., Jones, M., McIntosh, C. L. and Roberts, W. C. (1982). Intracuspal hematomas in bioprosthetic valves: pathologic findings and clinical implications. *Circulation*, **66** (Suppl. 1), I-167
89. Ferrans, V. J., Boyce, S. W., Billingham, M. E., Spray, T. L. and Roberts, W. C. (1979). Infection of glutaraldehyde-preserved porcine valve heterografts. *Am. J. Cardiol.*, **43**, 1123
90. Downham, W. H. and Rhoades, E. R. (1979). Endocarditis associated with porcine valve xenografts. *Arch. Intern. Med.*, **139**, 1350
91. Keys, T. F. and Hewitt, W. L. (1973). Endocarditis due to micrococci and *Staphylococcus epidermidis*. *Arch. Intern Med.*, **132**, 216
92. Magilligan, D. J., Quinn, E. L. and Davila, J. C. (1977). Bacteremia, endocarditis and the Hancock valve. *Ann. Thorac. Surg.*, **24**, 508
93. Angell, W. W. and Angell, J. D. (1980). Porcine valves. *Prog. Cardiovasc. Dis.*, **23**, 141
94. Navia, J. A., Haller, J. D., Gimenez, C. *et al.* (1982). Low profile bioprosthesis for cardiac valve replacement: hydraulic and hemodynamic studies. *Med. Instr.*, **16**, 57
95. Navia, J. A., Gimenez, C., Meletti, I. and Liotta, D. (1984). Thromboembolism with low profile bioprosthesis. *Europ. Heart J.*, **5** (Suppl. D), 95
96. Gallo, I., Figueroa, A. and Duran, C. M. (1985). Early clinical results with the Xenomedica porcine bioprosthesis. *Thorac. Cardiovasc. Surg.*, **33**, 248
97. Senning, A. (1967). Fascia lata replacement of aortic valve. *J. Thorac. Cardiovasc. Surg.*, **54**, 465
98. Ionescu, M. I. and Ross, D. N. (1969). Heart valve replacement with autologous fascia lata. *Lancet*, **2**, 1
99. Ionescu, M. I., Ross, D. N., Deac, R., Grimshaw, V. A., Taylor, S. H., Whitaker, W. and Wooler, G. H. (1970). Autologous fascia lata for heart valve replacement. *Thorax*, **25**, 46
100. Myers, W. O. and Miller, D. R. (1969). Autogenous fascial aortic valves in dogs. *J. Thorac. Cardiovasc. Surg.*, **57**, 805
101. McEnany, M. T., Ross, D. N. and Yates, A. K. (1972). Valve failure in seventy-two frame-supported autologous fascia lata mitral valves: two-year follow-up. *Surgery*, **63**, 199
102. Editorial (1976). Obituary for fascia lata heart valves. *Br. Med. J.*, **1**, 115
103. Zerbini, E. de J. and Puig, L. B. (1979). The dura mater allograft valve. In Ionescu, M. I. (ed.) *Tissue Heart Valves*. p. 253. (London: Butterworths)
104. Puig, L. B., Verginelli, G., Belotti, G., Kawabe, L., Frack, C. C. R., Pileggi, F., Decourt,

L. V. and Zerbini, E. J. (1972). Homologous dura mater cardiac valve: preliminary study of 30 cases. *J. Thorac. Cardiovasc. Surg.*, **64**, 154

105. Nuno-Conceicrao, A., Puig, L. B., Verginelli, G., Iryia, K., Bitttencourt, D. and Zerbini, E. J. (1975). Homologous dura mater cardiac valves. Structural aspects of eight implanted valves. *J. Thorac. Cardiovasc. Surg.*, **70**, 499

106. Stolf, N. A., Puig, L. B. and Zerbini, E. J. (1980). Late results of replacement of cardiac valves by dura-mater allografts. *Int. J. Artific. Organs*, **3**, 104

107. Allen, D. J., Highison, G. J., Didio, L. J., Zerbini, E. J. and Puig, L. B. (1982). Evidence of remodeling in dura mater cardiac valves. *J. Thorac. Cardiovasc. Surg.*, **84**, 267

8
Bovine Pericardial Xenograft Bioprostheses

IONESCU–SHILEY PERICARDIAL BIOPROSTHESIS

In 1970 Dr M. I. Ionescu started testing glutaraldehyde-stabilized pericardial xenografts. Initially, limited numbers of the valves were created in his own laboratory in Leeds, England and used for single valve replacements only[1]. After clinical testing[2], the Ionescu–Shiley bovine pericardial xenograft valve[3,4] was marketed from 1976 by Shiley Incorporated.

The Ionescu–Shiley valve consists of bovine pericardium mounted on a Dacron cloth-covered titanium stent. The sewing ring consists of porous Dacron fabric covered with a thin layer of Dacron cloth. All valve sizes have the same sewing ring configuration. The valve is available in standard and low profile varieties (Figure 8.1).

The pericardium is obtained from 6–18-month-old calves. Sterile procedures are used from the time the pericardium is harvested. Soluble antigens are removed by incubating the pericardium in a balanced electrolyte solution. Thereafter it is stored at 4°C for 2 weeks in 0.5% phosphate buffered glutaraldehyde. This treatment aims to reduce or eliminate antigenicity and prevent collagen denaturation by forming irreversible covalent cross-links between the amino groups of collagen and glutaraldehyde[3]. A single strip of pericardium (Figure 8.2) is used per prosthesis, and the tissue is stitched to the outside of the stent to maintain an excellent orifice-to-annulus diameter ratio. The strut posts of small valves are splayed 9 degrees outward to maintain the full central orifice.

The valves manufactured in Ionescu's own laboratory between 1971 and 1976 underwent little quality control[4] and no standardization of thickness and pliability of the cusps was attempted. Early valves were pretreated with sodium metaperiodate and ethylene glycol prior to fixation in a simple dilution of commercially available, non-purified glutaraldehyde. The latter has an unknown and unstable proportion of monomers and polymers. Monomeric glutaraldehyde is not an effective fixative. Solutions containing high concentrationsof very long-chain glutaraldehyde polymers are poor fixatives due to the reduced number of active aldehyde groups available for cross-linking. Pure solutions of relatively short-chain polymers appear to provide optimal fixation.

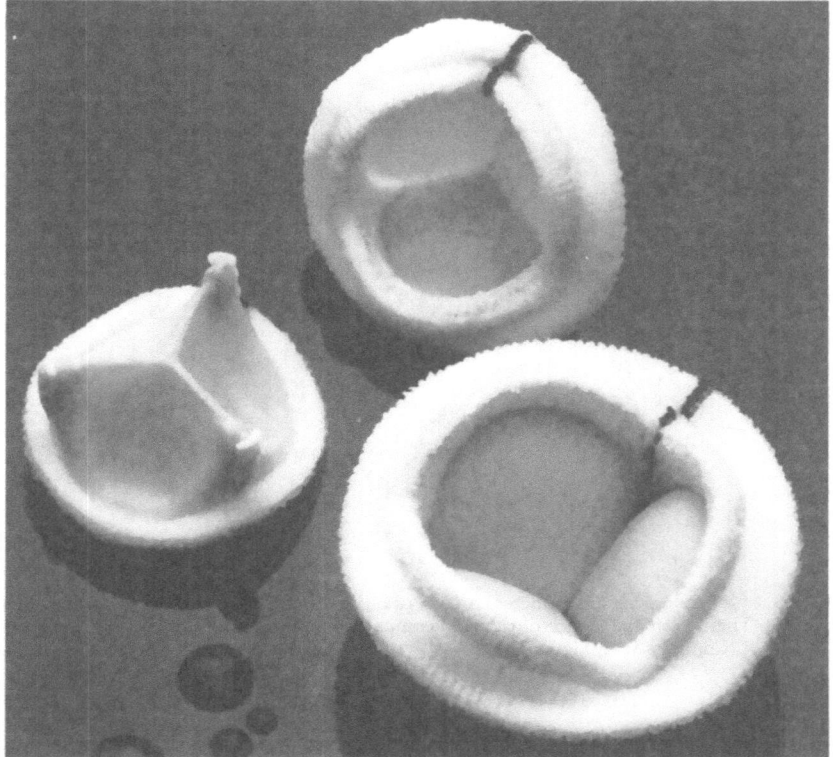

Figure 8.1 Ionescu–Shiley low-profile pericardial xenograft (family photo). (Picture courtesy of Shiley Inc.)

Since 1976 the pericardial xenografts produced by Shiley Laboratories have been treated with a solution of 'purified glutaraldehyde' containing the optimal proportion of monomers and polymers and an ideal cross-link density achieved by controlling the concentration and pH of the solution, as well as its temperature and the exposure time. The completed bioprosthesis is transported and stored in 4% buffered formaldehyde to maintain sterility.

The valve has a low thrombogenicity without anticoagulants, an absence of catastrophic failure, good haemodynamic function and lack of haemolysis. However, the narrow unpadded sewing ring predisposes to paravalvular leakage after aortic valve replacement[3,4]. While the valve appears to give good service in the aortic position, the 3-year reoperation rate of nearly 12% after mitral valve replacement, and the established poor durability record of other tissue valves[3] in this position leaves a question mark over this prosthesis for mitral valve replacement. As with any stent-mounted bioprosthesis, looping of a suture around a stent-post may lead to prosthetic stenosis (see Colour Plate R). Figure 8.3 shows a highly unusual form of prosthetic stenosis due to failure to remove the manufacturer's stent-restraining sutures.

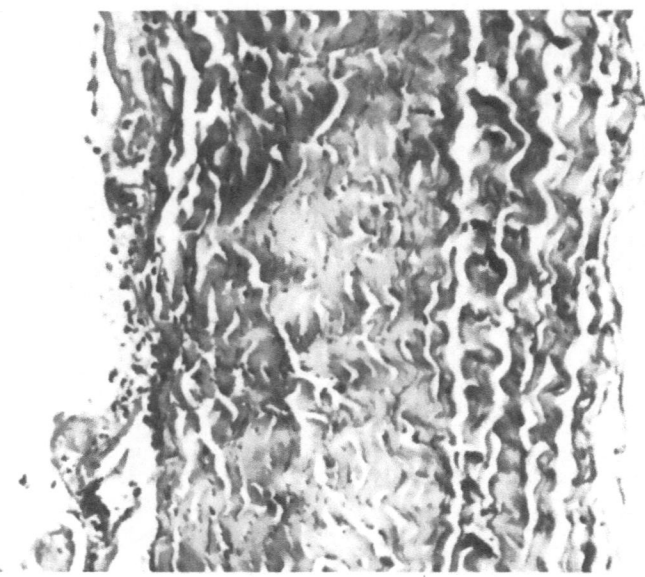

Figure 8.2 Histological appearance of a cusp of an Ionescu–Shiley bovine pericardial valve prosthesis. There is an abundance of collagen compared to the scanty fibrosa of porcine aortic valve cusps. (Compare with Figure 7.4 a)

Published experience[5-7] with follow-up periods of up to 10 years[8] records a low incidence of valve-related complications. Calcification of the prosthesis militates against its use in children[9]. Gallo et al.[10] reported that their patients with Ionescu–Shiley valves showed a higher incidence of primary tissue failure than those with glutaraldehyde-preserved porcine xenografts in the aortic position at 7 years' follow-up. Others have reported that the Ionescu–Shiley mitral bio prosthesis may fail suddenly[11]. Fatal bioprosthetic regurgitation immediately after mitral and tricuspid valve replacements with Ionescu–Shiley bioprostheses has been reported[12]. Brais et al.[13] followed up patients with Ionescu–Shiley prostheses for up to 6 years and found that their results compared favourably with results obtained with other bioprostheses. Silverton et al.[14] found a significantly lower rate of embolism (0.55% per annum) compared with mitral valve replacements with porcine xenografts (2.9–5.3%).

CARPENTIER–EDWARDS PERICARDIAL BIOPROSTHESIS

The bovine pericardial valve produced by American Edwards Laboratories differs from the Ionescu–Shiley valve in the following respects (see Chapter 3 also):

1. The frame is totally made of flexible Elgiloy wire rather than rigid titanium. Thus both the orifice and the supports are flexible, which reduces the

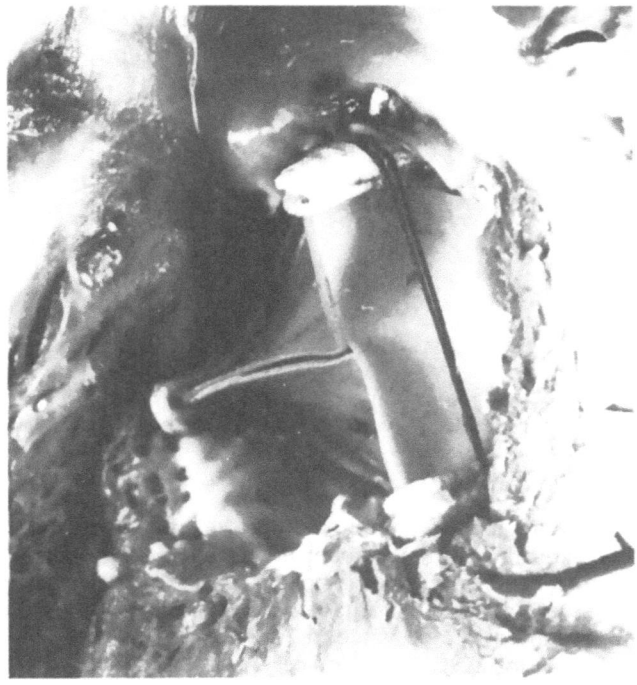

Figure 8.3 Referred heart containing an Ionescu–Shiley mitral valve prosthesis, which had been implanted in a patient at another hospital. The patient did not survive the operation. The surgeon had neglected to remove the stent-restraining sutures applied by the manufacturer

loading shock and stress on tissue that can result from constant leaflet motion.

2. The pericardium is treated with 0.625% glutaraldehyde rather than a 0.5% concentration.
3. There are different sewing ring arrangements for the aortic and atrioventricular prostheses.
4. The valve is transported and stored in glutaraldehyde rather than formaldehyde.

The pericardial tissue is mounted completely inside the stent to reduce the potential for abrasion between the stent and leaflets during opening and closing. Early results of the third-generation Carpentier–Edwards bioprosthesis are favourable[15].

MITROFLOW MEDICAL PERICARDIAL BIOPROSTHESIS

Bovine pericardial heart valve prostheses have recently been constructed by Mitral Medical International Inc., of Wheat Ridge, Colorado, USA. Mitral Medical of Canada Ltd is presently marketing this prosthesis. These valves

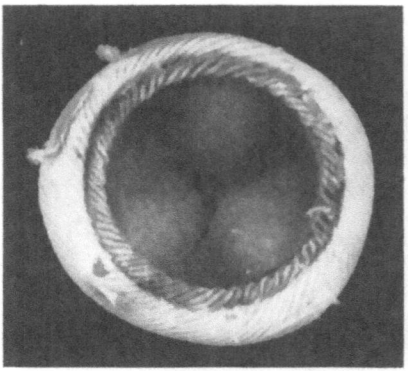 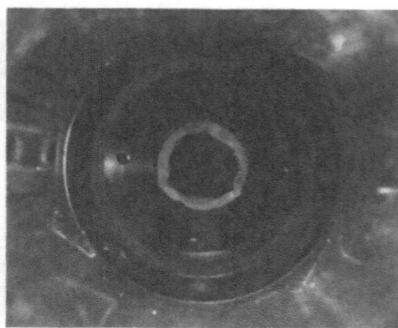

Fig. 8.4   Fig. 8.5

Figure 8.4   Inflow aspect of Mitroflow bovine pericardial valve prosthesis
Figure 8.5   Mitroflow pericardial heart valve in pulse duplicator; outlet view shows that leaflets open to form a cylinder

(Figure 8.4), which are made from glutaraldehyde-treated bovine pericardium, have been evaluated in a canine model in the USA and in baboons *(Papio ursinus)* at Groote Schuur Hospital, Cape Town[16,17]. The valves have been implanted in a few thousand patients worldwide. Investigational device exemption was granted for the valve in America in January 1985.

The stent is made of Delrin 500, an acetyl homopolymer with low 'creep' properties and good flex and shock absorbance. The sewing ring is moulded from Dow Corning medical grade silicone and contains 40% tungsten powder

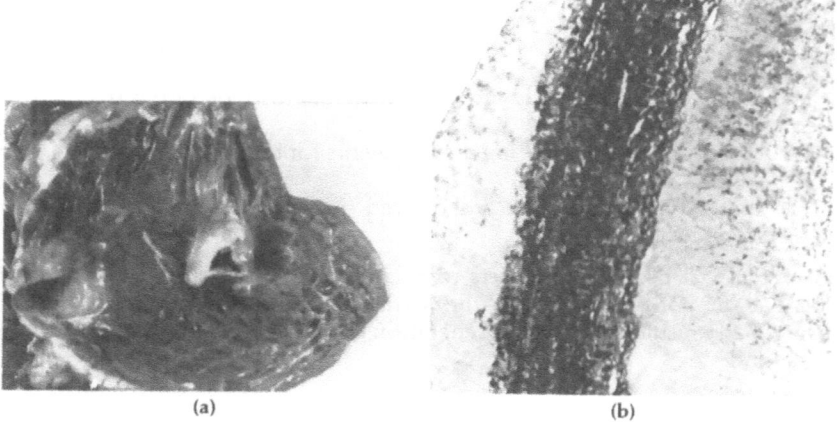

(a)   (b)

Figure 8.6   (a) Host tissue overgrowth has produced stenosis and incompetence of Mitroflow bovine pericardial valve which had been implanted in the mitral position in a baboon for 86 days. Scanty thrombus is also present. (b) Host tissue (myofibroblasts and collagen) has grown over both aspects of this cusp in a Mitroflow valve, which had been implanted in a baboon for 47 days. (Haematoxylin–eosin, × 80)

to render it radiopaque. Dacron fabric covers the stent and sewing ring so that there is a single seam and no exposed knots. The leaflets are constructed from a single piece of bovine pericardium. The larger valves have a thicker tissue. The tissue is mounted on the outside of the covered stent and the leaflets open to form a full cylinder (Figure 8.5).

The pericardium is orientated so that the mesothelial covered side forms the outflow aspect of the valve cusps, in order to lower the risk of thrombosis. Unlike the Ionescu–Shiley prosthesis there are no sutures tethering the leaflets at the commissures. Careful operative technique is recommended, including rinsing of the prosthesis prior to implantation to prevent the aldehydes producing tissue necrosis and paravalvular leaks.

Experimental implantation of Mitroflow valves in the baboon[16,17] showed no apparent advantage over the Ionescu–Shiley valve with regard to postoperative transvalvular gradients, thrombosis (Colour Plates S and T), and tissue overgrowth (Figure 8.6).

MEADOX–GABBAY PERICARDIAL BIOPROSTHESIS

This unicuspid pericardial heart valve was developed by Dr S. Gabbay of New Jersey, and is based on the theory that movement will prevent cuspal calcification. The single cusp, which is the only moving component of the valve, closes against an immobile pericardial baffle. Initial results in 66 patients followed up for 16 months have been good.

BICUSPID MITRAL BIOPROSTHESIS

At Guy's Hospital, London, a bicuspid bioprosthesis was prepared by mounting glutaraldehyde-processed porcine pericardium onto commercially available Brownlee–Yates stents. Evaluation of the prosthesis in dogs revealed significant closing reflux[18]. It was concluded that any stented biscuspid valve has to be tailored so that parts of the tissue can assume the function of the chordae tendineae to minimize the closing reflux.

HANCOCK PERICARDIAL BIOPROSTHESIS

This glutaraldehyde-fixed pericardial valve is treated by a calcification-retarding process which has yet to be proven clinically.

ABIOMED POLYMERIC PROSTHESIS

The Abiomed polymeric trileaflet heart valve prosthesis was originally designed for use in valved conduits. Flow studies indicate that it has improved leaflet motion and pressure drop characteristics compared to the Carpentier–Edwards porcine and Ionescu–Shiley pericardial valves. The Abiomed valve is, however, more stenotic than the St Jude Medical and Medtronic–Hall low-profile valves at normal cardiac outputs[19].

CALCIFICATION OF GLUTARALDEHYDE-PRESERVED XENOGRAFTS IN YOUNG PATIENTS

Stent-mounted glutaraldehyde-preserved porcine aortic valves (GPVs) have been used in hundreds of thousands of cardiac valve replacements since 1971. Late calcific degeneration of GPVs occurs commonly in long-term valve

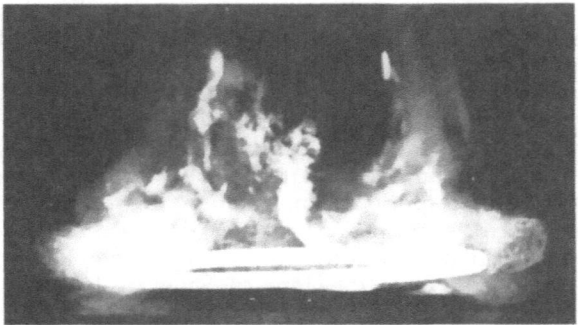

Figure 8.7   Radiograph of a heavily calcified Hancock porcine aortic valve prosthesis

replacements and often results in bioprosthetic failure[20-22]. Calcification is more common in the young[23,24]. At Groote Schuur Hospital, between 1975 and 1980, 670 GPVs have been inserted in 568 patients in the aortic and mitral positions[25]. Of these, 81 were Hancock and 589 were Carpentier–Edwards prostheses. Fifty-four of the Groote Schuur Hospital patients were under 16 years of age at the time of implantation. Most of these young patients have required reoperation within 3 years for prosthetic calcification (Figure 8.7) and severe stenosis. Pressure gradients across the calcified valves have varied from 12 to 63 mmHg with calculated orificial areas of 0.3–1.0 cm^2. Four patients died before reoperation and postmortem revealed severely calcified, stenotic prostheses. Colour Plate O shows the calcified xenograft of one of the first patients in the world to have this complication documented[20]. Tissue valves are no longer used in young patients.

Pathology

Calcification involved all three cusps in each xenograft. In most instances the calcified area was enclosed by a superficial layer of non-calcified cuspal tissue (Figure 8.8). The zones of the cusp undergoing calcification showed well-preserved collagen and the ghost outlines of pre-existing cuspal fibroblasts. Calcification mostly spared the portions of the cusps near the free margins. In a few areas, especially near the commissures, the calcification was present as calcified excrescences, which breached the otherwise smooth cuspal surface.

Calcified areas stained positively with the von Kossa and alizarin red stains after mild decalcification prior to routine tissue processing. Calcified zones also stained positively with empirical histological stains for fibrin (Martius scarlet blue and picro-Mallory methods). However, immunoperoxidase staining of the sections for fibrinogen often revealed scanty fibrin thrombus on the outflow portion of the cusps, but the calcified zones, as well as the remainder of the cuspal substance, were negative for fibrinogen. The results with the empiric stains were interpreted as non-specific, false-positive staining. Stains

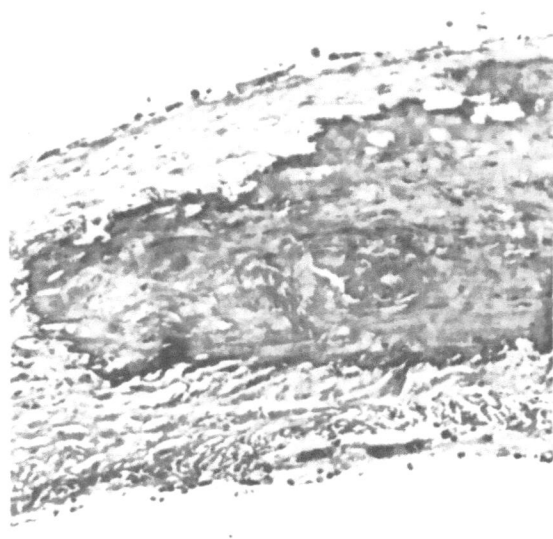

Figure 8.8 Histological section of a cusp of a calcified Hancock valve. Calcification involves the core of the cusp and spares the superficial portions of the cusp. (Haematoxylin–eosin, × 150)

for micro-organisms were uniformly negative.

Light microscopy of the xenograft valves revealed patchy, dystrophic cuspal calcification. Apart from calcification, the xenografts appeared no different from other non-calcified xenografts examined at various periods after implantation. Electron microscopy was performed upon seven of the calcified xenografts using samples from macroscopically non-calcified areas. Ultrastructural evidence of early calcification (Figure 8.9) was observed in three of the seven valves. In two of the three valves the earliest sign of calcification was observed in the interstitium adjacent to collagen fibres and fibroblast-like cells. In one valve early calcification was starting within the cytoplasm of a fibroblast-like cell.

Comment

Calcification of GPVs is a major problem in young persons. Calcification of xenografts in adults has been reported less frequently[26]. The reason for the discrepancy between the two age groups is not clear. None of our young patients with calcified GPVs had evidence of infective endocarditis, nor an abnormal calcium metabolism, although all had an elevated alkaline phosphatase level in keeping with their age. In addition to the age distribution, another unusual feature is the fact that the calcification mainly involves the core of the cusps and often spares the superficial portions.

Possible reasons for calcification of glutaraldehyde-preserved porcine

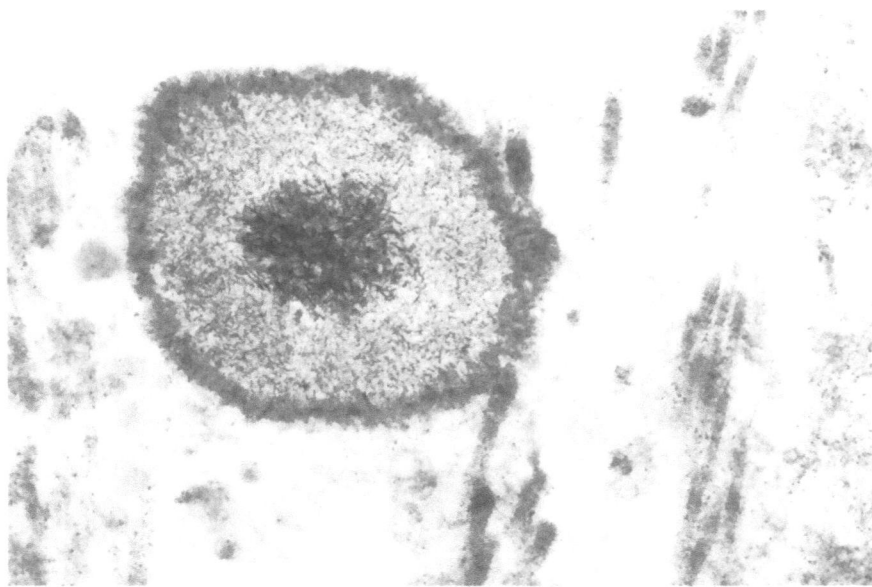

Figure 8.9 Early calcification within Hancock cuspal interstitial tissue is seen as a central, densely stained nidus within an aggregate of hydroxyapatite crystals. (Uranyl acetate and lead citrate, × 28 800)

xenografts include the different calcium metabolism of young persons[27], infection of the xenograft[28], the presence within the cusp of a calcium-binding amino acid[24], and the repeated flexing of the cusps[29]. Glutaraldehyde is a notoriously poorly penetrating fixative[25]. Cross-linking of the surface layers makes it progressively harder for glutaraldehyde to penetrate the tissue bulk in conventional reactions carried out at pH 7, and this can lead to incomplete fixation of the tissue. The superficial zones of the cusps, which are usually free of calcification, are the sites of the cusps that are fixed earliest and best by the glutaraldehyde solution. The observed pathology is in keeping with the concept that alterations favouring subsequent calcification develop in the imperfectly fixed core of the xenograft cusps.

In addition to the Hancock and Carpentier–Edwards prostheses, other glutaraldehyde-preserved porcine aortic valve prostheses, e.g. the Angell–Shiley bioprosthesis, appear to suffer from a similar problem of calcification in young hosts[30]. Mineralization has emerged as one of the most important causes of late failure of contemporary bioprostheses[31,32]. Bovine pericardial bioprostheses develop calcific obstruction significantly earlier than do porcine valves[33]. Most young persons with glutaraldehyde-treated bioprostheses have required early reoperation because of calcification. The policy at Groote Schuur Hospital has been to follow these young patients at 3-monthly intervals and to perform cardiac catheterization if they exhibit any symptoms of reduced effort tolerance, auscultatory features of prosthetic stenosis or pulmonary hypertension, electrocardiographic signs of progressive rightward axis deviation, or radiological evidence of pulmonary congestion. The cause of the bioprosthetic cuspal calcification still awaits final elucidation.

Experimental models in animals may provide more information in this regard. Levy et al.[34] found, in a study of subcutaneous implants of GPVs in rats, that glutaraldehyde fixation of porcine aortic leaflets was a prerequisite for the calcification of GPV implants. These authors point out that while specific steps in the glutaraldehyde treatment that promote the calcification are not known, the specific types of cross-links formed may be responsible. The pyridinium cross-link, which is one of the major types of glutaraldehyde-induced cross-links, is directly analogous to similar compounds found in bone-derived collagen and the desmosine residues of elastin. New observations portray calcification processes as similar whether occurring normally or pathologically[35]. The maximum concentration of calcium achieved in an experimental study[36] was similar to that previously encountered in failed clinical porcine bioprosthetic heart valves.

The unsolved problem for the manufacturers of xenograft bioprostheses is how such calcification may be prevented on a long-term basis. Most chemical methods used to date in the preparation procedure of GPVs have included materials to prevent precipitation or to compete with calcium for active sites. Most of these approaches show good short-term results, which diminish as the anti-calcific agent leaches from the tissues. Others have used adsorbed sodium dodecyl sulphate, surfactant, sodium borohydride, special buffers or infiltration of the tissue matrix by natural or synthetic polyelectrolytes. Ethanehydroxydiphosphonate prevents calcification of bioprosthetic cusps implanted subcutaneously in rats[37].

Porcine mitral valve calcification has been identified as a cause of intravascular haemolysis in children, and the presence of haemolysis may be used to gauge such dysfunction. It has been suggested that some systemic emboli in porcine valve recipients may not be due to intracardiac or prosthetic thrombosis, but to detachment of fragments of degenerative, calcified xenograft cuspal tissue.

REFERENCES

1. Ionescu, M. I. and Tandon, A. P. (1979). The Ionescu–Shiley pericardial xenograft heart valve. In Ionescu, M. I. (ed.) *Tissue Heart Valves*. p. 201 (London: Butterworths)
2. Ionescu, M. I., Tandon, A. P., Mary, D. A. S. and Abid, A. (1977). Heart valve replacement with the Ionescu–Shiley pericardial xenograft. *J. Thorac. Cardiovasc. Surg.*, **73**, 31
3. Lefrak, E. A. and Starr, A. (1979). *Cardiac Valve Prostheses*. (New York: Appleton-Century-Crofts)
4. Technical information on the Ionescu–Shiley pericardial xenograft heart valve. (1977). (Irvine, California: Shiley Laboratories)
5. Ionescu, M. I. and Tandon, A. P. (1980). Long-term clinical and hemodynamic evaluation of the Ionescu–Shiley pericardial xenograft heart valve. *Artif. Organs*, **4**, 13
6. Ghosh, S. C., Larrieu, A. J., Ablaza, S. G. and Grana, V. P. (1983). Spontaneous disruption of Ionescu–Shiley bovine pericardial xenograft in the mitral position. *J. Thorac. Cardiovasc. Surg.*, **86**, 784
7. Gonzalez-Lavin, L., Chi, S., Blair, T. C., Jung, J. Y., Fabaz, A. G., McFadden, P. M., Lewis,

B. and Daughters, G. (1983). Five-year experience with the Ionescu–Shiley bovine pericardial valve in the aortic position. *Ann. Thorac. Surg.*, **36**, 270

8. Ionescu, M. I., Chidambaram, M., Hasan, S. S. *et al.* (1982). Ten years experience with the Ionescu–Shiley pericardial xenograft heart valve. *Nippon Kyobu Geka Gakkai Zasshi*, **30**, 488

9. Walker, W. E., Duncan, J. M., Frazier, O. H. Jr., Livesay, J. J., Otto, D. A., Reul, G. and Cooley, D. A. (1983). Early experience with the Ionescu–Shiley pericardial xenograft valve. Accelerated calcification in children. *J. Thorac. Cardiovasc. Surg.*, **86**, 570

10. Gallo, I., Nistal, F., Revuelta, J. M., Garcia-Satue, E., Artinano, E. and Duran, C. G. (1985). Incidence of primary tissue valve failure with the Ionescu–Shiley pericardial valve. Preliminary results. *J. Thorac. Cardiovasc. Surg.*, **90**, 278

11. Gabbay, S., Bortolotti, U., Wasserman, F., Tindel, N., Factor, S. M. and Frater, R. W. (1984). Long-term follow-up of the Ionescu–Shiley mitral pericardial xenograft. *J. Thorac. Cardiovasc. Surg.*, **88**, 758

12. Lester, W. M. and Roberts, W. C. (1985). Fatal bioprosthetic regurgitation immediately after mitral and tricuspid replacements with Ionescu–Shiley bioprostheses. *Am. J. Cardiol.*, **55**, 590

13. Brais, M. P., Bedard, J. P., Goldstein, W., Koshal, A. and Keon, W. J. (1985). Ionescu–Shiley pericardial xenografts: Follow-up of up to 6 years. *Ann. Thorac. Surg.*, **39**, 105

14. Silverton, N. P., Abdulali, S. A., Yakirevich, V. S., Tandon, A. P. and Ionescu, M. (1984). Embolism, thrombosis and anticoagulant haemorrhage in mitral valve disease. A prospective study of patients having valve replacement with the pericardial xenograft. *Europ. Heart J.*, **5**, 19

15. Relland, A., Perier, P. and Lecointe, B. (1985). The third generation Carpentier–Edwards bioprosthesis: early results. *J. Am. Coll. Cardiol.*, **6**, 1149

16. Rose, A. G. (1984). The pathology of heart valve replacement by valvular prostheses. *MD thesis*, University of Cape Town

17. Hassoulas, J., Rose, A. G. and Reichart, B. A. (1986). Experimental evaluation of the Mitroflow pericardial heart valve in a baboon model. II. Pathology (Submitted for publication)

18. Bodnar, E., Bowden, N. L., Drury, P. J., Olsen, E. G., Durmaz, I. and Ross, D. N. (1981). Bicuspid mitral bioprosthesis. *Thorax*. **36**, 45

19. Galioto, F. M. Jr., Midgely, F. M., Kapur, S., Perry, L. W., Watson, D. C., Shapiro, S. R., Ruckman, R. N. and Scott, L. P. (1982). Early failures of Ionescu–Shiley bioprosthesis after mitral valve replacement in children. *J. Thorac. Cardiovasc. Surg.*, **83**, 306

20. Rose, A. G., Forman, R. and Bowen, R. M. (1978). Calcification of glutaraldehyde-fixed porcine xenograft. *Thorax*, **33**, 111

21. Schoen, F. J., Collins, J. J. and Cohn, L. H. (1983). Long-term failure rate and morphologic correlations in porcine bioprosthetic heart valves. *Am. Heart J.*, **51**, 957

22. Dunn, J. M. (1981). Porcine valve durability in children. *Ann. Thorac. Surg.*, **32**, 357

23. Kutschke, L. M., Oyer, P. and Shumway, N. (1979). An important complication of Hancock mitral valve replacement in children. *Circulation*, **60** (Suppl. 1), I-98

24. Sanders, S. P., Levy, R. J., Freed, M. D., Norwood, W. I. and Castaneda, A. R. (1980). Use of Hancock porcine xenografts in children and adolescents. *Am. J. Cardiol.*, **46**, 429

25. Curcio, C. A., Commerford, P. J., Rose, A. G., Stevens, J. E. and Barnard, M. S. (1981). Calcification of glutaraldehyde-preserved porcine xenografts in young patients. *J. Thorac. Cardiovasc. Surg.*, **81**, 621

26. Angell, W. W., Angell, J. D. and Kosek, J. C. (1982). Twelve-year experience with glutaraldehyde-preserved porcine xenografts. *J. Thorac. Cardiovasc. Surg.*, **83**, 493

27. Silver, M. M., Pollock, J., Silver, M. D., Williams, W. G. and Trusler, G. A. (1980). Calcification in porcine xenograft valves in children. *Am. J. Cardiol.*, **45**, 685

28. Nunez, L., de la Llana, R., Aguado, M. G., Iglesias, A., Larrea, J. L. and Celemin, D. (1983). Bioprosthetic valve endocarditis: indicators for surgical intervention. *Ann. Thorac. Surg.*, **35**, 262

29. Bruck, S. D. (1981). Possible causes for the calcification of glutaraldehyde-treated tissue heart valves and blood contacting elastomers during prolonged use in medical devices: a physico-chemical view. *Biomaterials*, **2**, 14

30. Lewis, B. S., Bakst, A., Rod, J. J., Rein, A., Gotsman, M. S. and Appelbaum, A. (1980).

Early calcification and obstruction of a mitral porcine bioprosthesis. *Ann. Thorac. Surg.,* **30,** 592

31. Schoen, F. J., Levy, R. J. (1984). Bioprosthetic heart valve failure: pathology and pathogenesis. *Cardiol. Clin.,* **2,** 717
32. Schoen, F. J., Hobson, C. E. (1985). Anatomic analysis of removed prosthetic heart valves: causes of failure of 33 mechanical valves and 58 bioprostheses, 1980 to 1983. *Hum. Pathol.,* **16,** 549
33. Fiddler, G. I., Gerlis, L. M., Walker, D. R. *et al.* (1983). Calcification of glutaraldehyde-preserved porcine and bovine xenograft valves in young children. *Ann. Thorac. Surg.,* **35,** 257
34. Levy, R. J., Schoen, F. J., Levy, J. T., Nelson, A. C., Howard, S. L. and Oshry, L. J. (1983). Biological determinants of dystrophic calcification and osteocalcin deposition in glutaraldehyde-preserved porcine aortic valve leaflets implanted subcutaneously in rats. *Am. J. Pathol.,* **113,** 143
35. Anderson, H. C. (1983). Calcific diseases: a concept. *Arch. Pathol. Lab. Med.,* **107,** 341
36. Schoen, F. J., Tsao, J. W. and Levy, R. J. (1986). Calcification of bovine pericardium used in cardiac valve bioprostheses. Implications for the mechanisms of bioprosthetic tissue mineralization. *Am. J. Pathol.,* **123,** 134
37. Levy, R. J., Wolfrum, J., Schoen, F. J., Hawley, M. A., Lund, S. A. and Langer, R. (1985). Inhibition of calcification of bioprosthetic heart valves by local controlled-release diphosphonate. *Science,* **228,** 190

9
Valve-containing Conduits

PULMONARY ARTERY AND VALVE SUBSTITUTES

Tubular conduits (Colour Plate U) containing valvular prostheses have been used as pulmonary artery and valve substitutes in complex congenital heart disease. In patients with transposition of the great arteries undergoing surgical correction, the finding of pulmonary obstruction too severe to be eliminated by excision is an indication for a Rastelli operation[1]. In this procedure the left ventricular flow is diverted via an intraventricular conduit through the ventricular septal defect into the aorta. The pulmonary artery is divided and the proximal (cardiac) stump is ligated. An extracardiac valved conduit restores continuity between the right ventricle and the distal pulmonary artery.

Kirklin and co-workers[2] used a composite conduit for repair of pulmonary valve and pulmonary artery atresia associated with a ventricular septal defect. The conduit consists of an artificial graft containing a homograft valve. The valve is inserted into a sleeve of knitted Dacron secured with three sutures proximally and distally. The knitted Dacron graft containing the homograft valve is then interposed between two woven Dacron grafts. The distal end of this composite graft is then fashioned according to the pathological features of the pulmonary arteries and is sutured distally. The proximal end of the graft is sutured to an opening in the right ventricle.

Artificial tube grafts containing valvular prostheses have also been used for the correction of other complex congenital cardiac diseases, e.g. a persistent truncus arteriosus (common aorticopulmonary trunk)[3]. Jonas et al.[4] suggest that the poor results in smaller children with porcine-valved, tightly woven Dacron conduits warrant a change to use of an alternative conduit.

LEFT VENTRICLE-TO-AORTA BYPASS

Valved tube grafts have been used to correct left-sided cardiac lesions[5]. The first fully reported clinical use of the double-outlet left ventricular concept for patients with severe aortic stenosis was that of Bernhard et al.[6]. Their patient also had hypoplasia of the aortic ring and of the ascending aorta.

Apico-aortic shunts (Colour Plate V) are used primarily in persons with complex forms of supravalvular or subvalvular aortic stenosis in whom complex surgery in the aortic root is to be avoided[5]. The conduits may also be used in patients with infective endocarditis, where insufficient tissue is left in the aortic ring for the suturing of a valve prosthesis.

Apico-aortic shunts need a rigid outlet connector to prevent occlusion of the apical outflow tract by myocardium. The conduits may differ with regard to the type of valve they incorporate and the location of the distal anastomosis. Tissue valves have been the most popular, because most conduits have been used in children in whom freedom from anticoagulants is an advantage. However, calcification and lack of long-term durability limit the use of such valves.

REPLACEMENT OF AORTIC VALVE AND ASCENDING AORTA .

As a safer procedure in patients with ascending aortic aneurysms and severe aortic incompetence, Bentall and De Bono[7] used a conduit consisting of a Starr–Edwards valve in a Teflon tube graft to join the aortic valve ring to the distal non-aneurysmal aorta. This technique obviates placing sutures in the often diseased aortic root. The coronary ostia are sutured to holes made in the tube graft. Lefrak and Starr[5] comment that this technique holds promise for patients with very small aortic valve rings who require aortic valve replacement.

Pathology of cardiac valvular prostheses situated within tube grafts

Table 9.1 lists 11 personally examined patients who came to autopsy with a variety of heart valve substitutes secured within tube conduit grafts made of woven Dacron. The group included only one later survivor. Seven out of the 11 patients were operated upon for congenital heart disease. Three patients had aortic aneurysms and one had an infected aortic valve prosthesis, which was excised. The tube graft linked the right ventricle to the main pulmonary artery in five patients, the right ventricle to the right pulmonary artery in one, the aortic root to the more distal aorta in four patients, and the left

Table 9.1 Autopsied patients with valved conduit tube grafts

Patient	Age, sex	Preoperative lesion	Survival (days)	Prosthesis	Cause of death
1	15,F	Infection	0	B–S	Leak
2	60,M	Aortic aneurysm	0	C–E	Unknown
3	2,F	Truncus	0	B–S	Pulmonary hypertension
4	39,M	Aortic aneurysm	0.125	B–S	Bleeding
5	24,F	Coarctation	5	Lill.	Unknown
6	7,M	TGA	9	B–S	Thrombosis
7	7,F	Tetralogy	10	B–S	Patch leak
8	39,M	Tetralogy	10	C–E	Right coronary artery stitch
9	34,M	Aortic aneurysm	20	S–E	Bleeding
10	18,M	DORV	24	B–S	Pulmonary hypertension
11	10,F	Truncus	2400	Han.	Pulmonary hypertension

M = male; F = female; TGA = transpostion of the great arteries; Han. = Hancock; DORV = double outlet right ventricle; C–E = Carpentier–Edwards; B–S = Bjork–Shiley; Lill. = Lillehei–Kaster; S–E = Starr–Edwards

ventricular apex to the distal aorta in one patient. The latter patient's death was due to a leak at the cardiac–tube graft anastomosis.

Comment

Complications of vascular grafts listed by Silver[8] include: (a) mechanical failure with rupture, haemorrhage or aneurysm formation; (b) kinking with graft stenosis or occlusion; (c) incomplete healing with detachment of the luminal surface thrombus (Figure 9.1) leading to graft stenosis; (d) infection, and (e) haemolysis. Fiore et al.[9] compared valved and non-valved right ventricular–pulmonary arterial extracardiac conduits in a canine experimental model. They showed that after 1 year the thickness of the neo-intimal lining (Figure 9.2) was threefold greater than in the valved conduits.

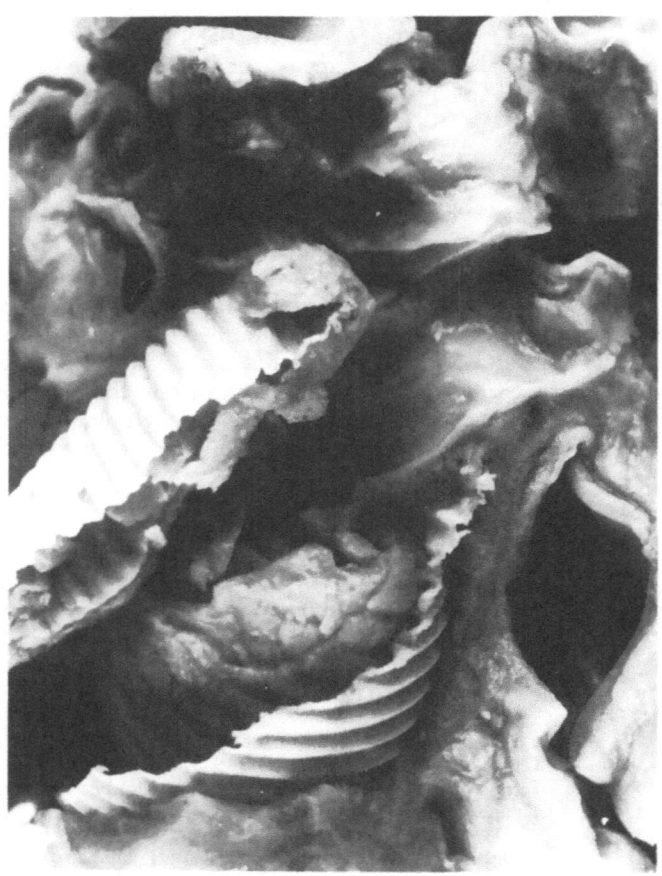

Figure 9.1 Partially detached thrombus is causing stenosis of tube graft linking right ventricle to main pulmonary artery

Semb et al.[10] reported good clinical results with the use of valved xenograft conduits to correct tricuspid atresia. Nath et al.[11] discuss the radiological evaluation of composite aortic grafts used to treat aneurysm of the ascending aorta. They found haemorrhage from the anastomotic sites to be the most important complication.

There are several clinical reports of intraconduit obstruction due to pannus formation[12-14]: infection has also occurred[15]. Proper conduit placement and intraoperative recognition of possible coronary artery compression by the conduit[16] are important in preventing significant ischaemic problems. Fatal coronary compression was encountered in only 0.35% of the 860 conduit operations performed at the Mayo Clinic[16]. Many totally asymptomatic patients may have severe right ventricular outflow tract obstruction produced by the conduit. It has been suggested that all patients with right ventricular conduits should have routine postoperative catheterization.

Porcine xenograft valves in conduits implanted in children have experienced the same problem with calcification that was noted in valves implanted orthotopically. Geha et al.[17] reported a 12% failure rate of extracardiac conduits, and Bisset et al.[18] encountered a 30% incidence of xenograft conduit failure over a shorter follow-up period. The latter authors concluded that although valved external conduits continue to play an important role in the treatment of complex congenital heart disease, a valved conduit with greater longevity is needed for use in children.

Incorporation of bioprosthetic heart valve cusps into valve rings is a recently described cause of wide-open regurgitation in right-sided valves and

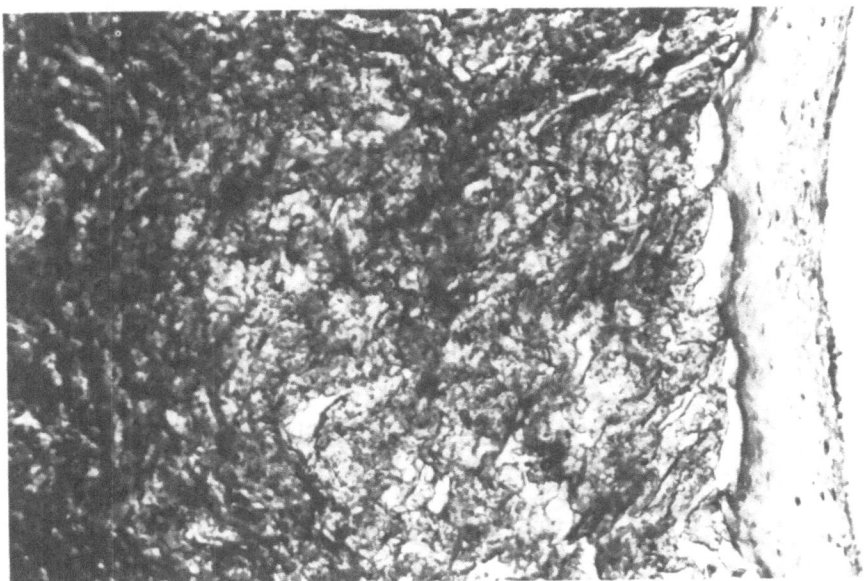

Figure 9.2 Neo-intimal lining (right) of a non-valved conduit

in valves within conduits[19]. Adhesive application of the cusps to valve rings and struts is the main pathogenetic process, with a contribution being made by cuspal retraction following fibrous ingrowth. Low-pressure and relatively non-pulsatile blood flow may facilitate the development of the permanently 'open' position of the valve cusps in right-sided heart valves.

REFERENCES

1. Rastelli, G. C., McGoon, D. C. and Wallace, R. B. (1969). Anatomic correction of transposition of the great arteries with ventricular septal defect and subpulmonary stenosis. *J. Thorac. Cardiovasc. Surg.*, **58**, 545
2. Kouchoukos, N. T., Bagerson, B. and Kirklin, J. W. (1971). Surgical treatment of congenital pulmonary atresia with ventricular septal defect. *J. Thorac. Cardiovasc. Surg.*, **61**, 70
3. Goor, D. A. and Lillehei, C. W. (1975). *Congenital Malformations of the Heart. Embryology, Anatomy, and Operative Considerations*. p. 164 (New York: Grune and Stratton)
4. Jonas, R. A., Freed, M. D., Mayer, J. E. and Castaneda, A. R. (1985). Long-term follow-up of patients with synthetic right heart conduits. *Circulation*, **72**, 1177
5. Lefrak, E. A. and Starr, A. (1979). *Cardiac Valve Prostheses*. (New York: Appleton-Century-Crofts)
6. Bernhard, W. F., Poirer, V. and La Farge, C. G. (1975). Relief of congenital obstruction to left ventricular outflow with a ventricular–aortic prosthesis. *J. Thorac. Cardiovasc. Surg.*, **69**, 223
7. Bentall, H. and De Bono, A. (1968). A technique for complete replacement of the ascending aorta. *Thorax*, **23**, 338
8. Silver, M. D. and Wilson, G. W. (1983). Pathology of cardiovascular prostheses including coronary artery bypass and other vascular grafts. In Silver, M. D. (ed.) *Cardiovascular Pathology*. Vol. 2, p. 1225. (New York: Churchill Livingstone)
9. Fiore, A. C., Peigh, P. S., Robison, R. J. *et al.* (1983). Valved and non-valved right ventricular-pulmonary arterial extra-cardiac conduits. An experimental comparison. *J. Thorac. Cardiovasc. Surg.*, **86**, 490
10. Semb, B. K., Sorland, S. J., Bjornstad, P. G. *et al.* (1981). Tricuspid atresia corrected with valved xenograft conduits. *Scand. J. Thorac. Cardiovasc. Surg.*, **15**, 241
11. Nath, P. H., Zollikofer, C., Castaneda-Zuniga, W. R., Velasquez, G., Formanek, A., Nicoloff, D. and Amplatz, K. (1979). Radiological evaluation of composite aortic grafts. *Radiology*, **131**, 43
12. Chun, P. K., Rocchini, A. P., Gibbs, H. R., Robinowitz, M., Green, D. and Virmani, R. (1981). Pannus formation in a Hancock-valved conduit resulting in proximal intra-conduit obstruction: late complication of Rastelli procedure for complete transposition of the great vessels with ventricular septal defect and pulmonic stenosis. *Am. Heart J.*, **101**, 855
13. Agarwal, K. C., Edwards, W. D., Feldt, R. H., Danielson, G. K., Puga, F. J. and McGoon, D. C. (1981). Clinicopathological correlates of obstructed right-sided porcine-valved extracardiac conduits. *J. Thorac. Cardiovasc. Surg.*, **81**, 591
14. Ben-Shachar, G., Nicoloff, D. M. and Edwards, J. E. (1981). Separation of neointima from Dacron graft causing obstruction. Case following Fontan procedure for tricuspid atresia. *J. Thorac. Cardiovasc. Surg.*, **82**, 268
15. Copeland, J. G., Morgan, C. M., Sahn, D. J., Allen, H. D. and Goldberg, S. J. (1983). Successful treatment of an infected right ventricular to pulmonary artery conduit. *Ann. Thorac. Surg.*, **35**, 308
16. Daskalopoulos, D. A., Edwards, W. D., Driscoll, D. J., Danielson, G. K. and Puga, F. J. (1983). Coronary artery compression with fatal myocardial ischemia. A rare complication of valved extracardiac conduits in children with congenital heart disease. *J. Thorac. Cardiovasc. Surg.*, **85**, 546
17. Geha, A. S., Laks, H., Stansel, H. C. Jr., Cornhill, J. F., Kilman, J. W., Buckley, M. J. and Roberts, W. C. (1979). Late failure of porcine valve heterografts in children. *J. Thorac. Cardiovasc. Surg.*, **78**, 351

18. Bisset, G. S., Schwartz, D. C., Benzing, G., Helmsworth, J., Schreiber, J. T. and Kaplan, S. (1981). Late results of reconstruction of the right ventricular outflow tract with porcine xenografts in children. *Ann. Thorac. Surg.*, **31**, 437

19. McManus, B., Fleming, W., Kugler, J., Murphy, S. and Rogler, W. (1986). Incorporation of bioprosthetic heart valve cusps into valve rings: an unrecognized cause of wide-open regurgitation in right-sided valves. (Abstract). Paper presented at the 75th Annual Meeting of the United States—Canadian Division of the International Academy of Pathology. New Orleans, 10–14 March

10
Miscellaneous Aspects of the Pathology of Heart Valve Replacement

PATHOLOGY OF THE ATRIOVENTRICULAR SYSTEM OF HIS–TAWARA IN PROSTHETIC HEART VALVE REPLACEMENT

The His–Tawara system should be examined in all cases of sudden death following heart valve replacement. In many such patients no cause of death is found, and death is commonly attributed to arrhythmia. A haematoma in the interatrial septum is common after mitral valve replacement. In some instances the haematoma (Figure 10.1) may extend downwards to the atrioventricular node and the bundle of His. The bundle[1] is also at risk during valve replacement as it penetrates the central fibrous body[2,3]. I have examined, using Hudson's method[4], the vulnerable proximal portion of the His–Tawara system of 36 patients who died following heart valve replacement (Tables 10.1 and 10.2). Twenty-seven of these 36 patients have been previously reported[5]. Fourteen control hearts from routine autopsies were also examined.

The findings in the patients who died less than 14 days after valve replacement (group A) are given in Table 10.1. Conduction system haemorrhage (Figures 10.1–10.3) was observed in 12 of these 22 patients, mainly within the bundle of His. In 11 of the 12 patients the blood tracked along the connective tissue within and around the conducting tissue in a manner similar to that described by Hudson[2]. The earliest death in the group B patients (Table 10.2) occurred 14 days after valve replacement, and the latest at 8 years. None of the group B patients showed evidence of recent conduction system haemorrhage. However, the haemosiderin deposits within the bundle branches of patients 23 and 24 probably indicate previous haemorrhage. Haemosiderin was also observed within the His bundle of patient 27, but this appeared to be related to trauma by a surgical suture, which passed through the conducting tissue. In most of the patients in group B the cause of death was readily apparent at autopsy, apart from three patients (numbers 27, 29 and 34) in whom the cause of death was unknown. In group A the cause of death was unknown in 11 of the 22 patients. Haemorrhage into the conducting tissue was present in only six of these 11 patients for whom no cause of death had been found at autopsy.

Table 10.1 Clinicopathological details of 22 early (less than 14 days) postoperative deaths (Group A)

Patient	Age (years), sex	Valves replaced	Prosthesis	Survival (days)	Histology of His–Tawara system			
					AVN	His bundle	LBB	RBB
1	9,M	Mitral	S–E	0	Haemorrhage	Haemorrhage	Normal	Haemorrhage
2	29,F	Aortic, mitral	S–E, UCT	0	Congestion	Haemorrhage	Haemorrhage	Normal
3	50,F	Aortic	C–E	0	Normal	Haemorrhage	Normal	Normal
4	82,F	Aortic	C–E	0	Normal	Normal	Normal	Normal
5	43,M	Mitral	UCT	0.125	Normal	Normal	Normal	Normal
6	46,M	Mitral	UCT	0.17	Normal	Normal	Normal	Normal
7	15,F	Aortic	UCT	0.3	Normal	Normal	Normal	Normal
8	16,M	Aortic, mitral, tricuspid	UCT × 3	0.4	Haemorrhage	Haemorrhage	Haemorrhage	Haemorrhage
9	58,F	Aortic	UCT	0.8	Congestion	Haemorrhage; suture material	Haemorrhage; suture material	Normal
10	42,F	Mitral	UCT	1.0	Normal	Normal	Normal	Normal
11	14,M	Aortic	Lill.	1.0	Normal	Normal	Congestion	Normal
12	31,M	Mitral, tricuspid	UCT, S–E	1.0	Normal	Haemorrhage	Normal	Haemorrhage
13	61,F	Aortic	Lill.	1.0	Normal	Normal	Normal	Haemorrhage
14	60,M	Aortic	UCT	1.5	Normal	Normal	Normal	Haemorrhage
15	41,M	Aortic	Lill.	1.5	Normal	Normal	Normal	Normal
16	28,F	Mitral	UCT	2.0	Not seen	Normal	Normal	Not seen
17	44,M	Mitral	S–E	2.0	Haemorrhage	Haemorrhage	Haemorrhage	Normal
18	66,M	Aortic	UCT	3.0	Normal	Haemorrhage	Not seen	Haemorrhage
19	47,F	Mitral	S–E	4.0	Haemorrhage	Haemorrhage	Haemorrhage	Not seen
20	22,M	Aortic, mitral	B–S, S–E	5.0	Haemorrhage; suture material	Normal	Normal	Normal
21	52,F	Mitral	UCT	5.3	Not seen	Normal	Normal	Normal
22	62,M	Aortic	SJM	12.0	Haemorrhage	Normal	Normal	Normal

M = male; F = female; S–E = Starr–Edwards; UCT = University of Cape Town; C–E = Carpentier–Edwards; Lill. = Lillehei–Kaster; B–S = Bjork–Shiley; SJM = St Jude Medical; AVN = atrioventricular node; LBB = left bundle branch; RBB = right bundle branch

Table 10.2 Clinicopathological details of 14 late (more than 14 days) postoperative deaths (Group B)

Patient	Age (years), sex	Valves replaced	Prosthesis	Survival (days)	Histology of His–Tawara system			
					AVN	His bundle	LBB	RBB
23	49,M	Aortic	UCT	15	Not seen	Abscess	Not seen	Iron
24	41,M	Aortic	UCT	42	Not seen	Iron	Iron	Not seen
25	40,M	Aortic	S–E	60	Normal	Normal	Normal	Normal
26	57,F	Aortic, mitral	UCT, S–E	165	Not seen	Normal	Normal	Normal
27	40,M	Mitral, tricuspid	UCT × 2	180	Suture material, iron	Iron	Normal	Not seen
28	35,M	Aortic	UCT	180	Normal	Normal	Normal	Normal
29	36,F	Mitral	UCT	300	Not seen	Normal	Normal	Normal
30	16,F	Mitral	S–E	330	Normal	Normal	Normal	Normal
31	23,F	Mitral	UCT	480	Normal	Normal	Normal	Normal
32	52,M	Aortic, mitral	UCT × 2	540	Not seen	Normal	Normal	Not seen
33	34,F	Mitral	UCT	730	Congestion	Normal	Not seen	Not seen
34	61,M	Aortic	UCT	1095	Not seen	Normal	Normal	Normal
35	27,F	Aortic, mitral	UCT,S–E	1825	Normal	Normal	Normal	Not seen
36	48,F	Mitral, tricuspid	UCT,S–E	2920	Normal	Normal	Normal	Normal

M = male; F = female; S–E = Starr–Edwards; UCT = University of Cape Town; C–E = Carpentier–Edwards; Lill. = Lillehei–Kaster, B–S = Bjork–Shiley; SJM = St Jude Medical; AVN = atrioventricular node; LBB = left bundle branch; RBB = right bundle branch

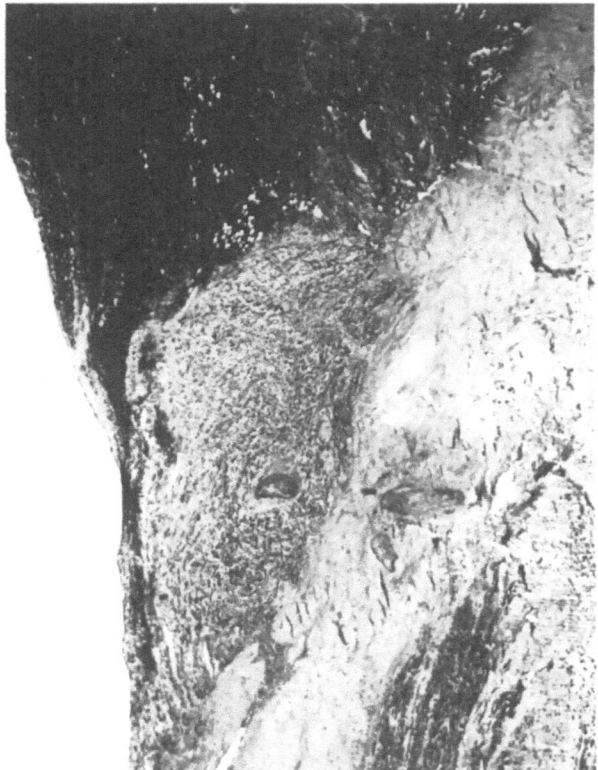

Figure 10.1 Darkly stained interatrial septal haematoma has extended down to reach the upper portion of the atrioventricular node. (Haematoxylin–eosin, × 60)

There was no sign of recent or old conduction tissue haemorrhage in the 14 control hearts. The conducting tissue haemorrhage, noted in group A patients, appeared separate in most instances from the larger and more obtrusive haemorrhage frequently observed in the interatrial septum following mitral valve replacement. In most hearts the conduction system haemorrhage was limited in extent, whereas in others it was more extensive and appeared to disrupt the conducting tissues. In some of these latter cases the haemorrhage was visible to the naked eye. Overall, 12 of the 22 group A patients showed haemorrhage at some site within the His–Tawara system.

Recent haemorrhage within the conduction system was only found in patients who died less than 2 weeks after heart valve replacement, and such haemorrhage is likely to be related to the operation. There appears to be no significant difference in the incidence of conduction tissue haemorrhage when one compares mitral and aortic prostheses. The central fibrous body and membranous septum constitute a continuous structure and are formed by the contiguous tricuspid, mitral and aortic valve rings[2]. The bundle of His

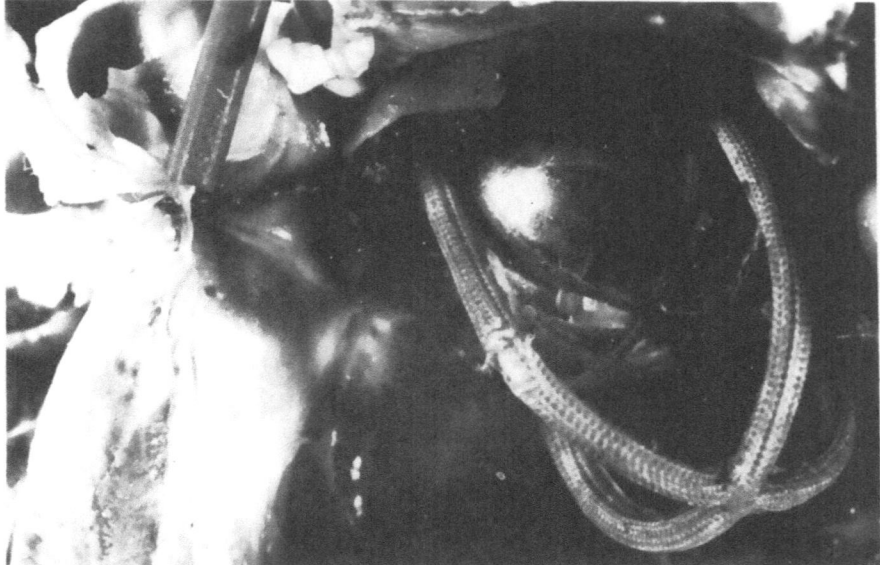

Fig. 10.2

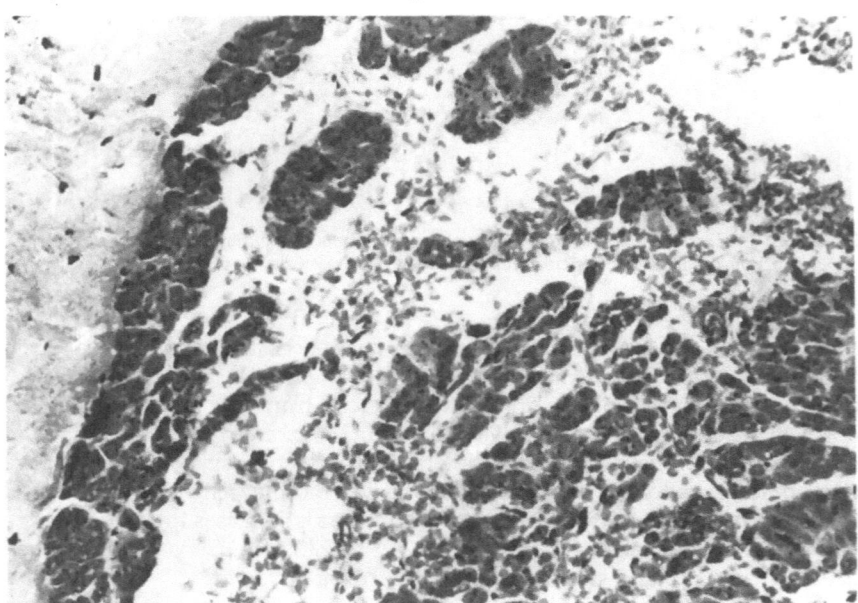

Fig. 10.3

Figure 10.2 Probe indicates haemorrhage within bundle of His at summit of interatrial septum. Patient died a few hours after mitral valve replacement with a Starr–Edwards valve prosthesis

Figure 10.3 Microscopical appearance of haemorrhage within the bundle of His. Same patient as shown in Figure 10.2 (Haematoxylin–eosin, × 43)

penetrates the central fibrous body, and is thus at risk in operations on these valves. The bundle is at greatest risk during aortic valve replacement[2]. Haemorrhage into the conducting tissues may result from either direct surgical trauma or anoxia.

Anoxia seems the likeliest cause of the conduction system haemorrhages noted in 11 of the patients in group A. The conduction tissue is the most heavily vascularized portion of the heart, and hypoxia produces capillary wall damage. Thus, hypoxia may be expected to produce selective haemorrhage into this area. Thung et al.[6] implicated hypoxia as a cause of haemorrhage into the cardiac conduction system, and emphasized the importance of adequate oxygenation in the post-thoracotomy patient. They also postulated that deposits of haemosiderin may remain within the conduction system, elicit scarring and produce arrhythmia.

Niles and Sandilands[7] found atrioventricular conduction system haemorrhage in 18 of 26 early deaths after valve replacement. Haemorrhage was also present in six of 36 late deaths. Most of their 24 cases of conduction tissue haemorrhage had shown an inadequate postoperative cardiac output, and they regarded the haemorrhages as a possible cause of fatal postoperative heart failure.

Study of the His–Tawara system in several patients who died after cardiac surgery for lesions not necessitating valve replacement (e.g. saphenous vein grafting of coronary arteries), but involving similar periods of time on cardiopulmonary bypass, also showed instances of haemorrhage into the His–Tawara system. This may indicate that the relative hypoxia of the bypass procedure is of greater significance than direct surgical trauma in the aetiology of such haemorrhage. A recent monograph describes the anatomy of the conduction system in various cardiac abnormalities[8].

Haemorrhage into the conduction tissue due to hypoxia is thus a common finding in patients dying 12 days or less after heart valve replacement. The clinical manifestation of haemorrhage into the atrioventricular conduction system is left bundle branch block followed by AV block and ventricular arrhythmia in the early postoperative period[9].

RENAL HAEMOSIDEROSIS IN PATIENTS WITH PROSTHETIC HEART VALVES

Haemolytic anaemia associated with an intracardiac prosthetic valve was reported for the first time by Rose et al.[10] in 1954. This complication was confirmed experimentally in dogs by Stohlman et al.[11] in 1956. While many subsequent reports dealing with the clinical and haematological aspects of haemolysis associated with intracardiac valve prostheses have been published, few refer to concomitant renal haemosiderosis[12–14], which is the anatomical indicator of intravascular haemolysis. When an excessive amount of iron is liberated into the blood by intravascular haemolysis it is deposited exclusively in the kidneys, and none is evident in the liver or spleen.

Haemolytic anaemia on a mechanical basis has been a particular problem in patients with mechanical valves[15]. Haemolysis is believed to result from two major factors: the 'hammer-and-anvil' effect resulting in damage to the erythrocytes by the occluder closing upon the metallic ring; and the abrasion or friction effect of a jet stream of blood against an irregular fabric surface. The first of these can be eliminated by having the occluder rest on small metallic struts rather than on a circular metal ring. The second may be reduced by having all parts of the valve except the sewing ring made of smooth, highly polished material. Studies on patients with native valvular heart disease, especially aortic stenosis[16] and incompetence[17], has revealed the presence of intravascular haemolysis. Mechanical haemolytic anaemia has also been reported after repair of ruptured mitral chordae tendineae[18]. Haemolysis resulted from the whiplash motion of the loose ends of the ruptured chordae and the disrupted suture material attached to the mitral valve apparatus.

The incidence and severity of renal haemosiderosis in a personally examined series of 105 autopsied patients with implanted prosthetic valves is given in Tables 10.3 and 10.4. Large (+ + +) amounts of iron (Figures 10.4 and 10.5) were present in the kidneys of nine of the 105 patients (8.6%). The haemosiderin granules were usually seen within the cells of the proximal convoluted tubules (Figure 10.5), but in some instances the iron was also present in the epithelial cells of the glomeruli. This distribution is similar to that observed by Roberts and Morrow[12]. Rarely, iron was seen lying free within Bowman's space or in the interstitium. No significant amount of iron

Table 10.3 Incidence and severity of renal siderosis in 105 autopsy patients with prosthetic heart valves

| | | Renal iron content | | |
Prosthesis	Nil	Scanty (+)	Moderate (+ +)	Abundant (+ + +)
UCT (n = 50)	22	17	7	4
Mixed (n = 17)	8	2	4	3
S–E (n = 14)	4	4	4	2
Lill. (n = 7)	7	0	0	0
B–S (n = 3)	2	1	0	0
Hanc. (n = 3)	3	0	0	0
C–E (n = 5)	3	2	0	0
SJM (n = 6)	4	0	2	0
Totals	53	26	17	9
Grand total = 105				

UCT = University of Cape Town; S–E = Starr–Edwards; Lill. = Lillehei–Kaster; B–S = Bjork–Shiley; Hanc. = Hancock; C–E = Carpentier–Edwards; SJM = St Jude Medical

was seen in the liver or spleen of any of these patients.

Renal haemosiderosis was absent in 31 of the 32 control patients who died with advanced rheumatic-type valvular deformities (Table 10.5). The only control patient showing renal siderosis was a 57-year-old white male who had mitral stenosis, trivial aortic stenosis and functional tricuspid incompetence. Cardiac symptoms had been present for 10 years. This same patient had large amounts of iron in his liver and spleen too, and as no blood transfusions had been given, this suggested a generalized haemosiderosis and indicated that the renal siderosis was not due to intravascular haemolysis.

Table 10.4 Data on patients with valve prostheses and abundant renal haemosiderosis

Patient	Age (years), sex	Prosthesis type	Postoperative survival (days)	Prostheses at autopsy	Cause of death
1.	41,M	UCT – Multiple	27	+ Thrombus	Coronary artery dissections
2.	20,F	UCT – Aortic	30	Normal	Cardiac failure
3.	48,M	UCT – Aortic	30	Infected	Brain infarct
4.	14,M	Mixed	150	+ Thrombus	Acute rheumatic fever
5.	39,F	UCT – Aortic + mitral	180	Infected	Brain infarct
6.	22,F	UCT – Mitral	330	Paravalvular leak	Brain infarct
7.	43,F	UCT – Multiple	720	Normal	Pneumonia
8.	24,F	S–E – Mitral	795	Cloth wear	Coronary artery embolus
9.	25,F	S–E – Mitral	2880	Cloth wear	Brain infarct

UCT = University of Cape Town; S–E = Starr–Edwards

Table 10.5 Autopsy incidence of renal siderosis in 53 control patients

Valve lesion	Renal iron content	
	Nil	Scanty
Mitral stenosis/incompetence	25	1
Aortic stenosis/incompetence	6	0
Routine autopsies (normal valves)	21	0

Comment

Significant (i.e. of moderate or severe degree) renal haemosiderosis was present in 26 of the 105 autopsy patients (25%) with valvular prostheses. Such siderosis was associated with severe sewing ring cloth wear, a paravalvular leak or thrombi on the prosthesis (infected in two). However, 12 patients showed no abnormality related to their prostheses.

All seven of Roberts and Morrow's[12] cases with renal siderosis had malfunctioning flexible Teflon aortic valves and haemolytic anaemia. Niles and Sandilands[13] encountered renal siderosis in four of 26 early deaths and in 17 of 36 late deaths following heart valve replacement with Starr–Edwards prostheses. The latter authors did not indicate the degree of the renal haemosiderosis, nor did they specify the state of the prosthetic valves in such patients. Both groups of authors agree that renal haemosiderosis does not impair renal function. The long-term effects of haemosiderinuria have not yet been adequately documented[19]. Some studies[20,21] have revealed haemolysis in patients whose prosthetic valves have shown no clinical evidence of incompetence. Postmortem renal siderosis may show clinically unapparent intravascular haemolysis.

Slight haemolysis is common with all mechanical valves[22]. Mechanical valves produce more severe haemolysis than xenograft valves with a similar degree of clinical incompetence[23]. Porcine xenograft valves do not seem to be associated with haemolysis unless complicated by a paravalvular leak[24]. Intravascular haemolysis may be associated with porcine mitral valve calcification in children[25]. Gallstones may result from even mild mechanical haemolysis[26].

Erythrocyte damage may not result simply from the mechanical trauma of poppet action on the red cells, but haemodynamic disturbances, such as turbulent blood flow and shearing stress resulting from rapidly changing velocity and pressure, may be the most important causes of traumatic mechanical damage. Urinary iron loss from continued intravascular haemolysis may even lead to chronic iron deficiency anaemia. Much less common after valve replacement is idiopathic haemolysis of the autoimmune type, with a positive antiglobulin test. Sulphinpyrazone may control cardiac valve-related haemolytic anaemia[27].

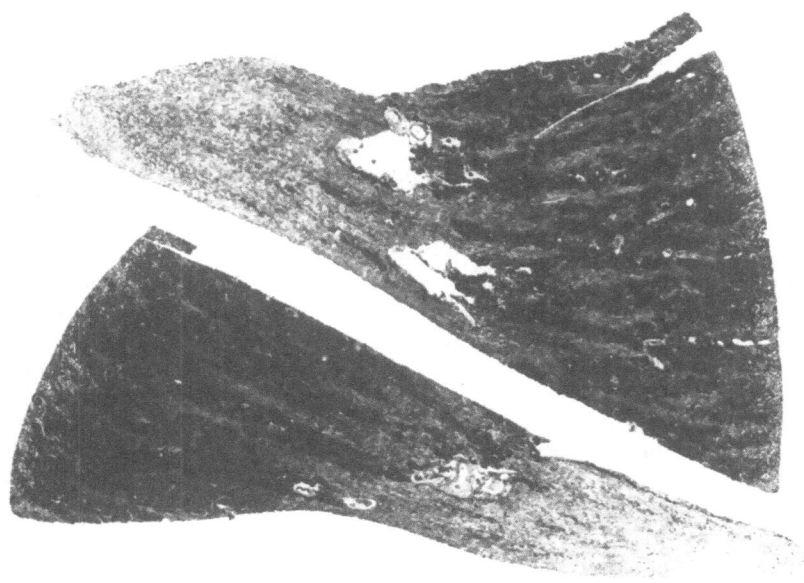

Fig. 10.4

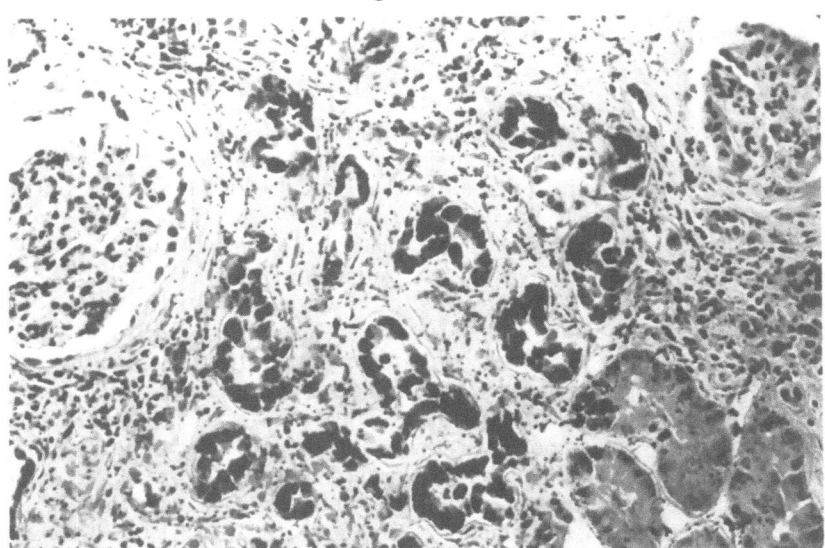

Fig. 10.5

Figure 10.4   Abundant (+ + +) renal cortical iron deposits in patient 1 with multiple UCT prostheses. (Perl's potassium ferrocyanide reaction)
Figure 10.5   Prominent iron deposits are seen within the epithelial cells of the proximal convoluted tubules. (Perl's potassium ferrocyanide reaction)

SUBVALVULAR LEFT VENTRICULAR FALSE ANEURYSM COMPLICATING MITRAL VALVE REPLACEMENT

Causes of left ventricular aneurysm[28,29] include myocardial infarction, trauma and rarities such as syphilis, tuberculosis, and mycotic aneurysms. False aneurysms may occur after non-fatal rupture of myocardial infarction (with adherent pericardium). Idiopathic aneurysms in the submitral, subaortic or apical regions of the left ventricle have been reported, predominantly from Africa. It has been suggested that the idiopathic aneurysms may develop because of defects in the attachment of the left ventricular myocardium or aorta to the fibrous mitral and aortic annuli.

Valve replacement surgery may cause a similar loss of atrioventricular continuity. Rupture of the heart at the atrioventricular sulcus (Figure 10.6) is a rare complication of excessive excision of the mitral annulus during mitral valve replacement[30-34]. Extension of valvular calcification into the annulus predisposes to this complication. Such disruption will lead to the formation of a subepicardial haematoma over the defect. Enlargement of the haematoma may compress the coronary sinus. In the absence of pericardial adhesions, rupture through the epicardium is likely with the production of cardiac tamponade. If the subepicardial haematoma undergoes organization instead of rupture, one may have the formation of a false cardiac aneurysm (Figure 10.7a,b), which communicates with the left ventricle through the mitral annular defect. Surgical repair of such an aneurysm diagnosed during life has been reported[35-38]. Similar aneurysm formation may complicate aortic valve replacement[39].

Comment

The left atrial myocardium is normally totally separated from the left ventricular muscle. It is the mitral ring together with the endocardium and epicardium that maintain the anatomical continuity between the left atrium and the left ventricle. It has been suggested[20,35] that rupture of the left atrioventricular sulcus during valve replacement is more likely to occur if mitral leaflet calcification involves the mitral ring too. Fibrous distortion of the posterior mitral leaflet, coupled with organized left atrial thrombus, may obliterate the exact limits of the annulus. Delayed rupture of the mitral annulus may also be produced by localized tissue necrosis resulting from prosthetic sewing ring sutures being placed too deeply into friable myocardium. In excising the mitral valve in a patient with a small left atrium, the exposure may be poor and a portion of the annulus may be inadvertently excised. After the valve is replaced and cardiopulmonary bypass is terminated, the stage is set for disruption of the atrioventricular sulcus.

Excessive removal of a laminated thrombus on the left atrial wall may also lead to perforation if excessive clearance is done, since the wall landmarks are often obscured. Selection of an oversized valve, resulting in a tight fit in the annular ring, may stretch or tear the annulus[35]. Re-excision of the annulus when removing a previously implanted mitral prosthesis may also lead to perforation. Wolpowitz et al.[36] recommend that in such cases the prosthesis

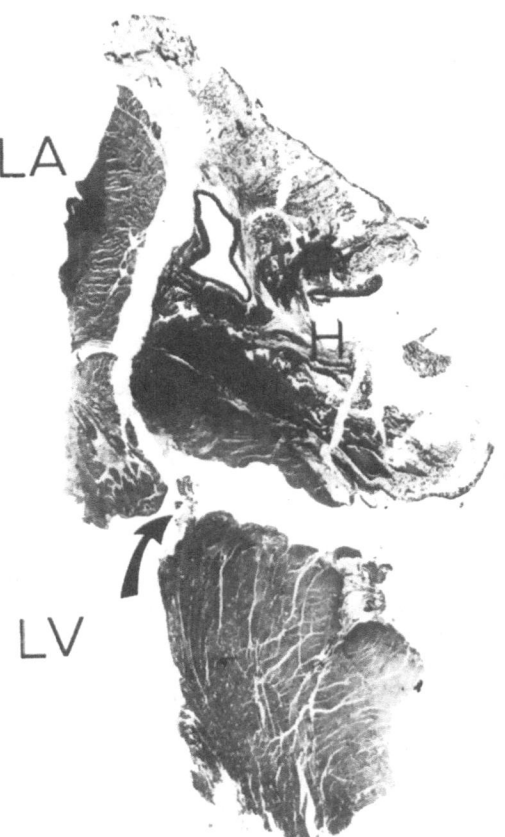

Figure 10.6 Subepicardial haematoma (H) overlies site of rupture (arrow) at junction of left atrium (LA) and left ventricle (LV), where excessive excision of the mitral valve ring has occurred during mitral valve replacement. External rupture of the haematoma caused fatal cardiac tamponade. (Haematoxylin–eosin, × 6)

should be excised between the sewing ring cushion and its metal frame. Firmly embedded prosthetic cloth is left behind for use of placement sutures as if it were the annulus. The use of a curved metal instrument to define posterior chordal attachments may also cause a perforation of the ventricle next to the atrioventricular junction. The postsurgical false aneurysm has the potential for expansion with pressure effects and perhaps rupture (either externally or into a cardiac chamber).

The type of left ventricular wall rupture associated with mitral valve replacement described above has been referred to as a type I rupture. A type II rupture occurs in the posterior mid-portion of the left ventricle[36,40,41]. Explanations for this problem[41] have included: (a) cutting too deep a plug and 'buttonholing' the ventricle during excision of the papillary muscle in a

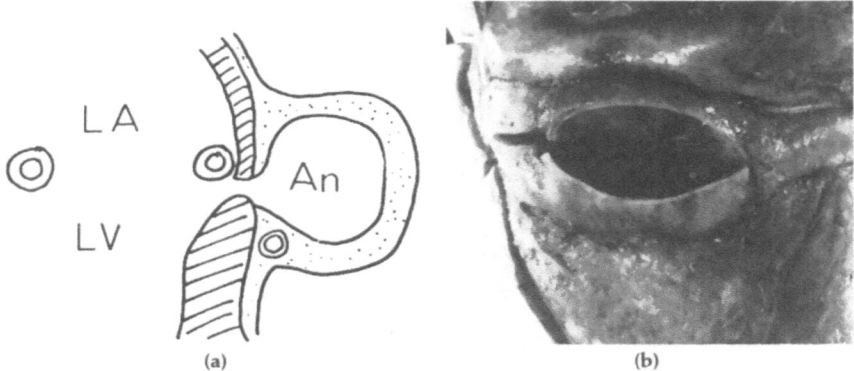

(a)   (b)

Figure 10.7 **(a)** Intra-epicardial false aneurysm communicates with left ventricle below sewing ring of mitral valve prosthesis. (From ref. 34; *Arch. Pathol. Lab. Med.* (1978), **102**, 285. Copyright 1978, American Medical Association. Reprinted by permission). **(b)** Deroofed submitral aneurysm in left atrioventricular groove on posterior aspect of the heart. Patient died of thromboembolism 4 years after mitral valve replacement

fragile, atrophic 'mitral ventricle'; (b) dissection of blood into the papillary muscle wound; (c) trauma from apical venting cardiotomy suckers[32]; (d) epicardial adhesions; (e) impingement of a prosthetic valve strut; (f) intrinsic myocardial disease; and (g) interruption of continuity between papillary muscle and mitral annulus. Cobbs *et al.*[41] suggest that a combination of factors may be important in the pathogenesis of this lesion. These factors include older patient age with associated coronary arterial disease, the size of the xenograft prosthetic valve, and the forceful central flow pattern of the Hancock valve. Cold- and potassium-induced cardioplegia render the heart more deformable and more liable to stretch-induced damage. The latter is favoured by excision of the mitral valve apparatus and too rapid weaning of the cardioplegic heart from bypass. Cobbs *et al.*[41] claim to have eliminated fatalities due to this complication by changing their operative technique to include a 30-minute period of empty beating after reversal of the cardioplegia.

False aneurysms may also be encountered at other sites after open-heart surgery. Jutrin *et al.*[42] described a false aneurysm of the right atrium, which appeared after open-heart surgery and appeared to be due to loosening of a right atrial suture. Because of the low pressure in the right atrium, the danger of rupture is low and conservative therapy is indicated. Becker *et al.*[43] reported a patient who presented 12 months post-aortic valve replacement with a false aneurysm near the aortic cannulation site. The patient refused surgery and died shortly afterwards. Autopsy revealed a smooth-walled 1 cm diameter defect adjacent to the cannulation site (presumably related to injury from a partial occlusion clamp). Weesner *et al.*[44] described left ventricular aneurysms associated with intraoperative venting of the cardiac apex in 32% of 50 children (average age 8 years) who were consecutively catheterized after surgical repair of congenital heart disease. The left ventricular apex had been vented by a sump during cardiopulmonary bypass in each patient. The aneurysms varied in size, but were generally small. The wall of the left

Table 10.6   Types and numbers (%) of infected prosthetic cardiac valves encountered among 275 patients with valve prostheses

University of Cape Town	16 (13.3%)
Lillehei–Kaster	2 (12.5%)
Bjork–Shiley	1 (6.7%)
Starr–Edwards	4 (8.5%)
St Jude Medical	4 (13.8%)
Mixed types of valves	3 (5.8%)
Carpentier–Edwards	1 (2.6%)

ventricular apex was thinner in patients with aneurysms than in age- and lesion-matched controls. All of the left ventricular aneurysm patients were asymptomatic during average follow-up of 4 years. The authors conclude that such aneurysms may be a potential source of complications and, where possible, they recommend alternative methods for venting the left ventricle.

INFECTIVE ENDOCARDITIS IN PATIENTS WITH PROSTHETIC HEART VALVES

Infective endocarditis (Colour Plate M, Figures 10.8 and 10.9) was encountered in 31 of 275 personally studied patients with valvular prostheses at autopsy. It accounted for 4.9% of the early deaths and 18.2% of the late deaths. Sixteen of the patients were females. The mean age of the patients was 41.9 years (SD = 13.6) with a range of 15–67 years. Mean postoperative survival was 332 days (SD = 657) with a range of 14–3285 days. Thirty patients had mechanical prostheses and only one had a tissue valve. The types of prosthetic valves affected are listed in Table 10.6. The diagnosis of prosthetic valve infection had not been suspected clinically in four patients (13%).

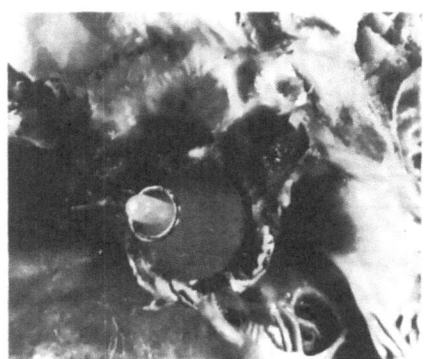
Fig. 10.8

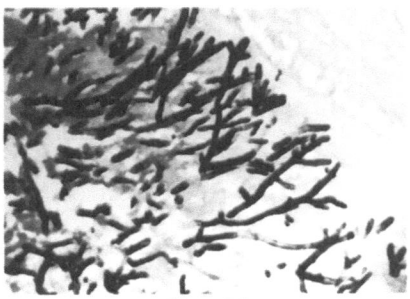
Fig. 10.9

Figure 10.8   Partial dehiscence of University of Cape Town aortic valve prosthesis due to infection with *Staphylococcus albus* alongside the sewing ring

Figure 10.9   Histological appearance of fungal infection within vegetation situated upon a mechanical valve prosthesis. Culture grew *Aspergillus niger*. (Methenamine silver stain, × 320)

Table 10.7 indicates the causative micro-organisms in the 31 patients with infected prostheses. The commonest pathogens were staphylococci, followed by Gram-negative bacilli and fungi. In all of the patients with mechanical valves the infection was situated at the site of attachment of the prosthetic sewing ring to the native valve ring. The one infected (Carpentier–Edwards) tissue valve had infected vegetations on the cusps with minimal juxta-sewing ring inflammation. Nearly all of the infected mechanical valves also had infected vegetations on the struts or cage. Ring abscesses were noted in almost one-third of cases (29%) and one patient developed complete heart block due to destruction of the bundle of His.

Three of the 31 patients with prosthetic valve infective endocarditis had a clinical history of preoperative infective endocarditis. None of the excised native valves showed histological evidence of infection. Seven patients with infected prostheses died due to prosthetic malfunction (five valves were partially detached, and two prostheses were severely obstructed by vegetations). Ten patients died of systemic embolism; four died of ruptured mycotic aneurysms, and 10 died of other causes, e.g. myocardial failure or pyaemic abscesses and toxaemia.

Comment

Not all bacteraemias in patients with prosthetic heart valves represent infection of the valve, particularly when there is no haemodynamic instability or evidence of valve dysfunction and when the bacteraemia is due to a Gram-negative bacillus. Parker et al.[45] noted bacteraemia in 3.6% of 890 patients after heart valve replacement in the hospital recovery period. Only two of the 32 bacteraemic patients developed endocarditis. Leitersdorf et al.[46] hypothesize that there is a close relationship between subclinical thrombo-endocarditis on the native valve and the early development of infective endocarditis on the implanted prosthesis. However, the organism presumed to be the cause of the prosthetic valve infective endocarditis (PVIE) was often different from the one isolated earlier as the cause of the natural valve endocarditis[47].

Table 10.7 Causative micro-organisms in 31 patients with prosthetic valve infective endocarditis

Organism	Group 1	Group 2	Total
Staphylococcus albus	0	7 (23%)	7 (23%)
Staphylococcus aureus	0	4 (13%)	4 (13%)
Candida albicans	2 (7%)	1 (3%)	3 (10%)
Candida parasilosis	0	1 (3%)	1 (3%)
Unidentified fungus	1 (3%)	0	1 (3%)
Klebsiella species	1 (3%)	0	1 (3%)
Diphtheroids	1 (3%)	1 (3%)	2 (7%)
Coliforms	0	1 (3%)	1 (3%)
Actinobacillus	0	1 (3%)	1 (3%)
Pseudomonas species	0	1 (3%)	1 (3%)
Bacillus cereus	0	1 (3%)	1 (3%)
Unknown	2 (7%)	6 (19%)	8 (26%)

Regarding the pathogenesis of fungal infection of heart valve prostheses, Robboy and Kaiser[48] made the controversial suggestion that foci of infection start on patches of neo-endocardium on the sewing cloth of the valve prosthesis, and that it is the neo-endocardium, rather than the cloth or metal of the prosthesis, which is the important predisposing factor. The early development of postoperative infective endocarditis is recognized as a distinct hazard and a unique clinical entity differing from non-surgical infective endocarditis in the following aspects: (a) different organisms are involved; (b) the typical clinical picture of infective endocarditis is frequently lacking; and (c) the fatality rate is unusually high.

Incidence

The incidence of infective endocarditis after cardiac surgery varies in different series. The incidence is higher after surgery requiring cardiopulmonary bypass than after 'closed' intracardiac procedures. The incidence of infective endocarditis after prosthetic valvular replacement varies among different medical centres and is determined by many factors[49], including the underlying condition of the patient at the time of operation, the skill of the surgeon, the type of prosthesis used, the duration of cardiopulmonary bypass, the sterility of the heart–lung machine and the operating theatre, the use of prophylactic antibiotics, the incidence of extracardiac postoperative infection and the length of the follow-up period after surgery. The incidence of early PVIE, defined as that occurring within 2 months after valve implantation, varies from 0 to 7.1% among different centres. The reported incidence of late PVIE for patients followed up for at least 6 months after surgery varies from 0 to 3.2% among different centres and the overall incidence of PVIE (all cases) varies from 0 to 9.5%, with an average of 2.3%[49].

Source of the organisms

Primary intraoperative contamination appears to be responsible for most postoperative endocarditis. Contamination of the heart–lung machine by diphtheroids and *Pseudomonas*[50] has resulted in endocarditis. The coagulase-negative *Staphylococcus*, which was the commonest cause of PVIE in our patients, is ubiquitous in the air of operating rooms and on human skin. Ankeney[51] performed 1555 intraoperative blood cultures during 383 open-heart operations and in 117 (7.5%) *Staphylococcus albus* was cultured; 153 (9.8%) grew a diphtheroid bacillus and 29 (1.9%) were other micro-organisms. Most positive cultures were obtained from the primed pump and the suction line during bypass, when the pump and blood were most exposed to air.

In addition to intraoperative contamination, the organisms may be introduced by diagnostic cardiac catheterization, the prolonged use of intravenous catheters, indwelling urinary catheters and contaminated blood. The valve prosthesis may become secondarily infected in all of the above circumstances. Finally, intrinsic contamination of the valve prosthesis itself is another potential source of infection[49]. Porcine aortic valves from one manufacturer have been contaminated by *Mycobacterium chelonei*, and at least two patients developed infective endocarditis[52].

Increased susceptibility to infection

Many of the organisms producing PVIE are of a 'low virulence'. Increased susceptibility to infection may result from both local and general factors. Elek[53] showed that the presence of silk sutures potentiated *Staphylococcus aureus* infection of the skin up to 10 000-fold. Similarly, foreign material placed within the heart increases the pathogenicity of bacteria and also makes infection difficult to eradicate by antimicrobial drugs. Cardiopulmonary bypass may reduce the host's resistance to bacterial infections and the phagocytic activity of neutrophils, as well as IgG and haemolytic complement, may be depressed after open-heart surgery.

Microbiology

The microbiology of PVIE is much different from that of natural valve infective endocarditis[54]. The types of micro-organisms involved in my 31 patients with PVIE are characteristic of the findings of others in PVIE. *Staphylococcus albus* is the single most important cause of both early and late PVIE, accounting for 27.4% of the early cases and 22.9% of the late cases[49]. *Staphylococcus albus* was the cause in 23% of our patients with PVIE overall. *Staphylococcus albus* has been inculpated in anywhere from 6% to 35% of reported cases of PVIE. *Staphylococcus aureus* is an important cause of early PVIE, accounting for 27.4% of the early cases and 22.9% of the late cases[49]. Streptococci, which are the most important group of aetiological agents in infective endocarditis of natural valves, are not an important cause of PVIE, accounting for only about 7.5% of early cases, and were not encountered in my autopsy patients. Streptococci account for about 37% of late PVIE[49], and presumably have the same sources as in patients with infected natural heart valves.

According to Wilson *et al.*[55], Gram-negative bacilli are the second leading cause of early-onset infections and are third in frequency among patients with late-onset PVIE. Gram-negative bacilli were the second most frequent pathogens in my 31 patients with fatal PVIE and accounted for 22% of the total. Gram-negative bacilli are a rare cause of infective endocarditis of natural valves except for intravenous drug abusers[54]. A wide variety of Gram-negative bacilli have been isolated in PVIE, including species of *Pseudomonas*[50], *Haemophilus*, *Escherichia coli*[50], *Alcaligenes faecalis* and *Eikenella corrodens*. Others include members of the genera *Klebsiella*, *Serratia*, *Enterobacter*[50], *Proteus*, and *Hafnia*. Miscellaneous bacteria causing PVIE include various species of diphtheroids, *Actinobacillus actinomycetemcomitans*, *Nocardia asteroides*, *Neisseria* species, *Mycobacterium chelonei*, *Brucella*, *Bacillus cereus*, *Kingella kingae*, Q fever and *Listeria monocytogenes*.

Fungal infections, which comprised 16% of my cases, are said by Watanakunakorn[49] to be responsible for 9.6% and 4.3% of the early and late cases, respectively. Norenberg *et al.*[56] reported a 13–20% incidence of fungal endocarditis following cardiac operations. *Candida albicans* plus other *Candida* species are important causes of PVIE. *Aspergillus* is reported to be the next most important cause of fungal PVIE[49,57]. Other fungi causing PVIE include *Histoplasma capsulatum*, *Cryptococcus neoformans*, *Mucor*, *Paecilomyces*, *Penicillium notatum*, and *Trichosporon cutaneum*.

Pathology

Although many reports are available on patients with fatal infective endocarditis of natural cardiac valves, there is limited information on the morphology of PVIE. PVIE may cause either obstruction or incompetence of the prosthesis[58–60]. Large ring abscesses may loosen the attachment of the prosthesis. Arnett and Roberts[61] analysed 22 necropsy patients with PVIE; as in my patients, *Staphylococcus* was the most frequent infecting organism. In each of their patients the infection was located behind the site of attachment of the prosthesis to the native valve ring. Prosthetic obstruction by vegetations occurred more commonly with an infected mitral valve prosthesis than with aortic prostheses. Anderson *et al.*[60] recorded a clinicopathological study of 22 patients with PVIE. Prosthetic valve dysfunction led to death in 45% of their patients, and embolic events killed 23%. Ring infection, often believed to be universally present, and a contraindication to surgery, was present in only 50% of their patients.

Specific aspects of PVIE include: fatal obstruction to left ventricular inflow[62], rupture of mycotic aneurysms[63], embolism[64], bioprosthetic endocarditis[65], or surgical management of prosthetic valve endocarditis[66]. There is no apparent relationship to specific prosthetic valve type or design with respect to incidence or organisms[67]. Usually the aortic site is involved more often than the mitral. The mortality rate is high, about 60% overall, being significantly higher for the early infection (73%) than for the late (45%). Since biomaterials themselves do not support the growth of infective organisms, the potentiation of infection by foreign bodies must involve an as yet poorly understood interaction of local physical and biological factors. An innovative approach to the prevention of PVIE is the incorporation of an antibiotic into the valve prosthesis, to be slowly released during function[68]. The principal guides to prognosis in PVIE are the patient's cardiac status and the nature of the infecting organism[69].

SMALL CORONARY ARTERIAL DISEASE

The small coronary arteries (SCA), which have a diameter less than 1 mm, are important because they include important anastomoses, supply the conduction tissues, and may be involved by occlusive lesions in a variety of systemic diseases. Twenty-seven of 275 personally examined patients (18.6%) with prostheses showed small coronary arterial abnormalities. Table 10.8 gives data regarding small coronary arterial disease in patients with valvular prostheses and in three groups of control patients. The majority of the small arteries in all three groups of patients examined showed no significant

Table 10.8 Small coronary arterial disease in patients with valvular prostheses and in three groups of control patients

	Patients with prostheses	Rheumatic fever		Routine autopsy patients
		Active	Healed	
No. of patients	275	13	26	20
No. of arteries	11 261	676	1008	758
Normal	90.8%	85.9%	86.6%	96.6%
Medial oedema	0.2%	6.7%	0.6%	0.4%
Longitudinal SMCs	0.1%	1.9%	1.1%	0.5%
Medial hypertrophy	0.9%	1.8%	1.8%	1.1%
Intimal fibrosis	2.3%	1.2%	1.6%	0.1%
Elastification	Nil	Nil	2.6%	Nil
Loss of mural demarcation	1.1%	0.7%	1.6%	0.1%
Fresh thromboemboli	1.4%	0.6%	1.5%	0.5%
Organized thromboemboli	2.7%	0.9%	2.4%	0.4%
Foreign body emboli	0.5%	Nil	Nil	Nil
Arteritis	Nil	0.3%	0.2%	Nil

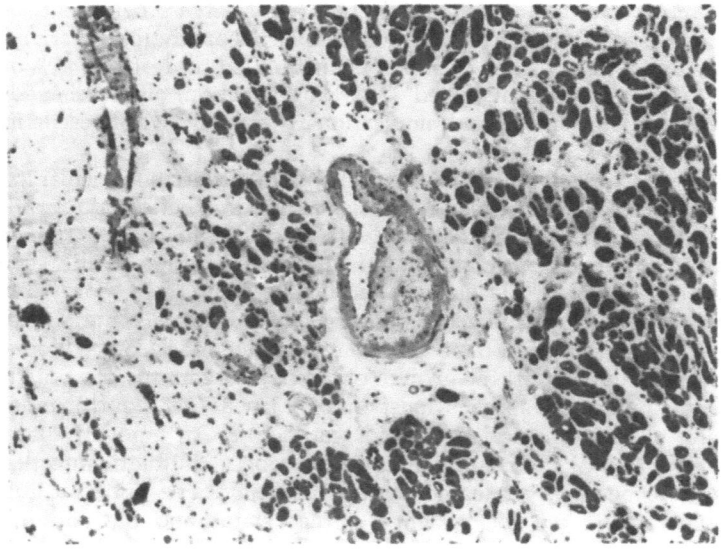

Figure 10.10 Organized thromboembolus in small coronary artery plus surrounding interstitial and replacement fibrosis of left ventricular myocardium. Patient died of myocardial failure a few days after aortic valve replacement. The myocardial changes antedated the valve surgery. (Haematoxylin–eosin, × 60)

abnormality. Organized thromboemboli (eccentric intimal thickening) (Figure 10.10) and concentric intimal fibrous thickening were the commonest abnormalities observed in SCA patients with prostheses, being present in 2.7% and 2.3% of arteries respectively. The incidence of thromboemboli in patients with valvular prostheses did not differ significantly from unoperated patients with healed chronic rheumatic valvular heart disease. Table 10.9 indicates the nature of the emboli encountered in patients with prostheses.

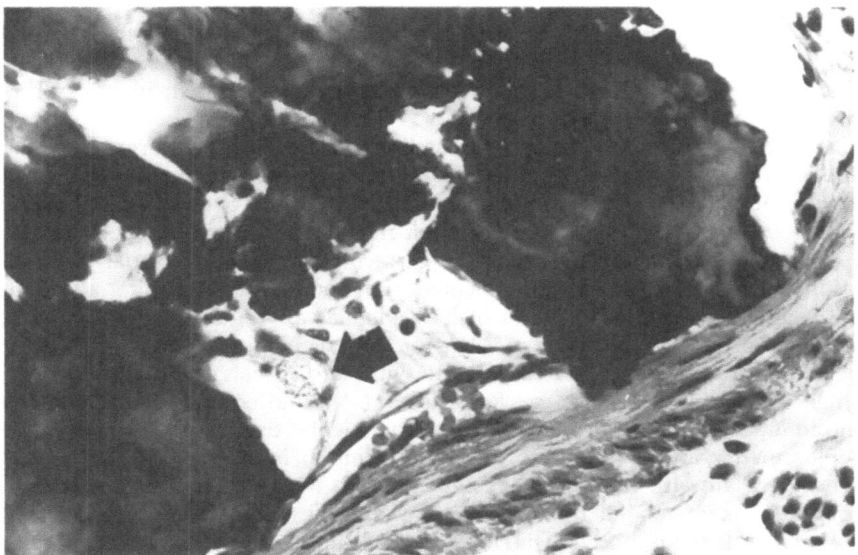

Figure 10.11 Small coronary artery contains calcific embolus plus a silicone embolus (arrow)

Comment

Small coronary arterial disease is not a major problem in patients with prosthetic heart valves. Only 13 of our 275 patients (4.6%) with implanted valvular prostheses showed small coronary emboli. The incidence of thromboembolism did not differ significantly from that noted in patients with rheumatic fever or routine autopsy controls. Foreign body emboli were confined to patients with prosthetic valves. Calcium embolism (Figure 10.11) may accompany surgical resection of calcified left-sided heart valves[70] or it may arise from a heavily calcified, ulcerated aortic valve as well as from a calcified valve after mitral valvotomy. There is a high risk of calcium

Table 10.9 Types of small coronary arterial emboli in 275 patients with implanted cardiac valvular prostheses

Type of embolus	No. of patients
Thromboembolus	
Fresh	11
Organized	8
Calcium	4
Atheromatous	1
Foreign	
Silicone	2
Fibres (? Teflon)	2
Unidentified	1
Total	29

microemboli in patients with a heavily calcified valve annulus who undergo valve replacement, since debridement of the calcified annular tissue is difficult. The use of microfilters in the bypass circuit has reduced the incidence of this complication.

Other types of foreign body microemboli related to cardiac surgery include cholesterol, suture material, silicone from the oxygenator pump[71], Teflon from prosthetic valves[72], and Dacron from the worn cloth covering of prosthetic valves. A diagnosis of cloth fibre emboli rather than thromboemboli may be favoured by the clinical manifestation of recurrent systemic arterial embolization more than 4 years after valve replacement and despite adequate anticoagulation[73]. Other emboli include platelet aggregates from the pump oxygenator, bone marrow/adipose tissue and air emboli.

In the present series 9% of patients with cardiac valvular prostheses had small coronary arterial disease. Roberts et al.[74] found embolic material in the intramural coronary arteries of 9% of patients dying after heart valve replacement. Silver[75] found foreign body emboli in about 10% of patients who died late after cardiac valve replacement. Many such emboli appeared as granulomata related to small coronary arteries, but without an obvious associated foreign body. The number of emboli and granulomata found increase and become more widespread in distribution if there has been wear of the prosthesis.

PATHOLOGY OF THE MAJOR CORONARY ARTERIES

Thromboemboli may be encountered within the coronary arteries of patients with valve prostheses; myocardial infarction is associated in a small percentage of patients. The thromboemboli usually lodge within epicardial coronary arteries (Figure 10.12), but occasionally they may be found in penetrating vessels, e.g. a septal perforator branch of the left anterior descending coronary artery (Colour Plate W). Postmortem angiography will help in detecting such cases.

Among 275 personally studied autopsy patients with prostheses, 17 showed epicardial coronary thromboemboli and six of the latter had myocardial infarcts. Seventeen patients (6%) had 75% or more reduction in luminal cross-sectional area of one or more of the major coronary arteries due to atherosclerosis (Figure 10.13). Seven patients underwent bypass grafting at the time of the valve surgery. Coronary atherosclerosis caused the death of only three of these patients. In more developed countries the incidence of atherosclerotic coronary disease is higher, e.g. 22% of the valve cases reported from America by Schoen et al.[76]. Valve replacement combined with coronary bypass grafting is time-consuming, and severely tests myocardial protection strategies. Lytle et al.[77] found that in-hospital mortality in such cases was increased by female sex, aortic insufficiency and advanced age.

Miscellaneous conditions were noted in 10 patients. Two had surgical sutures penetrating their left circumflex coronary artery. In an early patient with a congenitally proximal bifurcation of the left main coronary artery the coronary perfusion cannula entered the left anterior descending branch only,

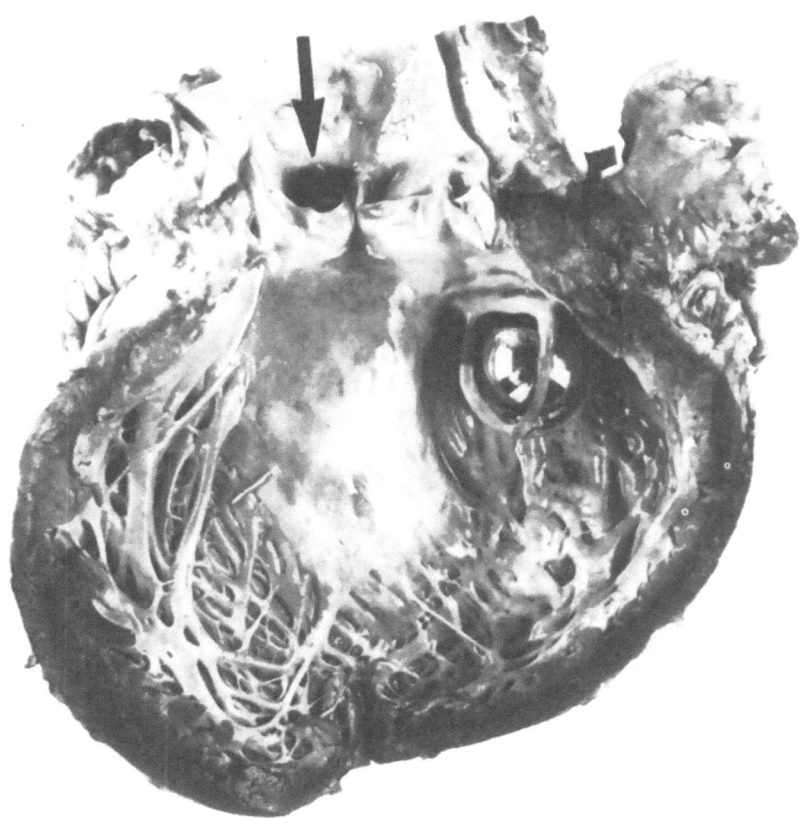

Figure 10.12 Sudden death 3.5 years after mitral valve replacement was due to thromboembolus (arrow) occluding ostium of right coronary artery. Starr–Edwards mitral valve prosthesis has host tissue covering sewing ring and portion of the cage struts. No thrombi were present on the prosthesis, but left atrial appendage contained abundant red thrombus similar in appearance to the thromboembolus

with occlusion of the non-perfused left circumflex coronary artery. Two patients with coronary arterial ostial stenosis both had coronary arterial bypass grafts performed. One patient had syphilis, and atherosclerosis caused the stenosis in the other. In a third patient a Lillehei–Kaster aortic valve prosthesis partially obstructed both coronary ostia; the patient did not survive the operation. Another patient had redundant suture material from the sewing ring of an aortic valve prosthesis protruding into the left coronary arterial ostium, but no significant obstruction resulted.

Three patients showed coronary arterial dissection; in one the coronary arterial involvement was due to extension of an aortic dissecting aneurysm. In a second patient coronary dissection complicated coronary angiography.

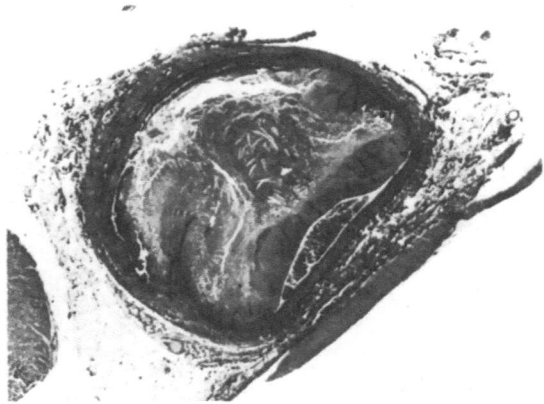

Figure 10.13 Grade 4 (> 75%) luminal narrowing of major coronary artery due to eccentric atherosclerosis. (Haematoxylin–eosin, × 10)

The dissection in the third patient was a complication of bypass grafting for atherosclerosis.

STATE OF THE MYOCARDIUM IN PATIENTS WITH PROSTHETIC HEART VALVES

Heart weights

Table 10.10 indicates the mean heart weights in early (group 1) and late (group 2) survivors following heart valve replacement (with 1 month postoperative survival as the cut-off point) and also compares the heart weights of patients with and without the clinical features of myocardial pump failure. Correction of the valvular defect(s) does not lead to reversal of the myocardial hypertrophy with prolonged postoperative survival. Valve prostheses are stenotic compared to natural valves and this may be a factor in the persistence of hypertrophy, especially with aortic valve replacement. Myocardial fibrosis due to rheumatic fever or ischaemia may also play a role. Little is known about the reversibility of myocardial hypertrophy. Patients

Table 10.10 Mean heart weights in patients with implanted prosthetic heart valves with reference to duration of postoperative survival and cardiac failure

Patients	Heart weights (g), mean, (SD)
Group 1 ($n = 114$)	646 (203)
Group 2 ($n = 121$)	660 (226)
Patients without failure ($n = 207$)	635 (208)*
Patients with failure ($n = 28$)	732 (202)*

*$p < 0.05$

dying with myocardial failure had significantly heavier hearts than those without failure ($p < 0.05$).

Myocardial necrosis

Myocardial necrosis may take one of four histological forms:

Coagulative necrosis[78]

The myocytes appear hypereosinophilic with lost cross-striations and nuclear detail, but the myocyte sarcoplasm remains intact for a prolonged period after its demise. Such necrosis may be regional (e.g. after coronary thrombosis) or global (due to diffuse subtotal major coronary arterial narrowing). The necrosis may also be categorized as transmural, subendocardial or subepicardial.

Contraction band necrosis

Contraction band necrosis (coagulative myocytolysis, myofibrillar degeneration)[79] is categorized by myocytes developing zones of supercontractions within their cytoplasm (Figure 10.14) in which there is a marked aggregation of myofilaments with clearing of the sarcoplasm on either side of the aggregate. This is the usual type of myocardial necrosis induced by catecholamine excess, and a similar artefact may be observed in endomyocardial biopsies taken from living patients.

Massive contraction band necrosis may produce the stone heart syndrome[80], which is analogous to rigor mortis in skeletal muscle and results from ATP depletion. The coronary arteries may be normal. At operation the heart is very firm to palpation, the ventricular cavity is minuscule (concentric hypertrophy) and no cardiac output can be obtained by manual massage. Prior to the institution of cold cardioplegia to protect the heart during cardiopulmonary bypass, the stone heart was an uncommon complication of ischaemic cardiac arrest, but it is virtually never seen these days. In experimental animals it is readily produced by global ischaemia of a normothermic heart; modern hypothermia prevents its occurrence. Isolated hearts given a calcium-free perfusion followed by a normocalcaemic reperfusion develop the ischaemic contracture within 5 minutes; hypothermia is again protective. Cardioplegia with myocardial cooling provides better myocardial protection than either alone[81].

Myocytolysis (Figure 10.15)

This is another form of myocyte necrosis, which may occur in association with coagulative necrosis or catecholamine excess and may follow contraction band necrosis. The sarcolemmal sheaths remain intact and there is vacuolization and dissolution of the cytoplasm and nucleus, leaving a honeycomb pattern

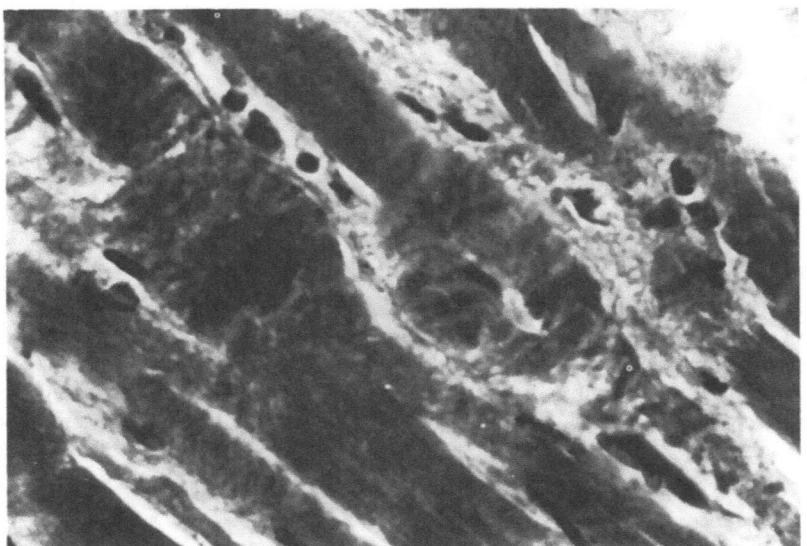

Figure 10.14   Myocytes show prominent cytoplasmic contraction banding. (Haematoxylin–eosin, × 600)

of empty sarcolemmal sheaths. A patchy mononuclear cellular infiltration may be present.

Subendocardial reperfusion-type haemorrhagic infarction

This condition (Colour Plate X) is usually seen in patients with severe postoperative myocardial failure after aortic or double valve replacement. Gotlieb *et al.*[82] list the following sequence of changes in this entity: contraction bands, subendocardial haemorrhages, coagulative necrosis, healing by granulation tissue, and fibrosis. The location of the lesion coincides with the vulnerable portion of the microcirculation.

I have studied 87 early survivors after valve replacement who were divided according to the form of intraoperative myocardial protection that was used[83]. The first group of 45 patients was treated with intraoperative coronary arterial perfusion with blood from the oxygenator pump machine with separate perfusion of the two coronary arteries, individual monitoring of pressure and flow, plus cooling of the beating heart to 32°C. The second group of 42 patients received cold cardioplegia and the heart was cooled down to about 15°C and arrested in diastole by potassium administration. The first three forms of myocardial necrosis described above occurred with equal severity in the two groups of patients.

Another aspect investigated was the state of the myocardium in patients who received intermittent versus continuous coronary arterial perfusion with

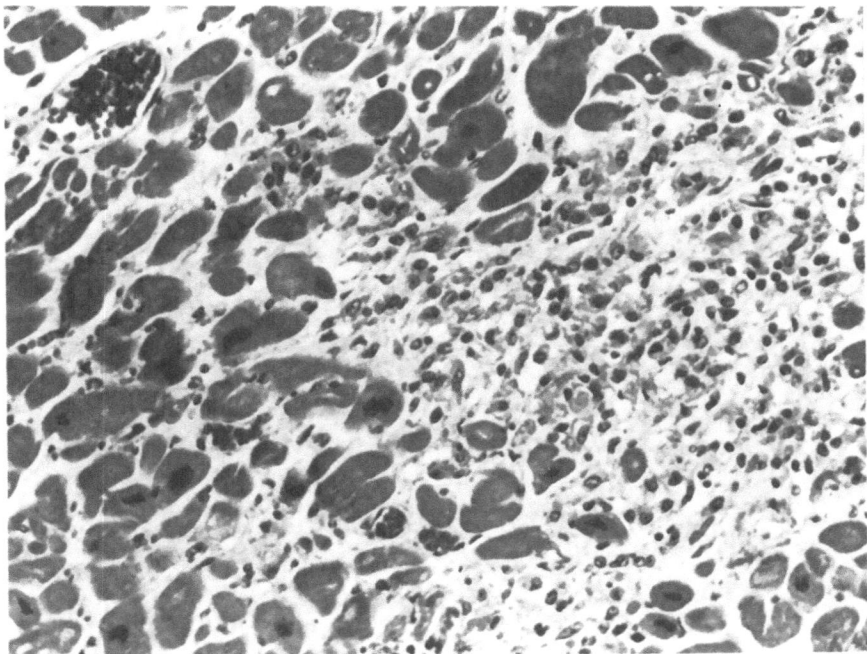

Figure 10.15 Zone of myocytolysis with early stromal collapse. (Haematoxylin–eosin, × 120)

blood during cardiopulmonary bypass; a similar evaluation was performed for patients with regularly beating hearts versus those whose hearts fibrillated continuously during bypass. No significant differences were found.

Myocardial fibrosis

Myocardial fibrosis[84] (Figure 10.16) may take one or more of the following forms:

1. *Replacement fibrosis* (Figure 10.17) in which groups of myocytes are replaced by collagen fibres.
2. *Interstitial fibrosis* appears as fine strands of connective tissue encircling and separating individual myocytes.
3. *Perivascular fibrosis* links up myocardial blood vessels and thereby delineates groups of myocytes.
4. *Plexiform fibrosis* is seen in areas of myocyte disarray similar to that seen in hypertrophic cardiomyopathy. Foci of collagenous fibrous tissue of irregular size and shape with jagged borders lie interlaced between the myocytes.

The severity of myocardial fibrosis can be assessed by morphometry, i.e. a volumetric analysis of tissue sections is achieved by point-counting. Such

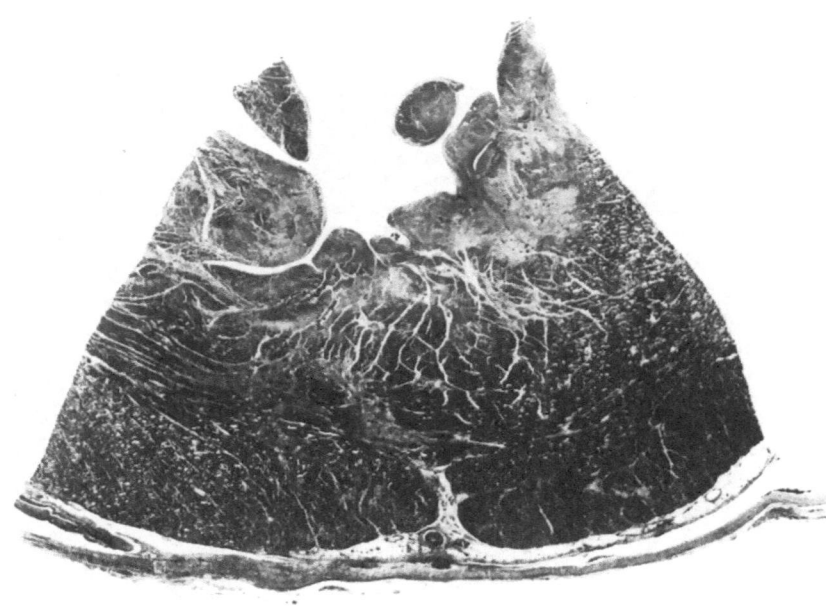

Figure 10.16 Subendocardial replacement fibrosis of left ventricle. (Elastic van Gieson, × 3.4)

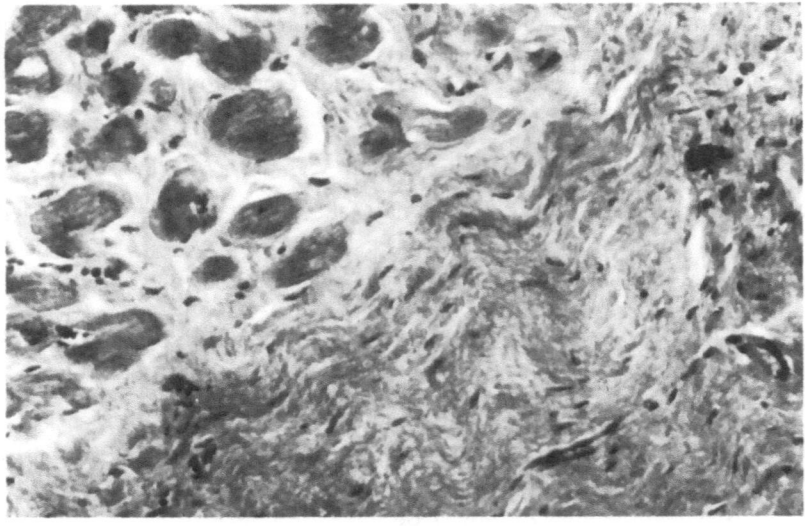

Figure 10.17 Replacement fibrosis of the myocardium (bottom right) merges with interstitial fibrosis (top left). (Haematoxylin–eosin, × 150)

an investigation showed no significant difference between autopsied patients with valve prostheses and unoperated controls with valvular disease[83].

POSTPERFUSION LUNG

Postperfusion lung is the name given to the 'adult respiratory distress syndrome' that may occur following heart valve replacement, particularly if there is a prolonged bypass period. The condition is characterized by oedema, fibrin exudation (hyaline membranes) within alveoli and microvascular thrombi. The pathogenesis of the condition is obscure; suggested causes include platelet and leukocytic microemboli in the pulmonary microcirculation with possible release of biologically active substances and circulatory obstruction. Resultant changes in surfactant levels may also play a role. The 'postperfusion lung' is characterized clinically by dyspnoea, arterial hypoxaemia with an increased alveolar–arterial oxygen difference, and increased fluid in the tracheobronchial tree[85]. Increasing pulmonary oedema may lead to a fatal outcome.

Baer and Osborn[86] encountered this complication in 70% of 41 patients dying after total cardiopulmonary bypass. They attributed the syndrome to overdistension of the left atrium during perfusion, anoxia, hypotension, foreign proteins or denatured blood elements. Kolff et al.[87] suggested that pulmonary damage during open-heart operations is usually due to temporary overfilling of the pulmonary vascular bed with blood, leading to capillary damage. The pulmonary lesions observed following extracorporeal circulation are similar to those found in adult respiratory distress syndrome caused by many other mechanisms and long-surviving patients may show pulmonary fibrosis. It is difficult to separate the histological changes of the postperfusion pulmonary syndrome from those induced in the lungs by respirator therapy.

Westaby[85] set out to determine which components of the bypass circuit may trigger the complement cascade. Nylon, polyurethane, polyethylene, polyvinyl chloride and polycarbonate form an important part of most bubble oxygenators and cardiotomy reservoirs. He found that all materials except polycarbonate activate complement to some extent, and nylon was especially potent in this regard.

REFERENCES

1. Hudson, R. E. B. (1983). The conducting system: anatomy, histology, pathology in acquired heart disease. In Silver, M. D. (ed.) *Cardiovascular Pathology*. p. 633. (New York: Churchill Livingstone)
2. Hudson, R. E. B. (1967). Surgical pathology of the conducting system of the heart. *Br. Heart J.*, **29**, 646
3. Zimmermann, J. and Bailey, C. P. (1962). The surgical significance of the fibrous skeleton of the heart. *J. Thorac. Cardiovasc. Surg.*, **44**, 701
4. Hudson, R. E. B. (1963). The human conduction system and its examination. *J. Clin. Pathol.*, **16**, 492
5. Rose, A. G. (1973). The bundle of His in prosthetic heart valve replacement. *S. Afr. Med. J.*, **47**, 136

6. Thung, N., Damman, J. F., Diaz-Perez, R., Thompson, W. M., Sanmarco, M. and Mehegan, C. (1962). Hypoxia as the cause of hemorrhage into the cardiac conduction system, arrhythmia, and sudden death. *J. Thorac. Cardiovasc. Surg.*, **44**, 687

7. Niles, N. R. and Sandilands, J. R. (1969). Pathology of heart valve replacement surgery: autopsies of 62 patients with Starr–Edwards prostheses. *Dis. Chest*, **56**, 373

8. Bharati, S., Lev, M. and Kirklin, J. W. (1983). *Cardiac Surgery and the Conduction System*. (New York: John Wiley)

9. Froysaker, T., Efskind, L. and Geruldsen, S. (1970). Haemorrhage in the interventricular septum after aortic valve surgery. *Scand. J. Thorac. Cardiovasc. Surg.*, **4**, 139

10. Rose, J. C., Hufnagel, C. A., Freis, E. D., Harvey, W. P. and Partenope, E. A. (1954). Hemodynamic alterations produced by plastic valvular prosthesis for severe aortic insufficiency in man. *J. Clin. Invest.*, **33**, 891

11. Stohlman, F., Sarnoff, S. F., Case, R. B. and Ness, A. T. (1956). Hemolytic syndrome following insertion of lucite ball valve prosthesis into cardiovascular system. *Circulation*, **13**, 586

12. Roberts, W. C. and Morrow, A. G. (1966). Renal hemosiderosis in patients with prosthetic heart valves. *Circulation*, **33**, 390

13. Niles, N. R. and Sandilands, J. R. (1969). Pathology of heart valve replacement surgery: autopsies of 62 patients with Starr–Edwards prostheses. *Dis. Chest*, **56**, 373

14. Rose, A. G. (1974). Renal haemosiderosis in patients with prosthetic heart valves. *S. Afr. Med. J.*, **48**, 721

15. Silver, M. D. (1969). Late complications of prosthetic heart valves: a pathologist's viewpoint. *Am. Heart J.*, **98**, 668

16. Roberts, W. C. (1966). Renal hemosiderosis (blue kidney) in patients with valvular heart disease. *Am. J. Pathol.*, **48**, 409

17. Rubinson, R. M., Morrow, A. G. and Gebel, P. (1966). Mechanical destruction of erythrocytes by incompetent aortic valvular prostheses. Clinical, hemodynamic and hematological findings. *Am. Heart J.*, **71**, 179

18. Gupta, S. C. and Suryaprasad, A. G. (1979). Mechanical hemolytic anemia after repair of ruptured chordae tendineae of mitral valve apparatus. *Angiology*, **30**, 776

19. Crexells, C., Aerichide, N., Bonny, Y., Lepage, G. and Campeau, L. (1972). Factors influencing hemolysis in valve prosthesis. *Am. Heart J.*, **84**, 161

20. Andersen, M. N., Gabrieli, E. and Zizzi, J. A. (1965). Chronic haemolysis in patients with ball-valve prostheses. *J. Thorac. Cardiovasc. Surg.*, **50**, 501

21. Roeser, W. H. P., Powell, L. W. and O'Brien, M. F. (1970). Hemolysis after heterograft and prosthetic valve replacement. *Am. Heart J.*, **79**, 281

22. Davies, L. G. (1970). Valve replacement. *Br. Heart J.*, **32**, 723

23. Roeser, W. H. P., Powell, L. W. and O'Brien, M. F. (1968). Red cell survival after heterograft valve surgery. *Br. Med. J.*, **4**, 806

24. Rao, K. R. P., Patel, A. R., Patel, R. N., Kumaraiah, V. and Towne, W. D. (1982). Erythrocyte survival in patients with porcine xenograft aortic and mitral valves. *South. Med. J.*, **75**, 296

25. Weesner, K. M., Rocchini, A. P., Rosenthal, A. and Behrendt, D. (1981). Intravascular hemolysis associated with porcine mitral valve calcification in children. *Am. J. Cardiol.*, **47**, 1286

26. Harrison, E. C., Roschke, E. J., Meyers, H. I., Edmiston, W. A., Chan, L. S., Tatter, D. and Lau, F. Y. K. (1978). Cholelithiasis: a frequent complication of artificial heart valve replacement. *Am. Heart J.*, **95**, 483

27. Woodruff, R. K. and Goble, A. J. (1985). Control of cardiac valve related hemolytic anemia by sulphinpyrazone. *Aust. N. Z. Med.*, **15**, 645

28. Chesler, E. (1972). Aneurysms of the left ventricle. *Cardiovasc. Clin.*, **4**, 187

29. Van Tassel, R. A. and Edwards, J. E. (1972). Rupture of the heart complicating myocardial infarction: analysis of 40 cases including nine examples of left ventricular false aneurysm. *Chest*, **61**, 104

30. Roberts, W. C., Bulkley, B. H. and Morrow, A. G. (1973). Pathologic anatomy of cardiac valve replacement: a study of 224 necropsy patients. *Prog. Cardiovasc. Res.*, **15**, 539

31. Bowes, V. F., Datta, B. N., Silver, M. D. and Minielly, J. A. (1974). Annular injuries following the insertion of heart valve prostheses. *Thorax*, **29**, 530

32. Feint, J. A., Richardson, J. P. and Clarebrough, J. K. (1975). Subvalvular left ventricular aneurysm following mitral valve replacement. *Aust. N.Z. J. Surg.*, **45**, 151

33. Casarotto, D., Bortolotti, U. and Thiene, G. (1977). Rupture of the posterior wall of the left heart at the atrio-ventricular groove following mitral valve replacement. *Acta Chir. Belg.*, **76**, 297
34. Rose, A. G. and Losman, J. G. (1978). Subvalvular left ventricular false aneurysm complicating mitral valve replacement. *Arch. Pathol. Lab. Med.*, **102**, 285
35. MacVaugh, H., Joyner, C. R., Pierce, W. S. and Johnson, J. (1969). Repair of subvalvular left ventricular aneurysm occurring as a complication of mitral valve replacement. *J. Thorac. Cardiovasc. Surg.*, **58**, 291
36. Wolpowitz, A., Barnard, M. S., Sanchez, H. and Barnard, C. N. (1978). Intraoperative posterior left ventricular wall rupture associated with mitral valve replacement. *Ann. Thorac. Surg.*, **25**, 551
37. Divineni, R. and McKenzie, F. N. (1983). Type I left ventricular rupture after mitral valve replacement. *J. Thorac. Cardiovasc. Surg.*, **86**, 742
38. Nili, M., Salomon, J. and Halevi, A. (1981). Left ventricular rupture after mitral valve replacement. Report of two cases and a review of the literature. *Scand. J. Thorac. Cardiovasc. Surg.*, **15**, 235
39. Pappas, G., Paton, B. and Davies, H. (1972). Nonmycotic subvalvar aneurysms after aortic valve replacement. *J. Thorac. Cardiovasc. Surg.*, **63**, 925
40. Silver, M. D. (1968). Erosion of the left ventricular wall caused by a ball-valve prosthesis. *Can. Med. Assoc. J.*, **99**, 1143
41. Cobbs, B. W. Jr., Hatcher, C. R. Jr., Craver, J. M., Jones, E. L. and Sewell, C. W. (1980). Transverse midventricular disruption after mitral valve replacement. *Am. Heart J.*, **99**, 33
42. Jutrin, I., Di Segni, E. and Krabel, G. (1979). False aneurysm of the right atrium. *Chest*, **75**, 629
43. Becker, R. M., Wexler, J. and Frater, R. W. (1981). False aneurysm of aorta secondary to partial occlusion clamp injury: diagnosis by nuclear flow study. *Chest*, **80**, 331
44. Weesner, K. M., Byrum, C. and Rosenthal, A. (1981). Left ventricular aneurysms associated with intraoperative venting of the cardiac apex in children. *Am. Heart J.*, **101**, 622
45. Parker, F. B. Jr, Greiner-Hayes, C., Tomar, R. H., Markowitz, A. H., Bove, E. L. and Marvasti, M. A. (1983). Bacteremia following prosthetic valve replacement. *Ann. Surg.*, **197**, 147
46. Leitersdorf, E., Friedman, G., Gozal, D., Appelbaum, A., Sacks, T. and Levij, I. (1982). Hypothesis: new concepts on the pathogenesis of early prosthetic valve endocarditis. *Med. Hypotheses*, **9**, 325
47. Ivert, T. S. A., Dismukes, W. E., Cobbs, C. G., Blackstone, E. H., Kirklin, J. W. and Bergdahl, L. A. L. (1984). Prosthetic valve endocarditis. *Circulation*, **69**, 223
48. Robboy, S. J. and Kaiser, J. (1975). Pathogenesis of fungal infection on heart valve prosthesis. *Hum. Pathol.*, **6**, 711
49. Watanakunakorn, C. (1979). Prosthetic valve endocarditis. *Prog. Cardiovasc. Dis.*, **22**, 181
50. Yeh. T. J., Anabtawi, I. N., Cornett, V. E., Stern, W. H. and Ellison, R. G. (1967). Bacterial endocarditis following open-heart surgery. *Ann. Thorac. Surg.*, **3**, 29
51. Ankeney, J. C. (1969). Staphylococcal endocarditis following open heart surgery related to positive intra-operative blood cultures. In *Prosthetic Heart Valves*. p. 719 (Springfield, Illinois: Charles C. Thomas)
52. Levy, C., Cutin, J. A. Watkins, A., Marsh, B., Garcia, J. and Mispireta, L. (1977). Mycobacterium chelonei infection of porcine heart valves. *N. Engl. J. Med.*, **297**, 667
53. Elek, S. D. (1956). Experimental staphylococcal infection in skin of man. *Ann. N.Y. Acad. Sci.*, **65**, 85
54. Watanakunakorn, C. (1977). Changing epidemiology and newer aspects of infective endocarditis. *Ann. Intern. Med.*, **22**, 21
55. Wilson, W. R., Danielson, G. K., Giuliani, E. R. and Geraci, J. E. (1982). Prosthetic valve endocarditis. *Mayo Clin. Proc.*, **57**, 155
56. Norenberg, R. G., Sethi, G. K., Scott, S. M. and Takaro, T. (1975). Opportunistic endocarditis following open-heart surgery. *Ann. Thorac. Surg.*, **19**, 592
57. Stulz, P., Hasse, J. and Mihatch, J. (1980). Candida endocarditis after heart valve replacement (successful management with reoperation and local disinfection). *J. Cardiovasc. Surg.*, **21**, 255

58. Roberts, W. C. and Morrow, A. G. (1966). Bacterial endocarditis involving prosthetic mitral valves. *Arch. Pathol.*, **82**, 164

59. Robinson, M. J., Greenberg, J. J., Korn, M. and Rywlin, A. M. (1972). Infective endocarditis at autopsy: 1965–1969. *Am. J. Med.*, **52**, 492

60. Anderson, D. J., Bulkley, B. H. and Hutchins, G. M. (1977). A clinicopathologic study of prosthetic valve endocarditis in 22 patients: morphologic basis for diagnosis and therapy. *Am. Heart J.*, **94**, 325

61. Arnett, E. N. and Roberts, W. C. (1976). Prosthetic valve endocarditis. *Am. J. Cardiol.*, **38**, 281

62. McAllister, R. G. Jr, Samet, J., Mazzoleni, A. and Dillon, M. L. (1974). Endocarditis on prosthetic mitral valves. Fatal obstruction to left ventricular inflow. *Chest*, **66**, 682

63. Bullock, R. and van Dellen, J. R. (1982). Rupture of bacterial intracranial aneurysms following replacement of cardiac valves. *Surg. Neurol.*, **17**, 9

64. Dayal, Y., Weindling, H. K. and Price, D. L. (1974). Cerebral infarction due to fungal embolus. A complication of Aspergillus infection on an aortic valve prosthesis. *Neurology*, **24**, 76

65. Downham, W. H. and Rhoades, E. R. (1979). Endocarditis associated with porcine valve xenografts. *Arch. Intern. Med.*, **139**, 1350

66. Heibig, J., Beall, A. C. Jr, Myers, R., Harder, E. and Feteih, N. (1983). Brucella aortic endocarditis corrected by prosthetic valve replacement. *Am. Heart J.*, **106**, 594

67. Schoen, F. J., Titus, J. L. and Lawrie, G. M. (1982). Bioengineering aspects of heart valve replacement. *Ann. Biomed. Eng.*, **10**, 97

68. Olanoff, L. S., Anderson, J. M. and Jones, R. D. (1979). Sustained release of gentamycin from prosthetic heart valves. *Trans. Am. Soc. Artif. Intern. Organs*, **25**, 334

69. Gayet, J. L., Etienne, J., Malquarti, V., Gruer, L. D., Didier, B., Chuzel, M., Champsaur, G., Chassignolle, J., Fleurette, J. and Delaye, J. (1984). Indices of effectiveness of medical and surgical treatment in 40 cases of prosthetic valve endocarditis. *Eur. Heart J.*, **5** (Suppl. C), 133

70. Larmi, T. K. I., Karkola, P., Kairaluoma, M. I., Sutinen, S. and Partanen-Talsta, A. (1977). Calcium microemboli and microfilters in valve operations. *Ann. Thorac. Surg.*, **24**, 34

71. Helmsworth, J. A., Gall, E. A., Perrin, E. V. *et al.* (1963). Occurrence of emboli during perfusion with an oxygenator pump. *Surgery*, **53**, 177

72. Niles, N. R. (1970). Teflon embolism from Starr–Edwards valves. *J. Thorac. Cardiovasc. Surg.*, **59**, 794

73. Shah, A., Dolgin, M., Tice, D. A. and Trehan, N. (1978). Complications due to cloth wear in cloth covered Starr–Edwards aortic and mitral valve prostheses — and their management. *Am. Heart J.*, **96**, 407

74. Roberts, W. C., Bulkley, B. H. and Morrow, A. G. (1973). Pathologic anatomy of cardiac valve replacement : a study of 224 necropsy patients. *Prog. Cardiovasc. Dis.*, **15**, 539

75. Silver, M. D. and Wilson, G. J. (1983). Pathology of cardiovascular prostheses including coronary artery bypass and other vascular grafts. In Silver, M. D. (ed.) *Cardiovascular Pathology*. p. 1225. (New York: Churchill Livingstone)

76. Schoen, F. J., Titus, J. L. and Lawrie, G. M. (1983). Autopsy-determined causes of death after cardiac valve replacement. *J. Am. Med. Assoc.*, **249**, 899

77. Lytle, B. W., Cosgrove, D. M., Loop, F. D., Taylor, P. C., Gill, C. C., Golding, L. A. R., Goormastic, M. and Groves, L. K. (1983). Replacement of aortic valve combined with myocardial revascularization: determinants of early and late risk for 500 patients, 1967–1981. *Circulation*, **68**, 1149

78. Crawford, T. (1977). *Pathology of Ischaemic Heart Disease*. p. 80 (London: Butterworths)

79. Baroldi, G. (1983). In Silver, M. D. (ed.) *Cardiovascular Pathology*. pp. 317–391. (New York: Churchill Livingstone)

80. Hutchins, G. M. and Silverman, K. J. (1979). Pathology of the stone heart syndrome. Massive myocardial contraction band necrosis and widely patent coronary arteries. *Am. J. Pathol.*, **95**, 745

81. Gay, W. A. (1980). Editorial: hypothermic cardioplegia. *Ann. Thorac. Surg.*, **30**, 517

82. Gotlieb, A., Masse, S., Allard, J. and Huang, S. (1977). Concentric hemorrhagic necrosis of the myocardium. *Hum. Pathol.*, **8**, 27

83. Rose, A. G. (1984). The pathology of heart valve replacement by valvular prostheses. *MD thesis*, University of Cape Town

84. Anderson, K. R., Sutton, M. G. St J. and Lie, J. T. (1979). Histopathological types of cardiac fibrosis in myocardial disease. *J. Pathol.*, **128**, 79
85. Westaby, S. (1983). Editorial: complement and the damaging effects of cardiopulmonary bypass. *Thorax*, **38**, 321
86. Baer, D. M. and Osborn, J. J. (1960). The post-perfusion pulmonary congestion syndrome. *Am. J. Clin. Pathol.*, **34**, 442
87. Kolff, W. J., Effler, D. B. and Groves, L. K. (1960). A review of four dreaded complications of open-heart operations. Causes, avoidance, and treatment of acidosis, overoxygenation, heart-block and pulmonary damage. *Br. Med. J.*, 16 April, 1149

11
Autopsy-determined Causes of Death Following Heart Valve Replacement

Despite numerous attempts, the perfect artificial heart valve has not yet been designed[1]. While there is a plethora of clinical and haemodynamic reports on various valve prostheses, scanty data have been published on the pathology of patients who die with prosthetic valves. Although more than 30 000 patients in the United States alone undergo this procedure each year, few studies have analysed the autopsy-determined causes of death in a large population of such patients[2]. Newer and better prosthetic valves are being continuously introduced[3]. The ultimate evaluation of a prosthesis can only be obtained from patients with implants. Identification of fatal complications following heart valve replacement is of the greatest importance in evolving means of lowering the postoperative mortality rate. Autopsy evaluation of a patient's cause of death is more accurate than a solely clinical assessment[4,5] since it gives substantial evidence as to whether or not the death was valve-related[6].

I reviewed the principal causes of death in 275 patients with heart valve prostheses (3% of 9291 autopsies) who were autopsied in the Department of Pathology, Groote Schuur Hospital and University of Cape Town from the beginning of 1962 up to the end of 1982[7]. Clinical records, autopsy reports and histological sections were available in all cases and 234 stored hearts were re-examined. In some cases possibly more than one explanation of the cause of death was valid, but a judgement was made as to which factor appeared to be the dominant cause. Although there may be some disagreement regarding a particular patient's principal cause of death, as long as the same person is making the judgement the information is useful in comparing one prosthesis, or one patient with a prosthesis, with another[8]. Other associated aetiological factors favouring a fatal outcome were also examined.

All patients with mechanical prostheses received anticoagulants (Warfarin sodium) permanently; patients with bioprostheses received anticoagulants for the first 3 postoperative months only. Rheumatic fever was the aetiological factor in 73% of operated patients. If a patient died within 2 weeks after a valve replacement reoperation necessitated by failure of a previously inserted valve prosthesis, then that patient's death was attributed to the original valve prosthesis. Such a situation was encountered in 12 of the patients studied.

An attempt was made to pinpoint a single principal cause of death for each patient after valve replacement using the approach of Roberts and Hammer[8]. The causes of early deaths (less than 1 month after surgery) were compared with the later deaths. Principal causes of death were classified as follows using a modification of the systematic approach of Silver and Wilson[9]:

1. Error in preoperative diagnosis, e.g. unrecognized significant associated valvular disease.
2. Error in operative technique. This may be related to the anaesthetic, to the extracorporeal circulation, or to the surgical technique, and it may affect the valvular prosthesis, the valve rings, blood vessels or the conducting tissues.
3. Valve prosthesis-related problems, e.g. thrombus, infected vegetations, anticoagulant-related complications, or design/structural problems inherent in the prosthesis.
4. Postoperative complications affecting non-cardiac organs.
5. Complications unrelated to valve surgery.
6. The final category consisted of those patients in whom no morphological cause of death was found.

This same classification of the principal causes of death was applied to pathological reports in the literature, which describe autopsy-determined causes of death in large groups of patients who died with valve prostheses. A few of the latter reports regarded early deaths as those occurring up to 2 months postoperatively. The pattern of organ infarcts in our patients with prostheses was analysed for each type of prosthesis and the incidence was compared with that observed in 103 non-operated subjects with valvular heart disease. The chi-square evaluation was performed upon data obtained by morphological assessment.

The 275 autopsy patients studied consisted of 142 males and 133 females. Their mean age was 35.8 years (SD = 18.2) with a range of from 1.5 to 82 years. The types of valvular prostheses implanted in the 275 patients are indicated in Table 11.1. The total patient-year survival was 684.1 years, and of this 565.5 years (83%) was due to patients with University of Cape Town (UCT) valves.

PRINCIPAL CAUSES OF DEATH

Tables 11.2 and 11.3 compare the principal causes of death in 275 patients with heart valve prostheses divided as to whether a mechanical or tissue valve prosthesis was present.

The percentages given in Table 11.3 refer to the percentage of all the principal causes of death for which that particular listed cause was responsible. Table 11.4 compares the incidence of prosthesis-related principal causes of death in the various types of prostheses studied. Table 11.5 and Figure 11.1 compare the early (less than 1 month postoperatively, group 1) and the late (greater than 1 month postoperatively, group 2) causes of death after cardiac valve replacement. Prosthesis-associated complications accounted for 13% of the early deaths and 61% of the late deaths. Deaths unrelated to cardiac surgery

Table 11.1 Types of cardiac valvular prostheses implanted in 275 autopsied patients

	Valve sites			
Valve type	Aortic	Mitral	Tricuspid	Multiple
Mechanical				
University of Cape Town	41	36	2	19
Lillehei–Kaster	9	7	—	—
Bjork–Shiley	12	1	—	1
Starr–Edwards	7	34	—	3
St Jude Medical	10	9	1	9
Tissue				
Hancock	1	8	—	3
Carpentier–Edwards	15	16	—	7
Mixed	—	—	—	24

Table 11.2 Principal causes of death in 275 patients with implanted prosthetic heart valves

Cause	Mechanical (n = 220)	Tissue (n = 50)	Total* (n = 275)
Error preoperative diagnosis	5 (2.3%)	0.0	5 (1.8%)
Error operative technique	25 (11.4%)	7 (14.0%)	35 (12.7%)
Prosthesis problem	89 (40.5%)	9 (18.0%)	98 (35.6%)
Postoperative complications	46 (20.9%)	5 (10.0%)	52 (18.9%)
Unrelated to cardiac operation	17 (7.7%)	11 (22.0%)	28 (10.2%)
Unknown	38 (17.3%)	18 (36.0%)	57 (20.7%)

*Includes five patients with mixed tissue and mechanical valves in the same heart

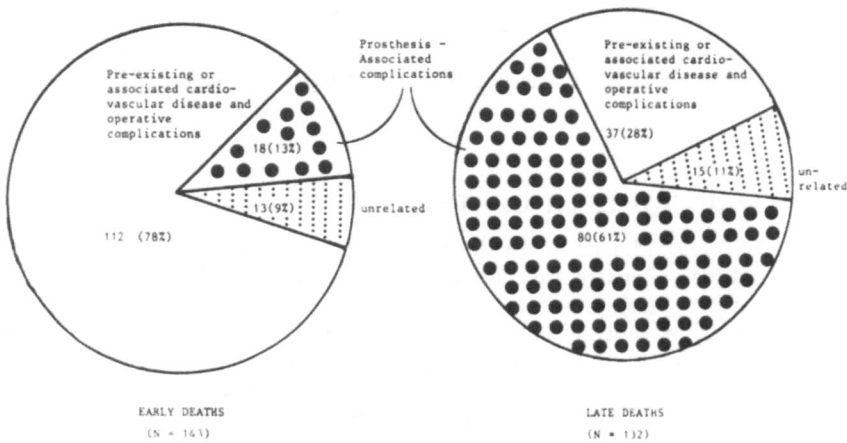

Figure 11.1 Early and late autopsy-determined causes of death after cardiac valve replacement at Groote Schuur Hospital, Cape Town, 1962–82

Table 11.3 Details of valve-related principal causes of death in two groups of patients with valve prostheses

Valve problems	Mechanical valves	Tissue valves
Thrombus-related	47 (21.4%)	3 (6.0%)
Infection	30 (13.6%)	1 (2.0%)
Design/structure	12 (5.5%)	5 (10.0%)

were responsible for 9.1% of the early and 11.4% of the late deaths. Thus, pre-existing or associated cardiovascular diseases (error in preoperative diagnosis), operative complications and deaths of unknown causes caused 77.9% of the early deaths and 27.6% of the late deaths.

THROMBOSIS ON THE PROSTHESIS AND THROMBOEMBOLISM

The number of prosthetic thrombi in patients with mechanical and tissue valves is compared in Table 11.6. The tissue valves showed significantly fewer thrombi and in general the latter were much scantier in amount than those observed on the mechanical prostheses. (Five patients with both mechanical and tissue valves in the same heart are excluded from Table 11.6.)

Table 11.7 indicates the number of organ infarcts in the mechanical and tissue valves. The differences between the mechanical and tissue valves are not significant with regard to infarcts in the systemic organs. The 'other' infarcts referred to in Table 11.7 include infarcts, e.g. of bowel and limbs. Tissue valves showed a significantly greater number of pulmonary infarcts. There was a significant difference in organ infarcts encountered in 275 patients with valvular prostheses compared with those recorded in 103 non-operated patients with natural valvular disease. Sixty of the control patients had predominantly mitral valvular disease and 43 had aortic valvular disease; 87% of the controls had chronic rheumatic-type valvular deformities. Patients with superimposed infective endocarditis were excluded. There was no significant difference in the incidence of renal infarcts between operated patients and controls. Patients with prostheses showed significantly more infarcts of other

Table 11.4 Principal causes of death in 275 patients with various types of prosthetic heart valves

Valve type	Non-prosthesis-related deaths	Prosthesis-related deaths
UCT $(n = 98)$	56 (57%)	42 (43%)
Lill. $(n = 16)$	9 (56%)	7 (44%)
B–S $(n = 14)$	13 (93%)	1 (7%)
S–E $(n = 44)$	21 (48%)	23 (52%)
SJM $(n = 29)$	20 (69%)	9 (31%)
Mixed $(n = 24)$	17 (71%)	7 (29%)
Han. $(n = 12)$	10 (83%)	2 (17%)
C–E $(n = 38)$	31 (82%)	7 (18%)

UCT = University of Cape Town; Lill. = Lillehei–Kaster; B–S = Bjork–Shiley; S–E = Starr–Edwards; SJM = St Jude Medical; Han. = Hancock; C–E = Carpentier–Edwards

Table 11.5 Early (group 1) and late (group 2) causes of death after cardiac valve replacement

	Group 1	Group 2
Error preoperative diagnosis	4 (2.8%)	1 (0.8%)
Error in operative technique		
Anaesthetic	9 (6.3%)	3 (2.3%)
Prosthesis dehiscence/disproportion	8 (5.6%)	4 (3.0%)
Pump/stone heart	7 (4.9%)	1 (0.8%)
Other	2 (1.4%)	1 (0.8%)
Inherent prosthetic problems		
Thrombosis	10 (7.0%)	40 (30.3%)
Infection	7 (4.9%)	24 (18.2%)
Design/structure	1 (0.7%)	16 (12.1%)
Postoperative complications		
General	31 (21.7%)	17 (12.9%)
Unique to cardiac surgery	4 (2.8%)	0
Unrelated to cardiac operation	13 (9.1%)	15 (11.4%)
Unknown cause	47 (32.9%)	10 (7.6%)
Totals	143	132

Table 11.6 Number of prostheses bearing thrombi in patients with mechanical and tissue valve prostheses

Prostheses	No. of patients with prosthetic thrombi	
Mechanical valves ($n = 220$ patients)	78	$\Big\} p < 0.01$
Tissue valves ($n = 50$ patients)	8	
Total ($n = 270$)	86	

organs, particularly of the brain and heart. Pulmonary infarcts were commoner in the non-operated patients, most of whom were in congestive cardiac failure.

Uncorrected valvular disease (Figure 11.2) was the commonest non-fatal associated abnormality, followed by a miscellaneous group which included mediastinal surgical emphysema, extradural abscess, acute pancreatitis, aortic dissection and subaortic stenosis due to a high-profile mitral prosthesis. Silicone embolism (Figure 11.3) was a feature of the earlier autopsies prior to the use of efficient filters during cardiopulmonary bypass. Fourteen patients had significant coronary arterial atherosclerotic narrowing, but death had been attributed to some other cause. Poor anticoagulant control led to internal bleeding (Figure 11.4) in some patients. Three patients were found to have an incidental malignancy at autopsy; a jejunal carcinoid tumour in one patient, and lung cancer and endometrial carcinoma respectively in the other two patients. There was no correlation between patients with poor anticoagulation control, dehiscence, infection or haemolysis with those who had specific prosthesis-related complications. One patient developed an oesophago-left atrial fistula due to a cautery electrode touching the lead of an oesophageal temperature-monitoring device during valve surgery (Figure 11.5).

Table 11.7 Organ infarcts in patients with implanted cardiac valvular prostheses and in non-operated controls with natural valvular disease

Organs	Patients with mechanical valves (n = 220)	Patients with tissue valves (n = 50)	All patients with valves (n = 275)	Non-operated patients (n = 103)
Kidney	64 (29%)	5 (10%)	69 (25%)	25 (24%)
Spleen	56 (26%)	3 (6%)	59 (22%)	17 (17%)
Brain	55 (25%)	3 (6%)	58 (21%)	14 (14%)
Heart	41 (19%)	6 (12%)	47 (17%)	6 (6%)
Other	25 (11%)	0	25 (9%)	6 (6%)
Lung	18 (8%)	5 (10%)	23 (8%)	25 (24%)

$p < 0.05$ $p < 0.01$

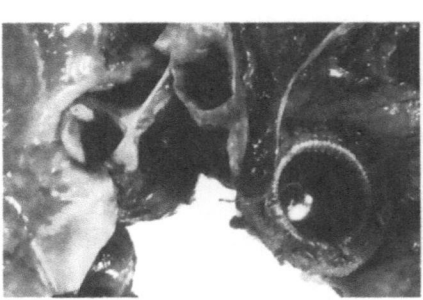 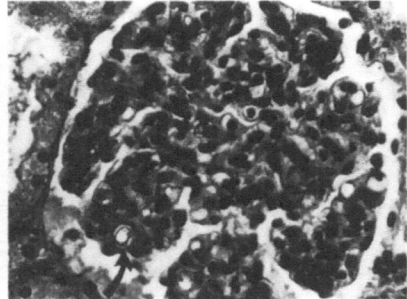

Fig. 11.2   Fig. 11.3

Figure 11.2 Acquired bicuspid aortic valve in a patient with a Starr–Edwards mitral valve prosthesis
Figure 11.3 Silicone embolus (arrow) from bubble oxygenator apparatus is trapped in a glomerular capillary. (Haematoxylin–eosin, × 82)

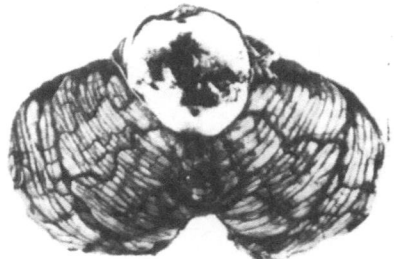 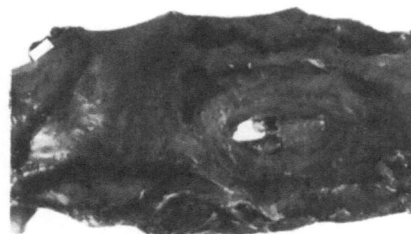

Fig. 11.4   Fig. 11.5

Figure 11.4 Pontine haemorrhage in a patient with a St Jude valve prosthesis who had received excessive anticoagulation
Figure 11.5 Oesophageal aspect of oesophago-left atrial fistula, which developed as a result of a cautery electrode touching the lead of an intra-oesophageal temperature-monitoring device during valve surgery. Thrombus which filled the defect at autopsy has been removed.

Comment

Table 11.8 compares the incidence of prosthesis-related deaths in the present series with that of other detailed pathological reports. The figures given for prosthesis-related complications in the reports cited in Table 11.8 are my own, being derived from study of the reports and an allocation as to the principal causes of death using the same categories used in the present study.

The means of the incidences of prosthesis-related causes of death in early and late survivors listed in Table 11.8 (my patients excluded) were as follows: early deaths, 16.7% (SD = 17.0) and late deaths, 45.4% (SD = 19.0). If the poorly durable Hufnagel trileaflet prosthesis[21] is excluded, then the means are 13.0% (SD = 11.9) and 41.8% (SD = 14.0), respectively. The longest follow-up period in the patients with the Hufnagel prosthesis was 58 months, so the high late mortality rate is not simply due to an unusually prolonged follow-up period. It should be noted that the simple percentage method lacks

Table 11.8 Incidence of early and late prosthesis-related causes of death after cardiac valve replacement

Reference	Valve (no. of patients)	Early (%)	Late (%)
Roberts and Morrow[10]	S–E (20)	–	25
Roberts and Morrow[11]	S–E (64)	48	30
Roberts and Morrow[12]	S–E (98)	9	30
Starr et al.[13]	S–E (32)	–	44
Herr et al.[14]	S–E (53)	15	64
Starr[15]	S–E (87)	–	58
Colapinto and Silver[16]	S–E,B–S (99)	10	–
Roberts et al.[17]	S–E (228)	10	54
Joassin and Edwards[18]	S–E (93)	8	–
Joassin and Edwards[19]	S–E (36)	–	36
Henze et al.[20]	B–S (20)	13	25
Fishbein et al.[21]	Huf. (20)	57	92
Fishbein et al.[22]	Han. (20)	7	33
Barnhorst et al.[23]	S–E (231)	8	35
Roberts and Hammer[8]	B–S (46)	9	62
Schoen et al.[2]	Mixed (279)	6	47
Present series	Mixed (275)	13	61

S–E = Starr–Edwards;   B–S = Bjork–Shiley;   Huf. == Hufnagel;   Han. = Hancock;
Mixed = various types of prostheses

the important meaning afforded by including the length of follow-up[24]. A shorter follow-up time tends to generate a lower mortality or late complication percentage than does a longer period of postoperative evaluation. The papers cited in Table 11.8 do not indicate follow-up periods in patient-years. In the present series the 275 autopsy patients with implanted heart valves had a total follow-up period of 684.1 patient-years.

This study is consistent with the accepted lower thrombogenicity (Table 11.6) of tissue valves (despite the absence of long-term anticoagulant therapy), as compared to mechanical valves. However, the incidence of systemic organ infarcts (Table 11.7) did not differ significantly between the two groups. Prosthesis-related problems (e.g. thrombosis, infection of the prosthesis, or design/structural problems) comprised the biggest single principal cause of death (36%) in the 275 patients with valve prostheses (see Table 11.2). This was followed in descending order of frequency by unknown causes, postoperative complications, errors in operative technique, diseases unrelated to the cardiac operation, and errors in preoperative diagnosis, which included unrecognized associated significant valvular disease. Separation of the principal causes of death in the patients according to whether a mechanical or a tissue valve had been implanted left one with 270 patients, once the five patients with both tissue and mechanical prostheses in the same heart had been excluded.

The commonest principal cause of death in the mechanical prosthesis group ($n = 220$) was prosthesis-related problems, whereas in the tissue valve group ($n = 50$) this cause ranked third in order of frequency (after unknown causes and diseases unrelated to valve surgery). In the mechanical valve group postoperative complications were the second commonest cause of death. There was an equal incidence of deaths attributable to errors in preoperative diagnosis. Analysis of the valve-related principal causes of death (Table 11.3) shows that thrombosis and infection were more important in the mechanical group, whereas structural failure was more common in the tissue valves. When the various types of prostheses are compared with one another with regard to prosthesis-related principal causes of death (Table 11.4), it is apparent that the University of Cape Town, the Lillehei–Kaster and the Starr–Edwards valve prostheses gave the worst results, whilst the Bjork–Shiley, Carpentier–Edwards, Hancock and St Jude Medical valve prostheses (in that order) showed fewer prosthesis-related fatal complications.

It would be incorrect to conclude that mechanical valves are superior to tissue valves. The limitation of the present study is that bioprostheses fail relatively late, but frequently, whereas the total experience with such valves in this study is only 28 patient-years. Also bioprosthetic failure is often slow enough to allow time for reoperation, unlike mechanical valves in which failure has rapidly lethal consequences.

Surprisingly, patients with mixed prostheses in the same heart showed only a 29% prosthesis-related fatal complication rate. Valve-related fatal complications were more frequently encountered with the Starr–Edwards ball-valves than with the pivoting/tilting-disc or bileaflet prostheses, viz. 54% versus 34%. There was a higher incidence of deaths due to errors in operative technique and death due to unknown causes in the non-ball-valve group. Roberts and Hammer[8] noted a similar difference in 'prosthesis-related' deaths between a group of patients with ball-valves and another group with tilting/pivoting-disc valves, which they ascribed to the higher incidence of disproportion with the ball-valves. In the present series patients with Starr–Edwards ball-valve prostheses had disproportion as the principal cause of death in only one instance, whereas thrombosis on the prosthesis appeared to be the major problem. Such thrombosis, often associated with thromboembolism, was the principal cause of death in 16 of 44 patients. The lower rate of disproportion in our patients with ball-valves may be related to the fact that these valves were inserted at a later time in most of our patients, by which time the surgeons had been alerted to this problem by the experience of others. Subjective observer error cannot be excluded as a factor either.

When all the patients with prostheses (both mechanical and tissue valves) are separated into early or late survivors, with 30 days postoperative survival as the cut-off point (Table 11.5), prosthesis-related fatal complications were seen in 12.6% of the early survivors and in 60.6% of the late survivors. Prosthetic thrombosis and its related complications was encountered more often as a principal cause of death in the late survivors (30.3%) than in the early survivors (7.0%), and so too were infection and problems related to prosthetic design or structure. Deaths due to unknown causes were commoner in patients who died less than 30 days post-operatively.

Few studies[2,8,10–23] give a detailed description of the principal causes of death (based on both clinical and autopsy findings) of patients with cardiac valve prostheses (see Table 11.8). The majority of these deal with patients with Starr–Edwards ball-valves. The series which most closely approximates the present one (mixed types of valve prostheses) is that of Schoen et al.[2]. Six per cent of their early deaths were prosthesis-related (compared to 13% of my patients) and 47% of their late deaths (compared to 61% of my patients) were due to prosthesis-related complications. These findings are consistent with the general trend found in the other detailed pathological reports cited in Table 11.8, with the exception of the report of Fishbein et al.[21] which reflects the poor durability of the Hufnagel trileaflet prosthesis, and that of Roberts and Morrow[10] which had an unusually high rate of early prosthesis-related complications. Chronic exposure to materials, such as Dacron, covering prosthetic valves may rarely locally induce a malignant tumour, e.g. a malignant fibrous histiocytoma[25].

REFERENCES

1. Hwang, N. H. C., Nan, X. Z. and Gross, D. R. (1983). Prosthetic heart valve replacements. *Crit. Rev. Biomed. Eng.*, **9**, 99
2. Schoen, F. J., Titus, J. L. and Lawrie, G. M. (1983). Autopsy-determined causes of death after cardiac valve replacement. *J. Am. Med. Assoc.*, **249**, 899
3. Wada, J. and Kasagi, Y. (1983). A new mechanical valve: SJM. *Int. Surg.*, **68**, 117
4. Cameron, H. M. and McGoogan, E. (1981). A prospective study of 1152 hospital autopsies: I. Inaccuracies in death certification. *J. Pathol.*, **133**, 273
5. Cameron, H. M. and McGoogan, E. (1981). A prospective study of 1152 hospital autopsies: II. Analysis of inaccuracies in clinical diagnoses and their significance. *J. Pathol.*, **133**, 285
6. Nicoloff, D. M., Lindsay, W. G., Arom, K. V. *et al.* (1983). Four and a half years experience with the St Jude prosthesis. In DeBakey, M. E. (ed.) *Advances in Cardiac Valves: Clinical Perspectives.* pp. 25-32. (New York: Yorke Medical Books)
7. Rose, A. G. (1986). Autopsy-determined causes of death following heart valve replacement. *Am. J. Cardiovasc. Pathol.*, 1986 (In press)
8. Roberts, W. C. and Hammer, W. J. (1976). Cardiac pathology after valve replacement with a tilting disc prosthesis (Bjork–Shiley type). A study of 46 necropsy patients and 49 Bjork–Shiley prostheses. *Am. J. Cardiol.*, **37**, 1024
9. Silver, M. D. and Wilson, G. J. (1983). Pathology of cardiovascular prostheses including coronary artery bypass and other vascular grafts. In Silver, M. D. (ed.) *Cardiovascular Pathology.* pp. 1225-1296. (New York: Churchill Livingstone)
10. Roberts, W. C. and Morrow, A. G. (1967). Late postoperative pathological findings after cardiac valve replacement. *Circulation*, **35,36** (Suppl. 1), I-48
11. Roberts, W. C. and Morrow, A. G. (1967). Causes of early postoperative death following cardiac valve replacement. Clinico-pathological correlations in 64 patients studied at necropsy. *J. Thorac. Cardiovasc. Surg.*, **54**, 422
12. Roberts, W. C. and Morrow, A. G. (1967). Topics in clinical medicine. Anatomic studies of hearts containing caged-ball prosthetic valves. *Johns Hopkins Med. J.*, **121**, 271
13. Starr, A., Herr, R. H. and Wood, J. A. (1967). Mitral replacement. Review of six years' experience. *J. Thorac. Cardiovasc. Surg.*, **54**, 333
14. Herr, R. H., Starr, A., Pierie, W. R., Wood, J. A. and Bigelow, J. C. (1968). Aortic valve replacement. A review of six years' experience with the ball-valve prosthesis. *Ann. Thorac. Surg.*, **6**, 199
15. Starr, A. (1971). Mitral valve replacement with ball valve prostheses. *Br. Heart J.*, **33** (Suppl.), 47
16. Colapinto, N. D. and Silver, M. D. (1971). Prosthetic heart valve replacement. Causes of early postoperative death. *J. Thorac. Cardiovasc. Surg.*, **61**, 938
17. Roberts, W. C., Bulkley, B. H. and Morrow, A. G. (1973). Pathologic anatomy of cardiac valve replacement: a study of 224 necropsy patients. *Prog. Cardiovasc. Dis.*, **15**, 539
18. Joassin, A. and Edwards, J. E. (1973). Causes of death within 30 days of mitral valvular replacement. Analysis of 93 cases. *Cardiovasc. Clin.*, **5**, 169
19. Joassin, A. and Edwards, J. E. (1973). Late causes of death after mitral valve replacement. Analysis of 36 cases. *J. Thorac. Cardiovasc. Surg.*, **65**, 255

20. Henze, A., Carlsson, S. and Bjork, V. O. (1973). Mortality and pathology following aortic valve replacement with the Bjork–Shiley tilting disc valve. *Scand. J. Thorac. Cardiovasc. Surg.*, **7**, 7
21. Fishbein, M. C., Roberts, W. C., Golden, A. and Hufnagel, C. A. (1975). Cardiac pathology after aortic valve replacement using Hufnagel trileaflet prostheses: a study of 20 necropsy patients. *Am. Heart J.*, **89**, 443
22. Fishbein, M. C., Gissen, S. A., Collins, J. J. Jr., Barsamian, E. M. and Cohn, L. H. (1977). Pathologic findings after cardiac valve replacement with glutaraldehyde-fixed porcine valves. *Am. J. Cardiol.*, **40**, 331
23. Barnhorst, D. A., Oxman, H. A., Connolly, D. C. *et al.* (1976). Isolated replacement of the mitral valve with the Starr–Edwards prosthesis. An eleven-year review. *J. Thorac. Cardiovasc. Surg.*, **71**, 230
24. Lefrak, E. A. and Starr, A. (1979). *Cardiac Valve Prostheses.* pp. 38-63 (New York: Appleton-Century-Crofts)
25. Holtzman, E., Schiby, G., Segal, P. and Priel, I. (1986). Malignant fibrous histiocytoma complicating mitral valve replacement. *J. Am. Coll. Cardiol.*, **7**, 956

Index

203